Lung Plague: Origins, Impact and Epidemiology of Contagious Bovine Pleuropneumonia

Lung Plague: Origins, Impact and Epidemiology of Contagious Bovine Pleuropneumonia

Robin A.J. Nicholas
Former Head of Mycoplasma Group, Animal and Plant Health Agency, Weybridge, Surrey, UK

Justin J. Kastner
Professor, Department of Diagnostic Medicine/Pathobiology, College of Veterinary Medicine, Kansas State University, Manhattan, Kansas, USA

CABI

CABI is a trading name of CAB International

CABI
Nosworthy Way
Wallingford
Oxfordshire OX10 8DE
UK

Tel: +44 (0)1491 832111
E-mail: info@cabi.org
Website: www.cabi.org

CABI
200 Portland Street
Boston
MA 02114
USA

T: +1 (617)682-9015
E-mail: cabi-nao@cabi.org

A catalogue record for this book is available from the British Library, London, UK.

ISBN-13: 9781800627512 (hardback)
9781800627529 (ePDF)
9781800627536 (ePub)

DOI: 10.1079/9781800627536.0000

Commissioning Editor: Alexandra Lainsbury
Editorial Assistant: Emma McCann
Production Editor: Helen Elliott

Typeset by Exeter Premedia Services Pvt Ltd, Chennai, India
Printed and bound in the UK by CPI Group (UK) Ltd, Croydon, CR0 4YY

Contents

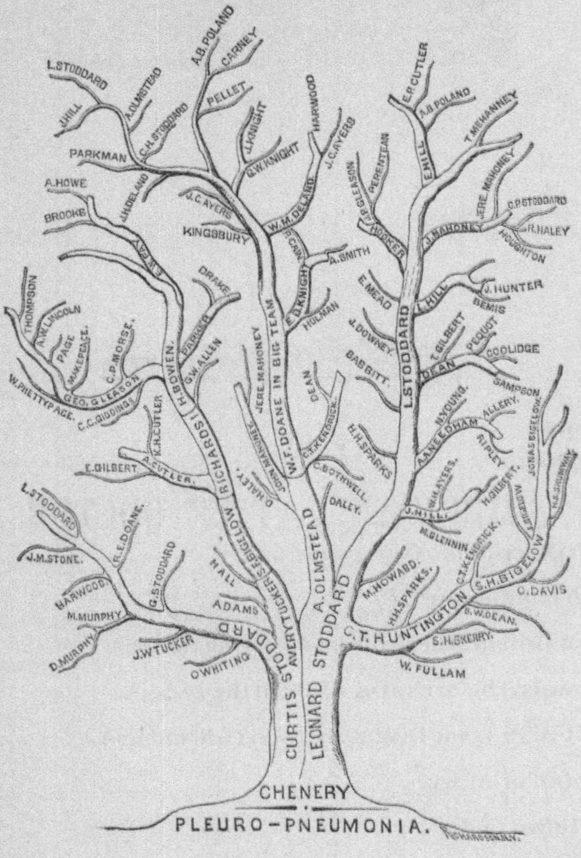

EXPLANATION.

The above cut represents the geneology of pleuro-pneumonia, as it occurred in Massachusetts, a few years ago. It commenced with Mr. Chenery's herd, and spread in the above order. The names are those of the parties whose herds took the disease by infection or contagion. (See article Pleuro-pneumonia.)

(14)

George H. Dadd (p 14 of Dadd, G. H., 1869). The American Cattle Doctor: A complete work of all the disease of cattle, sheep, and swine, including every disease particular to America, and embracing all the latest information on the Cattle Plague and Trichina, New York, Orange Judd Company, 1888 reprint; public domain; Engraver: Richardson N.Y.; image courtesy of the Richard L. D. & Marjorie J. Morse Department of Archives and Special Collections, Kansas State University.

Preface

Known variously as lung plague, lung sickness, pleuro-pneumonia, 'pleuro' in English, and a host of other names in affected countries, contagious bovine pleuropneumonia (CBPP), one of the great historical plagues of cattle, has severely affected herds on five continents. First mentioned about 500 years ago in Europe, CBPP spread silently in infected animals to most parts of the world but was eradicated from much of it in the last century. However, it persists in many countries in sub-Saharan Africa – in particular Angola, Zambia and Ethiopia – though little is known of its prevalence in central Africa where surveillance is poor. Indeed, following the COVID-19 pandemic, attempts to control it using vaccines and movement restrictions have deteriorated further to dangerously low levels. Unconfirmed reports also place the disease in isolated parts of Asia which needs to be investigated.

Research on CBPP has vacillated over the years, increasing significantly following an upsurge in outbreaks – especially (and some non-Europeans would say typically) those seen in Europe in the late 20th century. That renewed interest spilled over to Africa for a period but has made very little overall impact on its prevalence there. Despite huge advances in veterinary medicine in the last 30 years, in many countries the vaccine and diagnostic test of choice remain the 70-year-old T1/44 vaccine and the century-old complement fixation test, respectively. In the meantime, the other dreaded scourge of cattle, rinderpest, has been eradicated, which perversely has had adverse implications for CBPP.

This book describes the characteristics and cause of CBPP, charts the spread of the disease from its beginnings in late medieval Europe to most corners of the world, describes how and where it was controlled and who the main characters were in the development of our understanding and control of the disease. Molecular genetic tracing has confirmed the origin of the causative pathogen to around 1700, give or take a century, which matches fairly well with reports of its first appearance in cattle herds in Europe.

From an authorship perspective, we have come to this book from different positions: Robin is a longtime researcher with experience of the disease in the laboratory and field, while Justin has strong interests and knowledge of the history and impact of livestock diseases, in particular CBPP, on international trade. Our interests merged with the discovery by Justin of archives testifying to a would-be trade dispute, happily averted, during the late 19th century and involving the USA and Great Britain; this dispute, birthed prior to the clear establishment of CBPP's aetiology, was rooted in disagreements on the results of post-mortem examinations and whether imported US cattle were affected by CBPP. Unusually, the two warring parties were not divided on national lines but on strongly held views of what gross lesions of CBPP should look like. To add to the confusion, both countries were heavily infected with CBPP at the time. While we (especially Robin) possess a robust 21st-century scientific understanding of CBPP, we have come to sympathize with our respective countries' forebears disagreeing so much; indeed, US and British veterinarians, bacteriologists, trade diplomats and livestock raisers were faced with a high-stakes disease and fast-moving circumstances with many considerations that demanded quick decision making. As distinguished British historian Derek Brewer puts it, 'The various aspects of life which in history we inevitably divide are to the living all one' (Brewer, 1963, p. 63). True to Brewer's point, those who made decisions about CBPP in the late 19th century did not consider *only* science or *only* economics or *only* politics; indeed, they had to consider all of these aspects when making difficult judgement calls about what was then a poorly understood disease.

An important inclusion in the book is a detailed account of the unexpected re-emergence of CBPP in southern Europe in the 1980s which has never been satisfactorily explained. During his career, Robin actively participated in a number of CBPP outbreak responses and preventative efforts in Europe and Africa. He has also read publications and spoken to many of the leading scientists at the time, from the countries involved, which has shed more light on these outbreaks. We review the evidence for the commonly held belief that CBPP entered Africa in a single animal from the Netherlands in the mid-19th century, with historical and molecular genetic reports that suggest there may have been other entry points. Very little was known about the impact of CBPP on China until relatively recently; indeed, official bodies up until the 1990s had believed China had not been affected. We know now that it greatly affected Mao Zedong's policy known as the Great Leap Forward. While the century-long infection in Australia by CBPP has been documented, its infection and successful eradication in New Zealand is not so well known. It is almost certain that reports of CBPP in India in the late 19th century were misdiagnosed, but in the late 1930s the disease unambiguously entered the small Indian state of Assam in the north-east of the country where it remained for several decades.

Wherever possible we have looked at primary sources, a good number of which were obtainable from collections held on both sides of the Atlantic. In the UK, these included the National Archives at Kew, the British Library in London, and the Surrey History Centre in Woking. In the USA, we consulted archives at the Center for Brooklyn History and Brooklyn Public Library in New York; Kansas State University Libraries in Manhattan, Kansas; and even the library and archives of an 18th century plantation (that of George Mason) at Gunston Hall in Mason Neck, Virginia. We are also grateful to a number of other European libraries including, but not limited to, Venice's Fondazione Querini Stampalia (Biblioteca Civica di Venezia). As we combed through these treasure troves, we marvelled at finding documents testifying to the pioneering work of real people engaged in good thinking and good practice. These included, but are not limited to, the forgotten work of Victorian-era travelling inspectors whose job was to check the health of livestock throughout Britain, the work of the Privy Council, reports from Parliamentary debates described in Hansard showing the serious effect that CBPP was having on the country in the late 19th century, and the courageous efforts of North American veterinarians (most of them British-trained) in addressing CBPP hotspots in such locales as Long Island, New York. While this book project was formally initiated in 2023, it also draws upon decades of previous adventures in, and on, laboratories, farms, universities and libraries. In this way, we each brought into this book project previously acquired insights, research findings and personal communications with colleagues in the CBPP community.

A recurring theme in this book is that of cooperation – between and among scientists and regulators. As such thought-leading institutions as the World Organisation for Animal Health (WOAH) maintain, cooperation is essential for ensuring the ongoing operation of agriculture generally, and animal agriculture specifically. The 12 chapters that follow illustrate the truth of WOAH's insistence, and bring to mind the rich heritage of past cooperation and the need for enduring partnerships in microbiology, immunology, and biosecurity management. Whether you are reading this as a microbiologist, veterinary pathologist, or agricultural enthusiast, we hope that you gain a new appreciation for a disease that has truly posed challenges for at least one-half of a millennium.

Robin A.J. Nicholas and Justin J. Kastner
Farnham, Surrey, and Manhattan, Kansas
14 February 2025

References

Brewer, D. (1963) *Chaucer in His Time*. Thomas Nelson and Sons Ltd, London.

Acknowledgements

Robin A.J. Nicholas:
Many mycoplasmologists, veterinarians, and historians have contributed unwittingly to this book following enjoyable conversations in delightful places. First, I would like to acknowledge and thank my friend and colleague Roger Ayling with whom I spent a great deal of time in the field, laboratory, restaurants and bars of Europe, Middle East, North America and Africa in the pursuit of mycoplasma diseases in a range of animal species. *You were great and reassuring company and I'm glad our friendship continues*. Second, I want to thank Federigo Santini, José Regalla and Rosario Gonçalves for opening up their countries to me during their CBPP outbreaks, and providing such warm hospitality that Italy and Portugal seem like second homes to me now. Third, my gratitude extends to the king of CBPP pathology, Massimo Scacchia, who drove me from Windhoek, Namibia, to Livingstone, Zambia, and back (about 3000 km) to see CBPP and taught me a great deal during this trip and at the many pathological demonstrations he led. I was always thankful when 'mio fratello' Guido Loria was able to join me on my trips – his wide pathological experience supplemented my meagre veterinary knowledge. I am also very grateful to Eugenio Scanziani, Lucia Manso-Silvan, Lucas Domínguez Rodríguez, Peter Koolmees and Christian de la Fe who provided important documents and informed opinions and showed no weariness with my frequently asked questions. Using her fluent German, Helen Steele somehow translated some invaluable Dutch texts and provided great summaries from them. My wife Chris Nicholas read and corrected all my chapters and provided the tea and biscuits that sustained me in my attic study. Finally, I am grateful to my co-author, Professor Justin Kastner, for showing me the wonderful world of the archives and true American hospitality.

Sadly, I would like to recognize posthumously two giants in the field: Otto Hübschle, CVO of Namibia, who did so much to enable us to carry out field research in the natural environment and showed us the beauties of the Caprivi; and Roger Windsor, who did so much to inform the CBPP community of the *in vivo* behaviour of the mycoplasma pathogen, which successions of researchers have had to re-learn. He also provided me with many 19th century papers as well as his very valuable unpublished doctoral thesis.

I dedicate this book to the next generation of Nicholases: Mia, Arthur and Roma.

Justin J. Kastner:
I have long maintained that the most powerful people at any university are, quite simply, the librarians. Without them, scholars like us would be left to our own devices – overwhelmed by mountains and oceans of printed and electronic material. One of the greatest events in the professionalization

of university life has been the advent – in the last century or so – of broadly educated and specifically competent 'library scientists', and I would like to thank several from this esteemed profession. On both sides of the Atlantic, several specialists, archivists, and library-science gurus have lent us their invaluable expertise and generous goodwill. Within the Kansas State University (KSU) libraries, we have more than a few to thank. Chief among them is Heather Etelamaki, collections specialist for the KSU College of Veterinary Medicine (CVM) library. Heather assisted on innumerable occasions with materials related to the contributions and development of veterinary scientists and institutions, while also helping us unearth several key gems held in the impressively curated historical collection at the KSU CVM library. While I worked most closely with Heather, I want to also express gratitude to Andi Warren, KSU CVM Librarian and Director. Other key players within the KSU Libraries community have included Dennis Ryan, who kindly permitted access to materials held at the Annex, while also permitting us to conduct a few on-site workshops at the Annex. For their help in giving access to legislative journals and government publications documenting various responses to animal disease outbreak events in the mid-19th century, I thank Cliff Hight, Roger Adams and Haileigh Jacobs, all based at the Richard L.D. and Marjorie J. Morse department of archives and special collections in KSU's Hale Library.

With the kind assistance of the KSU Department of Diagnostic Medicine/Pathobiology (DMP) and the CVM business office, I have received logistical support for travel to a number of libraries and archives outside of Manhattan, Kansas. Page Simpson (accountant in the CVM business office) has been the 'MVP' in this regard, helping arrange travel, executing payments of archival fees, and guiding me through a new university travel platform. Research trips involved travel to consult collections and librarians in New York (Dee Bowers, Archives Manager at the Center for Brooklyn History, Brooklyn Public Library; and Michelle from the collections department in lower Manhattan's South Street Seaport Museum); Virginia (Dr Kate Steir, Senior Curator and Head of Collections, Gunston Hall); Minnesota (staff members from the Gale Family Library, Minnesota Historical Society); and Maryland (staff members at the National Library of Medicine on the NIH campus in Bethesda). In the UK, Robin and I benefited from the assistance of library specialists at the National Archives at Kew, as well as the Surrey History Centre in Woking. We also thank Dr Derek Mosier (Head, DMP), along with DMP office colleagues Brandy Nowakowski and Plern Kongsamut, for making it possible for Robin to travel to Kansas, work on our project, and deliver a DMP seminar on his career of working with CBPP.

While not librarians, other noteworthy scholars and friends have helped me during this project. These wonderful people provided guidance, inspiration and practical help on many fronts. They include the late J. Fred Smithcors, arguably the most influential pioneer of the history of veterinary medicine within the American academic community; I am perpetually grateful to have met Fred and his late wife Ann when, as a new KSU faculty member 20 years ago, I met at their home to get Dr. Smithcors's take on the history of CBPP. On both a professional and personal note, I continue to give thanks for my family's dear friend Jacqueline Williams, the brilliant and kind-hearted great-granddaughter of Professor William Williams (who played a key role in the late 19th century CBPP-related trade disputes). At KSU, I am indebted to Dr Howard Erickson, Professor Emeritus, who has carried the standard for the history of veterinary medicine in the CVM. Other long-time colleagues and friends – including, but not limited to, Drs Jason Ackleson, Marco Patruno, and Ellyn Mulcahy – have been key confidants throughout this project and have helped me involve students in many of this its research trips. Finally, I thank my fellow veterinary-history enthusiasts affiliated with the American Veterinary Medical History Society, the Veterinary History Society, and the World Association for the History of Veterinary Medicine; their journals, conferences and networks have helped me clarify much of what appears in these pages.

Supremely, I thank Dr Robin Nicholas, who initiated this joy-filled collaborative project. From sitting next to each other in archives to sharing our screens in Zoom meetings, Robin has illuminated for me the storied world of CBPP. I am grateful for our in-person visits (one in Kansas, and one in Surrey) which provided us the chance to research, write, dine and – every time – laugh together.

These occasions facilitated our collaboration and deepened our friendship, one that we are delighted to share with our respective families.

Speaking of families, I hereby dedicate this book to my wife Susie, our son Ian, our daughter Sally, and my parents Curtis and Rebecca; I love, respect and admire you all so much!

Milestones of CBPP

1523	First convincing description of CBPP appears in John Fitzherbert's *Boke of Husbandrie* in England
1550	Agostino Gallo describes CBPP-like 'polmonera' in Italy
1570	In Paris, *L'agriculture et maison rustique* (Jean Liebault's French translation of Charles Estienne's original work) is published; it mentions 'au mal de poulmon', likely CBPP
1695	Valentini (Michael Bernhard) reports a respiratory disease that killed many cattle in Germany
1713	A respiratory ailment assumed to be CBPP appears Germany, Switzerland, Italy, and Holland, killing 200,000 cattle within ten years
1758	England's Thomas Hale of the Royal Society refers to 'disorders of the lungs'
1766	Bourgelat differentiates CBPP ('murie', later termed 'la péripneumonie' or 'péripneumonie contagieuse') from other respiratory diseases
1773	Albrecht von Haller recommends slaughter to control
1824	Russia experiences one of several CBPP outbreaks, likely from previous spread courtesy of Napoleon's Grand Armée, which had transported food-producing animals, including cattle, all over Europe
1829	CBPP devastates the Russian army during its invasion of Turkey; unable to feed its soldiers, Russia is compelled to sign a peace treaty
1833	Professor Lecoq of the École Vétérinaire de Lyon publishes a report of an outbreak in France; Britain's William Youatt, editor of The *Veterinarian*, takes notice and disseminates Lecoq's insights to his students and colleagues
1839	CBPP introduced into County Cork, Ireland, through Dutch dairy cattle imports
1840	While previously suspected, Delafond confirms contagiousness of CBPP
1842	Liberalization of trade in Great Britain leads to more CBPP introductions

1843	USA infected with CBPP via a Dutch cow aboard an English ship; purchased by milkman Peter Dunn of Brooklyn, Long Island, which would remain a CBPP 'hotbed' for decades
1851	Australia infected from Britain by a single infected heifer
1852	Willems begins crude vaccination
1854	CBPP infects South Africa from Holland
1856	CBPP, termed 'Lungenseuche', breaks out in the Mecklenburgh region of Germany
1859	In the USA, Mr Winthrop Chenery of Massachusetts imports several Dutch cows, leading to a major CBPP outbreak across several New England states
1860	CBPP kills over 100,000 cattle in Britain
1866	In Britain, the Central and Associated Chambers of Agriculture is created; its founders lay the groundwork for an eventual Board of Agriculture and ministry
1868	Dr James Law, a Scottish veterinarian and protégé of Dr John Gamgee, emigrates to New York to become the first veterinary professor in the USA
1868	US Commissioner of Agriculture Horace Capron hires Dr John Gamgee to investigate Texas Fever in the American West; Gamgee's later report highlights major CBPP concerns in the eastern states
1877	Speaking at St James's Hall, John Gamgee decries 'the legacy of Free-trade legislation' as the culprit of CBPP's spread in Britain
1879	CBPP discovered in American cattle landed in Liverpool, leading to trade-related and disease-diagnosis controversies
1880	US Commissioner of Agriculture William G. Le Duc hires Harvard's Dr Charles Lyman to investigate the true prevalence of CBPP; gathering data from veterinary correspondents across the country, Dr Lyman creates a map differentiating between infected and non-infected counties
1886	An upsurge in CBPP cases in Scotland is attributed to Irish cattle imports
1888	In Britain, a departmental committee considers testimony about the merits of adopting inoculation for CBPP; their 300-page report definitively eschews inoculation and reiterates the country's 'stamping out' policy
1892	CBPP eradicated from the USA
1894	The Humanitarian League, an animal welfare activist group, advocates for better shipping regulations to reduce both the spread of disease and animal discomfort
1898	CBPP eradicated from Great Britain
1898	Nocard and Roux isolate the causative agent of CBPP, publishing their groundbreaking article, 'Le Microbe de la Péripneumonie', in the *Annales de l'Institut Pasteur*
1902	CBPP eradicated from Hungary
1910	Borrel names the pathogen *Asterococcus mycoides* because of its fungal-like nature
1921	China infected from Australia
1930	Complement fixation test (CFT) developed for antibody testing herds

1938	CBPP breaks out in Assam
1950s	Sheriff and Pierce develop T1/44 vaccine in Kenya
1955	Pathogen renamed *Mycoplasma mycoides* subsp. *mycoides* small colony variant (SC) to distinguish it from closely related goat mycoplasma which produced larger colonies
1980–1983	Re-emerges on the Spanish–French border and appears in Portugal
1990	Italy re-infected after 100 years freedom
1994	First use of polymerase chain reaction (PCR) for detecting CBPP
1996	Botswana eradicates CBPP after first outbreak for 40 years
1997	Re-emergent strains show inability to oxidize glycerol and partial loss of genome
1998	ELISA developed for mass screening of herds
1999	Last case of CBPP seen in Europe
2004	Genome of pathogen, *Mycoplasma mycoides* subsp. *mycoides* SC, sequenced
2010	Pathogen renamed *Mycoplasma mycoides* subsp. *mycoides*
2012	Genetic analysis reveals that the emergence of the causative mycoplasma likely occurred approximately 300 years ago

Contributors

Robin A.J. Nicholas, Former Head of Mycoplasma Group, Animal and Plant Health Agency, Weybridge, Surrey, KT15 3NB, UK. Email: robin.a.j.nicholas@gmail.com

Justin J. Kastner, Professor, Department of Diagnostic Medicine/Pathobiology, College of Veterinary Medicine, Kansas State University, Manhattan, KS 66506, USA. Email: jkastner@ksu.edu

1 Lung Plague: Description, Cause and Control

Abstract

Contagious bovine pleuropneumonia (CBPP), variously known in English as lung plague, lung fever and pleuropneumonia, is one of the great historic plagues of cattle along with Foot and Mouth Disease, tuberculosis and rinderpest. The causative agent of CBPP is the wall-less degenerate bacterium called *Mycoplasma mycoides* subspecies *mycoides* (previously known as *mycoides* small colony (SC)) and was the first mycoplasma to be isolated late in the 19th century. The pathogen attacks the lungs and pleural membranes that line the thoracic cavity, causing fever and respiratory distress such as laboured breathing, coughing and nasal discharge. Its main pathological features are the presence of serofibrinous deposits, interstitial pneumonia, interlobular oedema and hepatization giving a marbled appearance of the lung in the acute and subacute phase and capsulated lesions called sequestra in the lungs of chronically affected cattle. Because it is highly contagious with a mortality rate of up to 50% in naïve herds, it causes significant economic losses, particularly to poorer farmers. CBPP is now considered the most important cattle disease in sub-Saharan Africa. The last reported occurrence of CBPP in Europe was in Portugal in 1999 but unconfirmed reports indicate it may still be present in parts of Asia.

Disease Definition

Hutyra *et al.* (1938) best defined the disease in the early 20th century, in the following:

> The disease is a specific contagious pneumonia of cattle usually running a subacute or chronic course, characterised by a serous inflammation of the interlobular lymphatics, croupous inflammation of the parenchyma of the lung, and subsequent anaemic necrosis of the affected parts of the lung, and usually accompanied by sero-fibrinous pleuritis. (Hutyra *et al.*, 1938, p. 455)

At the time of writing, the authors could only describe the causative pathogen as 'a specific polymorphous micro-organism'.

Host Species Affected

Domesticated cattle (*Bos taurus*) and the humped zebu cattle (*Bos indicus*) are the main species affected by CBPP in sub-Saharan Africa but differences in the susceptibility of cattle breeds to CBPP have long been known. In Kenya, the improved Boran zebu breed had fewer clinical signs and less severe pathology than the small East African zebu when experimentally infected with the same challenge material. The small Côte d'Ivoire zebu breed and the Masai breed of Tanzania are believed to be resistant. In the 19th century, Dutch and Flemish cattle were reported to be more susceptible than Swiss cattle. In Australia, the Anglo-Normandy dairy cattle were more prone to experimental infection than Hereford beef cattle. Portuguese Frisian cattle, known locally as the Turina breed, were proportionately more likely to develop CBPP than local breeds such as the 'Galega' or 'Mirandesa' (Regalla *et al.*, 1996). Clearly, selecting the most resistant breed could do much to limit the damage to cattle production.

During the Italian outbreaks of 1990–1993, a herd of nearly 2000 Asian water buffalo (*Bubalus bubalis*) in Foggia Province, bred for the production of mozzarella cheese, became infected by contact with cattle introduced from the north. Of five seropositive but clinically normal buffaloes, only one, a five-year-old female, had CBPP lesions from which *Mycoplasma mycoides* subsp. *mycoides*, the pathogen of CBPP, was isolated. Santini *et al.* (1992) concluded that buffalo should be considered poorly susceptible to CBPP and pose little risk to cattle. In Australia, this species became feral following its introduction

DOI: 10.1079/9781800627536.0001

in the 19th century and was more susceptible to experimental infection than the African buffalo (*Syncerus caffer*) (Masiga *et al.*, 1996). An outbreak of CBPP in the Brussels Zoo in the late 19th century spread to bison though it is not clear whether it was the American bison (*Bison bison*) or the European bison (*Bison bonasus*) or how severe the disease was (Blancou, 2000).

Reports have appeared over the last 50 years implicating the role of small ruminants as carriers of the disease, but little direct field evidence exists so these must be treated with caution. Infections are rarely reported in small ruminants today and even when they are, it is unlikely that they could transmit disease to cattle. In a rare case, *M. m. mycoides* was isolated from sheep and goats with pneumonia and mastitis during the Portuguese outbreaks of 1983–1999, but in a region where CBPP had not been reported. Experimental infection of healthy sheep with this strain and one from cattle with CBPP failed to lead to any significant pathology or immune response (Gonçalves *et al.*, 2002) suggesting a negligible role for small ruminants in the epidemiology of CBPP.

In China, natural disease was reported in yaks (*Poephagus grunnien* formerly *Bos grunnien*) as well as dzomos (*P. grunnien* x *B. primigenius taurus*) which are a yak–domestic cattle hybrid. While strains of *M. m. mycoides* isolated from China are closely related to those from Africa and Australia, they appear to have a wider host range albeit by experimental infections. During the development of an attenuated live vaccine for CBPP, the Ben-1 strain was first adapted to rabbits which generated small quantities of pleural fluid; this material was then passaged in healthy sheep to increase antigen yield (Xin *et al.*, 2012. The sheep initially showed an increased respiratory rate and an elevated temperature after three days and became recumbent. Post-mortem examination revealed large quantities of pleural fluid which were used as a vaccine for cattle after further passaging in sheep. Due to an unacceptable level of adverse reactions in yaks, production was switched to Tibetan sheep or argalis (*Ovis ammon*) which showed no ill effects. This type of vaccine production would not be allowed for animal welfare concerns in most parts of the world today. Whether African strains could produce lesions in sheep and related species has not been reported so far.

Hyslop (1958) showed that rabbits, guinea pigs, golden hamsters and mice could all be infected with the CBPP pathogen (previously called *Asterococcus mycoides*) by most inoculation routes, though the subcutaneous route in mice was the most effective. The mycoplasma could be passaged 50 times subcutaneously in mice without reducing its virulence in cattle. Subculturing the mouse-grown strain in chick embryos reduced its virulence for cattle after only 20 passages and showed more promise for vaccine development. Mouse culture was used for a time in Kenya to isolate the pathogen from clinical samples before faster and more acceptable *in vitro* diagnostic methods superseded it.

Pathogen

It is surprising that rodents have not been used more in developing experimental models for mycoplasma infection. Their first use was by students of the great Louis Pasteur, Edmond Nocard and Emile Roux, in 1898 (Fig. 1.1a,b), to isolate the unknown cause of CBPP; these researchers enclosed infected clinical material in semi-permeable collodion sacs which were placed in the peritoneal cavities of rabbits (Nocard and Roux, 1990). The turbidity of the sac contents increased over 2–3 weeks to reveal many small, motile, opalescent bodies. These microbes were smaller than any previously described and cultures could be propagated in a mixture of peptone broth and mammalian serum (Bové, 1999). Inoculating the fifth passage into cattle confirmed the unnamed organism as the cause of CBPP.

Later, the same procedure for culturing the pathogen proved successful in the abdominal cavity of cattle. However, this largely impractical practice was superseded by methods outside the animal body in which the organism was propagated on agar-enriched broth containing cattle or rabbit serum (Hutyra and Marek, 1912). *In vitro* growth was much quicker with colonies appearing within 2 to 3 days. In liquid broth, the microbes formed 'short, fine spirillar formations', according to Bordet in 1909, while a year later Borrel and co-workers reported: 'coccal, streptococcal and morula-shaped bodies in stained preparations; also serpiginous and bifurcating filaments, and mycelial and asteroid

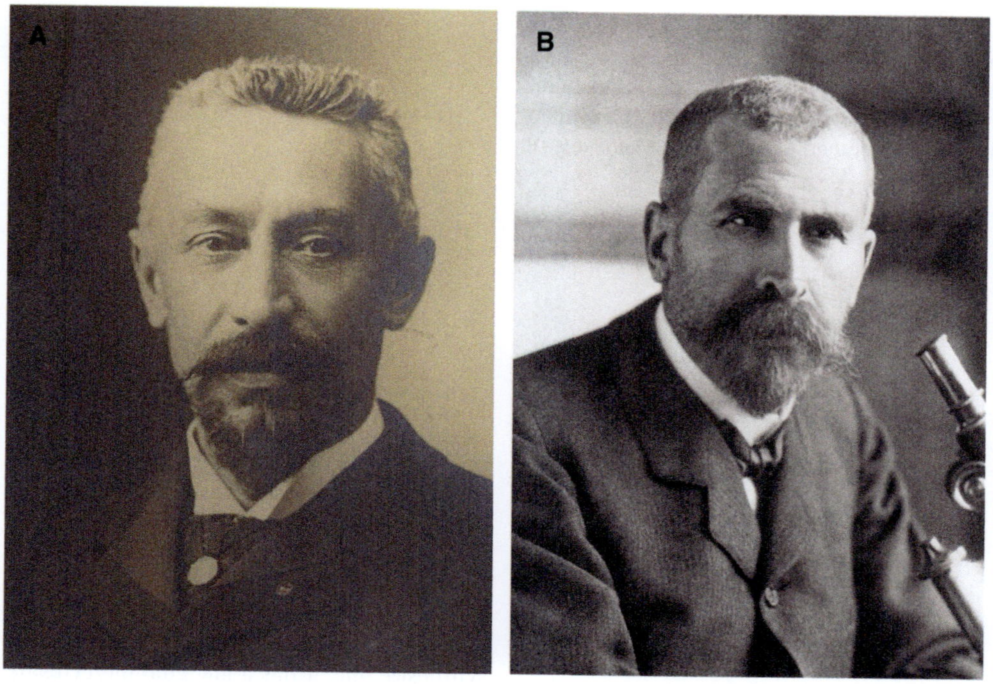

Fig. 1.1. Edmund Nocard (A) and Emile Roux (B) isolated the CBPP pathogen in 1898. (A: from Photothèque Biu santé Paris, 2015, CC-PD via Wikimedia Commons.) (B: from Pasteur Institute, 1900, CC-PD via Wikimedia Commons.)

formations enclosed in a mucoid envelope' (Hutyra *et al.*, 1938).

By the early 1900s, the major characteristics of the pathogen were known, including its very small size, its requirement for serum in the culture medium and, most characteristically, its production of fried egg-shaped colonies on a solid medium. In the next decade, it was shown to be highly pleomorphic, a fact later discovered to result from it having no cell wall but instead possessing a thin, soft skin known as the plasma membrane.

These filamentous organisms could pass through filters normally used to retain bacteria, so Nocard and Roux (Bové, 1999) and many others believed they were 'ultra-viruses'. Later, Professor John McFadyean at the Royal Veterinary College in London believed, wrongly as it turned out, that they were a form of fungal-like schizomycetes because they looked to have mycelia. As a result, this led to some confused nomenclature: *Asterococcus mycoides* by Amédée Borrel in 1910, *Micromyces pleuro-pneumoniae contagioise* by Paul Frosch, *Mycoplasma peripneumoniae* by Julian Nowak, and *Borrelomyces peripneumoniae* by the Australian group led by Arthur William Turner in the 1930s who classified it as *Borrelomycetales*, a new order of the Schizomycetes.

Using a medium originally developed for anaerobes but buffered and supplemented with bovine serum, Turner intensively studied the mycoplasmas' morphology, describing the relatively non-filtrable long, branching mycelium-like filaments from which very small filterable particles were produced. Turner *et al.* (1935) also showed that these organisms could be detected and stained in infected lungs as long as the fixative formalin was avoided. Once more was known of their bacterial properties, these microbes were renamed *Mycoplasma mycoides* subsp. *mycoides* small colony (SC) variant (Freundt, 1955) to differentiate them from a closely related pathogen of goats which produced larger colonies *in vitro*. The CBPP agent was finally named *Mycoplasma mycoides* subsp. *mycoides* (Firrao and Brown, 2011) following further analysis.

Mycoplasma. mycoides subsp. *mycoides* is a small, simple, self-replicating degenerate bacterium, (Figs 1.2–1.4) and is distinguishable from walled bacteria by several unique properties. As a member of the Class *Mollicutes*, it lacks a cell wall and the genetic machinery to synthesize one; it has a low guanine/cytosine content (less than 30%); and it has a small genome and, consequently, produces small numbers of synthesized proteins (Nicholas *et al.*, 2008). *M. m. mycoides*, is facultatively anaerobic, growing well in both anaerobic and aerobic environments at a pH of 7.6–7.8. It usually grows well in sealed liquid broth cultures, especially if the broth level is a few inches deep to allow for an oxygen or air gradient. Gentle aeration increases the growth rate and yield of *M. m. mycoides*. In actively growing cultures, *M. m. mycoides* is filamentous which is the result of genetic division preceding cytoplasmic division. At the end of growth, however, short-beaded filaments predominate and, ultimately, only coccoid bodies are seen.

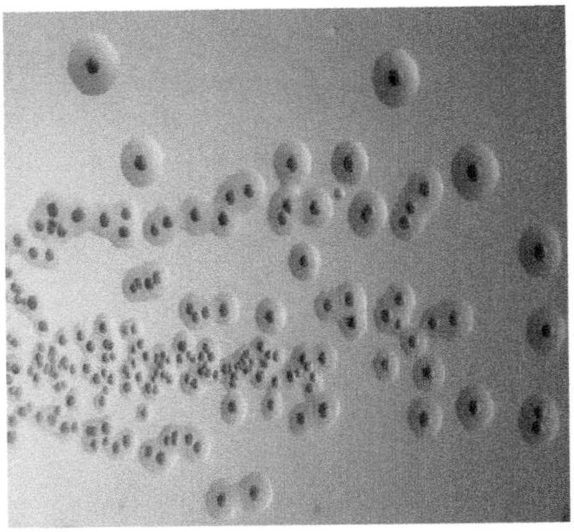

Fig. 1.2. Colonies of the CBPP pathogen: *Mycoplasma mycoides* subsp. *mycoides* growing on semi-solid medium showing fried egg appearance. (Photo courtesy of Dr Lucia Manso-Silvan, CIRAD, Montpellier.)

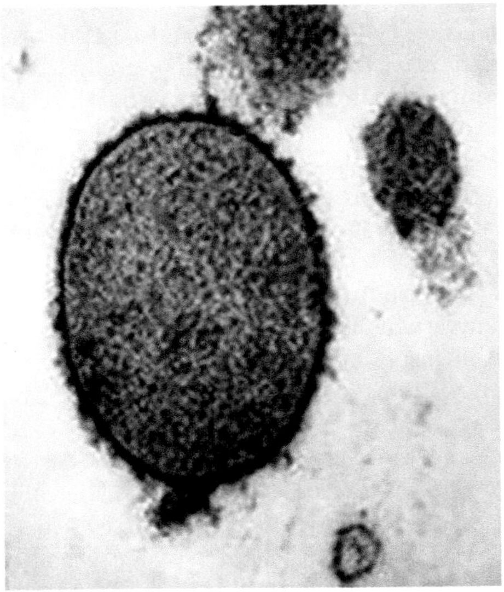

Fig. 1.3. Thin section electron micrograph of *Mycoplasma mycoides* subsp. *mycoides* showing galactan on outside of the triple-layered membrane enclosing ribosomes and nucleic material. (Photo source: Robin Nicholas.)

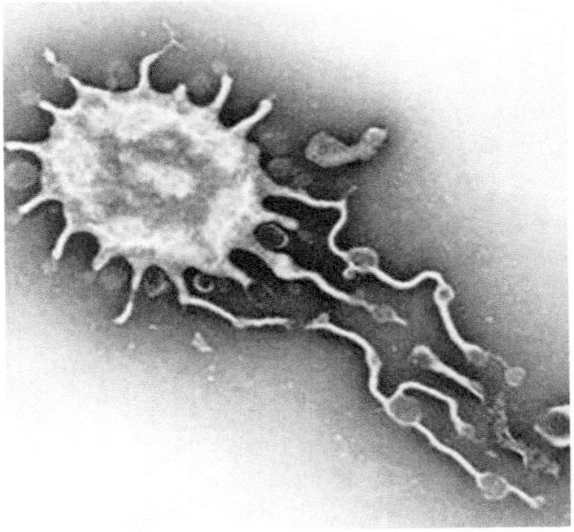

Fig. 1.4. Negative contrast electron micrograph of *Mycoplasma mycoides* subsp. *mycoides* showing pleomorphic nature. (Photo source: Robin Nicholas.)

M. m. mycoides is a member of the *Mycoplasma. mycoides* cluster, which consists of five important ruminant pathogens, which share immunological, genetic and biochemical features. The decision to omit the 'SC' (small colony) from the name was taken in 2011 when it became clear that there were sufficient differences between SC and the other member of the subspecies previously referred to as LC (large colony) to merit separation; LC became incorporated into the subspecies *capri* with which it was indistinguishable biologically and clinically (Shahram *et al.*, 2010). Molecular analysis of over 100 strains of the *M. mycoides* cluster, including the mycoplasmas responsible for contagious caprine pleuropneumonia and contagious agalactia, indicated that its origin probably dates to about 8000 BCE coinciding, according to Fischer *et al.* (2012), with the domestication of livestock by early Neolithic people, enabling the spread and diversification of these mycoplasmas.

M. m. mycoides is not intrinsically difficult to culture *in vitro*, unlike many other fastidious mollicutes, but requires a complex peptone medium with glucose, supplemented ideally with pyruvate as an additional energy source supplemented with porcine serum and buffered with HEPES (Nicholas *et al.*, 2008). It can grow under aerobic and anaerobic conditions, the optimum being at 37°C with 5% CO_2. The mycoplasma can be isolated from the lungs of CBPP-affected cattle relatively easily from the interface between diseased and healthy-looking lung tissue and directly from pleural fluid seen in the thorax of affected animals. Isolation from nasal swabs is more inconsistent. Pretreatment of cattle with antimicrobials can negatively impact isolation rates.

Molecular Biology and Epidemiology

Several *M. m. mycoides* strains have been fully sequenced, showing very low diversity among genomes. As an example, the genome of the Italian strain 57/13 showed an overall identity of 99% compared with the type strain PG1. The genome of the 57/13 strain consisted of a single chromosome of 1,192,498 bp, and 1077 protein-encoding genes were identified of which 332 encode for hypothetical proteins conserved among other *M. m. mycoides* isolates. Just over a quarter of the genes were unique to *M. m. mycoides* while about 10% had no known function (Di Teodoro *et al.*, 2020).

The lack of sequence variation among *M. m. mycoides* strains even between African and European isolates strongly suggests a recent emergence of this subspecies. A combination of next-generation sequencing and Bayesian analysis by Dupuy *et al.* (2012) dated the most recent common ancestor of *M. m. mycoides* to around the end of the 17th century (give or take 100 years) possibly emerging following infection of cattle by the goat pathogen *M. m. capri*, due to a change to, and intensification of, mixed livestock farming.

Molecular epidemiological studies were initially hampered by the very close homogeneity of strains but have now shed light on the spread of CBPP worldwide. Using a molecular typing method called multilocus sequence (MLST) analysis of 20 *M. m. mycoides* strains divided African strains into three distinct groups (Yaya *et al.*, 2008): Central and East African; West African; and Southern African. Variable number tandem repeat (VNTR) analysis appeared more discriminatory and showed clear differences between strains from Southern and East Africa (McAuliffe *et al.*, 2007).

In the 1980s, CBPP re-emerged in Southern Europe after an apparent absence of about a decade. Isolates from these new outbreaks were very closely related (Gosney *et al.*, 2011). Remarkably, comparative analysis of the new European isolates with African strains showed that these recent European strains did not oxidize glycerol, resulting in little hydrogen peroxide production attributable to the lack of the enzyme L-*α* glycerol phosphate oxidase (Houshaymi *et al.*, 1997). In contrast, African strains produced copious amounts of this toxic oxygen radical. Subsequently, genetic analysis revealed a genomic segment of 8.8 kb, present in African strains, which was completely missing in these new European strains; within this region was a copy of the *lppB* gene, a potential virulence factor, and the glycerol uptake gene. A single European strain from outbreaks in France in 1967 before the re-emergence did not have this deletion. There has been no satisfactory explanation for this deletion, but the result appears to have had some effect on the virulence of these European strains. The last case of CBPP in Europe was seen in 1999 in Portugal but continues in over 20 countries in sub-Saharan Africa.

Virulence Factors

The identification of factors playing key roles in the pathogenicity of *M. m. mycoides* is hindered by the high cost of experimental infection studies using cattle and the absence of any small animal models in which the disease can be reproduced. Nevertheless, experimental infections have shown virulence differences among African strains while morbidity and mortality are generally lower in European disease outbreaks than in African ones. However, the pathological lesions seen in natural outbreaks in both Africa and Europe are very similar and follow the same pattern: during new outbreaks, many cattle show acute and subacute lesions while chronic lesions, sequestra, predominate in later outbreaks. The lack of mortality and overt morbidity seen in European outbreaks is due, in part, to better husbandry, a less hostile environment in which to feed (usually cattle are housed much of the year) and better health and rapid access to antimicrobial treatment (Nicholas *et al.*, 2008).

The production of hydrogen peroxide and other active oxygen species by *M. m. mycoides* are important factors in mycoplasma pathogenicity causing cytotoxic damage to host cells (Houshaymi *et al.*, 1997). The mycoplasma also has a carbohydrate capsule, composed of a galactose sugar, which contributes to pathogenicity by promoting binding to host tissue surfaces and enhancing resistance to phagocytosis. In addition, there is some evidence that the capsule of *M. m. mycoides* might have a direct toxic effect on host cells and its structural similarity to bovine pneumogalactan further suggests that it might induce auto-immune reactions. Membrane-located lipoproteins and variable surface proteins are believed to facilitate evasion of the host immune response and also cause harmful immunopathological effects. A more recently discovered virulence mechanism is the MIB-MIP system whereby the mycoplasma can degrade host antibodies (Jores *et al.*, 2020). All or some of these factors may contribute to virulence at different times or circumstances.

Survival in the Host and Environment

It was believed that *M. m. mycoides* was poorly resistant in the environment particularly in arid regions seen in many parts of Africa and its survival mainly depended on the infection of susceptible animals. In damper regions like Europe and Assam, especially in housing, mycoplasmas might be able to survive for longer. McAuliffe *et al.* (2006) discovered that mycoplasmas could produce protective coats called biofilms under stressful conditions like other bacteria. In the biofilm state, *M. m. mycoides* can survive for extended times compared to conventionally grown cells and are more resistant to heat, chemicals, osmotic shock and oxidative stress (McAuliffe *et al.*, 2008). Proteomic analysis also revealed several over-expressed proteins in the biofilm-grown cells not evident in planktonic cells which were thought to make the mycoplasmas more resistant to host defences as well as making them more virulent. These researchers concluded that biofilm could represent the natural state in the environment and, more crucially, in the host which could account for the chronic nature of mycoplasma infections.

Incubation Period

One of the longest incubation periods recorded for natural disease must be that of the cow named ‘St Bees’ that made the three-month sea journey from London to Melbourne in 1858. But how attentive the crew were in recognizing the clinical signs among the other cattle accompanying the heifer is not known but this single animal on arrival infected Australia with CBPP, a disease which would take over a century to eradicate.

Various periods have been reported for the minimum and maximum limits of incubation. A very wide range of 2–8 months was reported during the CBPP outbreaks in Assam in the 1940s (Shirlaw and Iver, 1946), which may be related to the damp conditions found there. Earlier, Turner and Campbell (1937) reported a range of 1–2 months from their experiences in Australia; while Provost *et al.* (1987), with a focus on African disease, estimated 3–6 weeks for the incubation period. In experimental infections, Regalla *et al.* (1996) reported disease signs appearing in cattle 40 days after contact with inoculated animals with overt disease persisting for nearly 3 weeks. Results from intubation experiments where infection is delivered directly to the lungs are not appropriate for determining incubation in the field, though the use of these ‘seeder’ animals provides excellent challenge to healthy contacts. There is no hard evidence for the excessively long incubation periods that litter the literature, which is usually accounted for by an undetected carrier.

Epidemiology

Infection is spread to a susceptible animal by the inhalation of expired breath laden with *M. m. mycoides* from an infected, usually coughing, animal invariably in the acute or subacute stage of disease (Masiga *et al.*, 1996). The role of the sequestrum in chronically infected cattle to transmit CBPP was long discounted by a series of experiments by Windsor and Masiga (1977) in East Africa. Thus, husbandry practices that promote close and repeated contact, along with poor ventilation, will enhance the spread of disease. In an infected herd, most animals at any given moment do not present clinical disease, and the appearance of disease in uninfected areas is usually associated with the introduction of an infected but symptomless animal. Cattle movement, either commercial, nomadic or transhumance, is usually the cause for the spread of CBPP between herds. The role of infected urine, foetal fluids and even nasal discharge, is negligible in disease transmission compared to aerosol transmission.

Infected bedding as a source of disease was advocated strongly by Daniel E. Salmon, chief of the USA's Bureau of Animal Industry in the late 19th century. Salmon made the following impassioned and bad-tempered response to a Dr Gadsden, after the latter claimed that large-scale disinfection of premises was unnecessary as 'mediate contagion' (i.e. direct transmission between cattle) was the only way the disease was propagated (Salmon, 1888–1889).

> The doctor [Gadsden] and his disciples have carried their case into the daily and weekly newspapers, and seem to consider it a most remarkable feat which they have succeeded in convincing people who under no circumstances have an opportunity of hearing the other side of the case, and who from total lack of scientific training would be incapable of reaching a logical conclusion if they had all the facts before them. (Salmon, 1888–1889, p. 63)

The debate had not been helped by Salmon's rejection (apparently for technical reasons) of Gadsden's paper at a conference on pleuropneumonia held in Philadelphia. Thus, forced to attend a meeting of stock growers in Kansas City, Missouri, Gadsden described the results of housing nearly 900 healthy cattle on heavily contaminated premises at the Shufeldt Distillery, Chicago in which none of the animals contracted CBPP. Salmon cried foul and believed some disinfection had taken place in the distillery but today it is believed that the environment plays little role in the transmission of disease though disinfection is still considered desirable.

In some carefully crafted experiments, Hudson (1971) finally confirmed Gadsden's findings that there was no practical risk of spreading infection by introducing healthy cattle into an environment which had previously held CBPP-infected stock nor could contaminated fodder spread the disease. He also emphasised that the risks of importing meat were negligible.

Clinical Diagnosis

Until the late 19th century, diagnosis of CBPP on living cattle was based on non-specific and often mild clinical signs. Rather overlooked was the use of a thermometer to measure temperature rise to separate healthy cattle from those incubating disease. The British Privy Council was concerned that the delay in slaughtering all infected cattle, required by the Animal (Amendment) Order of 1873, was impeding the eradication of CBPP from Britain. In a letter written in 1874, the council instructed that cattle from a suspect herd must be separated into two groups based on internal body temperature (Privy Council, 1874). Cattle with temperatures above 103°F (39.4°C) were to be slaughtered immediately and the rest monitored weekly. While not a specific test, its use would certainly accelerate the culling of cattle where CBPP was highly suspected.

Clinical Disease

There is considerable variation in the degree of signs seen in cattle affected with CBPP, ranging from the hyperacute through acute, to chronic and subclinical forms. Respiratory distress and coughing, evident on stimulation of resting animals, are the main signs of CBPP. Experimental reproduction of the disease is difficult but can be achieved by bronchial intubation or contact infection with an intubated animal which often gives the most natural response; only small lesions have been reproduced with aerosol inhalation of low passage *M. m. mycoides*.

Hyperacute Form

The clinical signs observed in the hyperacute form are greatly accelerated. The pathological signs are usually characteristic with marked pleural adhesion accompanied by exudative pericarditis (Provost *et al.*, 1987). Affected animals may die within a few days of exhibiting classical respiratory signs.

Acute Form

The early stages of the disease are indistinguishable from any other severe pneumonia with pleurisy. Animals show dullness, anorexia, and irregular rumination with moderate fever, and may show signs of respiratory distress. Coughing is usually persistent and is slight or dry (Done *et al.*, 1995). Sometimes body temperature rises from 40 to 42°C and the animal prostrates with difficulty of movement. As the lung lesion(s) develop, the signs become more pronounced with increased frequency of coughing and the animal may stand with back arched, head extended, and knee joints abducted (Fig. 1.5). Because the pleurisy is so painful, it is rare for animals to go off their feet until just before death. While classical respiratory signs may be evident in calves, the causal agent often localizes in the joints with attendant arthritis and involvement of tendons. Complications accompanying this disease in calves may also include valvular endocarditis and myocarditis.

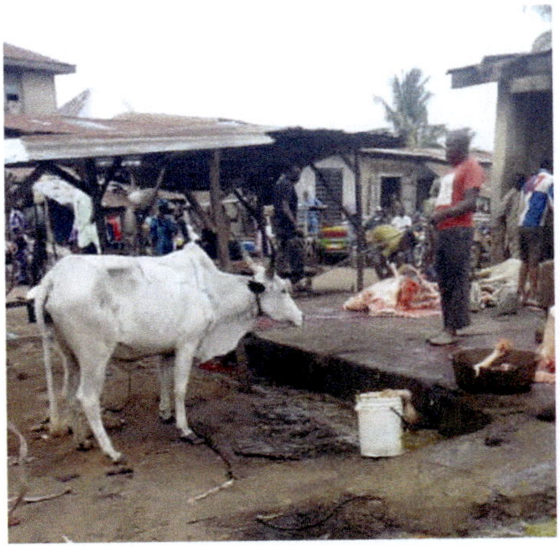

Fig. 1.5. Cow with CBPP showing respiratory distress and anorexia. (Photo source: Robin Nicholas.)

Subacute and Chronic Forms

In the subacute form, signs may be limited to a slight cough, only noticeable when the animal is exercised. CBPP in Europe, unlike that caused in Africa where mortality rates are typically 10–70% in epizootics, is characterized by low morbidity and low or non-existent mortality with the majority of infected cattle showing chronic lesions; this is characteristic of endemic disease (Regalla, 1984). These differences are perhaps because European cattle are healthier, better fed, subjected to less physical stress and are often permanently housed throughout the year (Nicholas and Palmer, 1994). In Italy during the early 1990s, less than 5% of cattle in an infected herd showed clinical signs (Guadagnini *et al.*, 1991). The use of antibiotics and anti-inflammatory drugs may help to mask clinical signs and to accelerate the formation of chronic lesions. In Africa, up to one-third of cases that recover from acute disease become potential carriers. During the CBPP outbreaks in Europe, the number of animals becoming carriers would undoubtedly have been higher than in Africa because of Europe's greater use of antimicrobial drugs (Nicholas and Palmer, 1994).

Gross Lesions

The lesions are mostly confined to the thoracic cavity and lungs, and lesions are usually unilateral, i.e. seen in one lung only. In a study of nearly 600 CBPP-affected lungs in Portugal, Nunes Petisca *et al.* (1990) showed 95% of lesions to be unilateral, which contrasts with infections caused by *Pasteurella haemolytica* where both lungs are usually affected. The diaphragmatic lobes were observed to be more commonly affected than the apical lobes. The thoracic cavity of affected animals may contain many litres of clear yellowish-brown fluid containing pieces of fibrin (Fig. 1.6). Caseous fibrinous deposits are observed on the parietal and visceral surfaces of the lungs (Provost *et al.*, 1987).

The interlobular septa of the affected lung show distension with amber-coloured fluid surrounding the distended lymphatics. This fluid separates the lung lobules which vary in colour with red, grey and yellow hepatization being evident indicating different stages of inflammatory lesions. Consolidation of the lungs with typical marbled appearance, sometimes accompanied by adhesion of the parietal and visceral surfaces is also characteristic (Fig. 1.7). In chronic or advanced cases, a sequestrum consisting of necrotic lung parenchyma surrounded by a fibrous capsule (Fig. 1.8), which varies in size between 1 and 10 cm in thickness, is formed (Santini *et al.*, 1992). It was believed that the sequestrum may constitute a source of infection to cattle when ruptured, particularly where the sequestrum is drained by a bronchus and forms an outlet for the dissemination of infected aerosol droplets. Such a mechanism would account for outbreaks of disease in closed herds but is more often due to a surreptitious introduction of an infected animal or an animal with a long-lasting hidden infection. Windsor and Masiga (1977), however, could not experimentally induce the breakdown of sequestra and believed that only acutely infected animals transmitted the disease. In acutely infected animals, one or more infarcts may be seen in the kidneys.

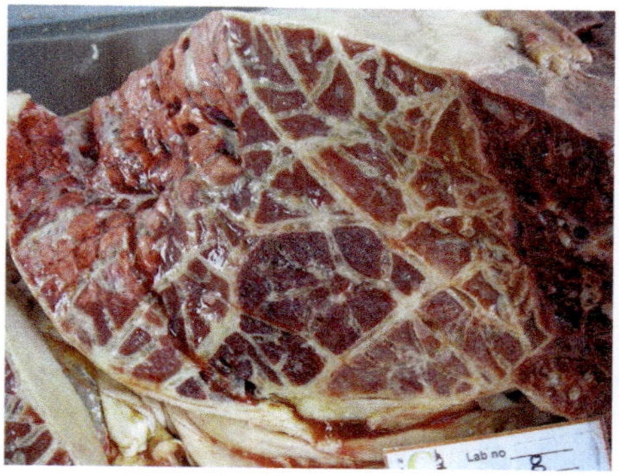

Fig. 1.7. Marbled lung showing greatly distended interlobular and areas of consolidation. (Photo source: Robin Nicholas.)

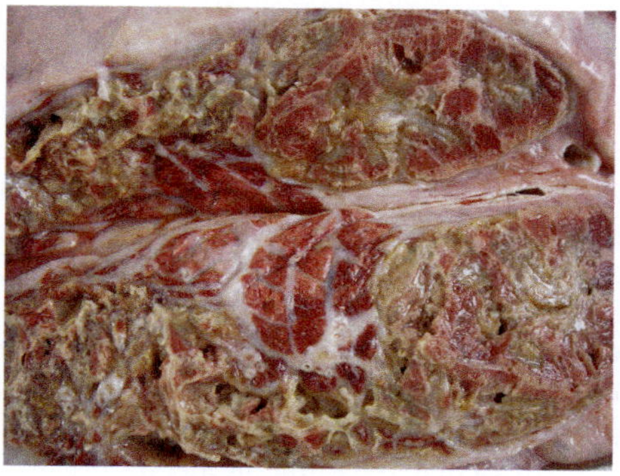

Fig. 1.8. Sequestra developing – showing lung tissue at various stages of necrosis surrounded by fibrotic capsule. (Photo source: Robin Nicholas.)

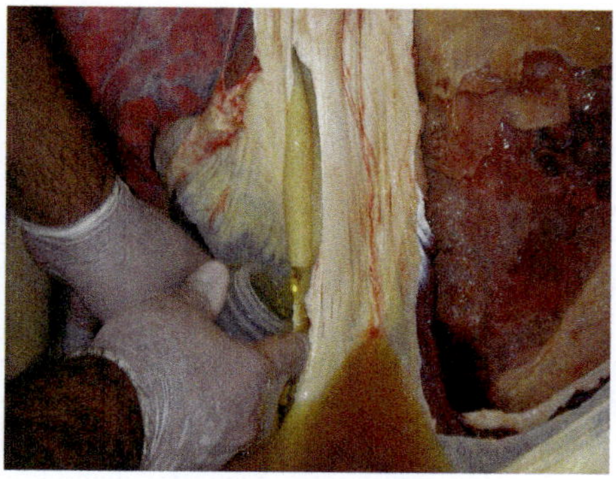

Fig. 1.6. Pleural fluid in the thoracic cavity of CBPP affected cow. (Photo source: Robin Nicholas.)

In addition to respiratory disease, affected calves may present exudative peritonitis, arthritis, bursitis and fibrinous arthritis of the carpal and tarsal joints (Provost *et al.*, 1987). Often, enlargement of the suprascapular lymph nodes may accompany these changes.

Histopathology

Early on in the course of disease, the CBPP lesion comprises a bronchiolar necrosis and oedema, progressing rapidly to an exudative sero-fibrinous bronchiolitis with extension to the alveoli and uptake of alveolar fluid into tissue spaces, lymph vessels and, ultimately, septal lymphatics ducts (Done *et al.*, 1995). These rapidly reach saturation, and the process is extended centrifugally to the tracheobronchial lymph nodes, and centripetally to the pleural lymphatic ducts. The mediastinal, sternal, aortic and intercostal lymph nodes may then become enlarged, oedematous or even haemorrhagic. With stasis, lymph vessels become thrombosed and, ultimately, fibrosed. The pulmonary lobules become consolidated with alveolar oedema, fibrin and inflammatory cells. Coagulative necrosis is common. *M. m. mycoides* can be isolated from or demonstrated in these lobules by immunohistochemistry.

Perivascular organization foci or 'organizing centres', found in the interlobular septa, are considered pathognomonic for CBPP (Ferronha *et al.*, 1988). They consist of a centre occupied by a blood vessel with proliferation of connective and inflammatory cells, surrounded by a peripheral zone of necrotic cells. Two types of foci have been recognized (Nunes Petisca *et al.*, 1988). Type I foci contain more proliferative cells in the central zone, which is larger than the peripheral zone and probably corresponds to the success of the host immune response in resolving the infection; immunoreactive antigen is associated with macrophages. In Type II foci, the proliferative cells are scarce, and the peripheral zone is relatively larger. Immunoreactive antigens can be seen in the central zone inside blood vessels, and it is thought that Type II foci indicate a failure of the immune response leading to aggravation of signs.

An immunocytochemical study of CBPP-infected Italian cattle (Scanziani *et al.*, 1997) showed that the severity of lung lesions

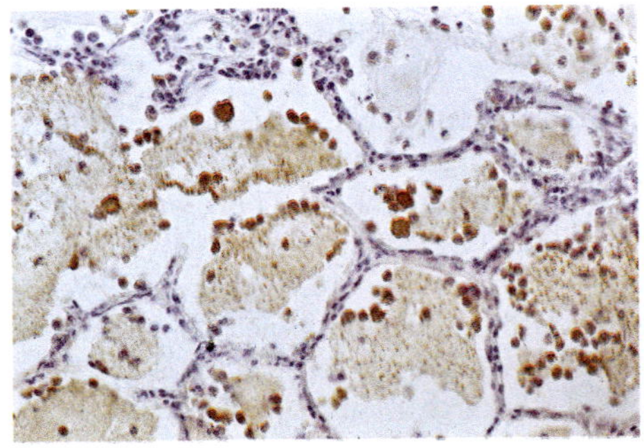

Fig. 1.9. Immunocytochemistry staining – lungs from a cow with acute CBPP. Alveolar spaces show positivity associated with the fibrinous exudate and inflammatory cells. The magnification is 400x. The primary antibody is a rabbit polyclonal (x400). (Photo courtesy of Professor Eugenio Scanziani.)

correlated with the severity of changes in the lymph nodes. In the acute stage of the disease, specific antigen was detected in the lobular periphery and in the cytoplasm of alveolar macrophages. In chronic lesions, immunoreactivity was seen in the fibrotic areas and in macrophages located in the lobular septa (Fig. 1.9)). Necrotic debris and macrophages located in the inner part of the sequestrum were specifically stained. Immunoreactive material was also seen in the centro-follicular areas of the broncho-associated lymphoid tissue structures and in the lymph node follicles. Furthermore, electron microscopy of the mediastinal lymph nodes of a chronically affected calf showed degenerating mycoplasmas and a few apparently intact mycoplasmas in the macrophages.

Differential Diagnosis

During the re-emergence of the disease in southern Europe in the 1980s, CBPP was present in cattle herds in all four affected countries, months, if not years, before it was diagnosed, despite respiratory signs being evident in many of the herds. Rapid use of antimicrobial medication by attending veterinarians would have suppressed clinical signs inhibiting accurate diagnosis. So, differentiating CBPP from other diseases requires attention to the onset of clinical signs, their severity, and the specific signs associated with respiratory distress. In housed conditions, cattle can be virtually dead on their feet before CBPP is recognized (Nicholas *et al.*, 1996). Today, once suspected, a tentative diagnosis can be achieved in minutes by pen-side tests, such as the latex agglutination test (LAT), without the need for a specialist laboratory. While not as sensitive as other tests, the LAT is able to detect a sufficient number of positive cattle to enable control measures to be initiated until the results are confirmed by laboratory-based tests.

Rinderpest could sometimes be confused with CBPP due to fever and discharges from the eyes, nose and mouth. Furthermore, lung lesions consisting of red areas of collapse, together with emphysema of lung lobules and the septa separating them, were seen in more chronic cases of rinderpest. Since the global eradication of rinderpest in 2011, this is no longer an issue. The more common diseases which may give rise to misdiagnoses include haemorrhagic septicaemia, also known as shipping fever, caused by *Pasteurella* and *Mannheimia* species. It was thought to be the disease, resembling CBPP, which almost led to a trade war between Britain and the USA in the late 19th century (see Chapter 5). It can produce lung lesions similar to the marbling seen in CBPP, fluid in the chest cavity and lung adhesion. Bovine respiratory disease caused by multiple bacterial and viral pathogens may also cause concern though, unlike CBPP, lesions are mostly seen in both lungs. More alarmingly, *Mycoplasma bovis* lesions can occasionally resemble the swelling of the interlobular septa (Fig. 1.10). Tubercular nodules caused by bovine TB can look like sequestra but are not so well defined and may be calcified.

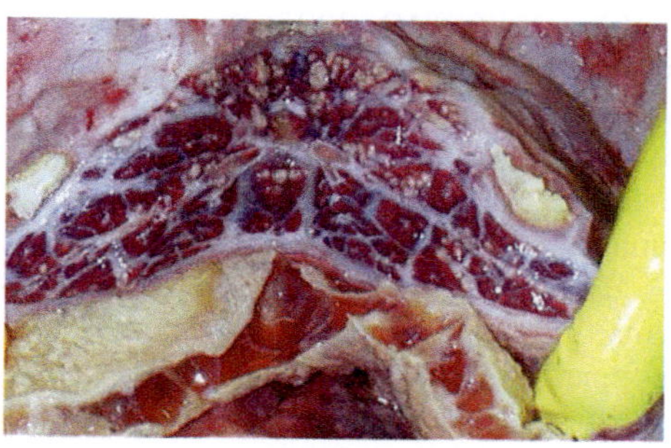

Fig. 1.10. Atypical lesion produced by Mycoplasma bovis resembling CBPP. (Photo source: Robin Nicholas.)

Immunisation and Vaccines

The internationally approved product is a live attenuated vaccine, T1/44, which has been in use for over 70 years (Olorunshola *et al.*, 2017). It suffers from a short duration of efficacy, adverse reactions and cold chain dependence. Endobronchial inoculation of the vaccine has been shown to lead to CBPP (Mbulu *et al.*, 2004). Furthermore, there were suspicions that this vaccine and its variants had lost efficacy and that the vaccination campaigns of 1995 and 1996 did not provide the expected levels of protection. In 1995, such were the doubts about the identity and potency of the widely used streptomycin-resistant variant T1/44-SR, that its use was discouraged (Tulasne *et al.*, 1996). Various suggestions were made to explain vaccine failure, including loss of immunogenicity, increased virulence of outbreaks and insufficient vaccine titres. March (2004) recommended changing the buffering of the vaccine, which was designed for the bivalent rinderpest-CBPP vaccine and probably had a deleterious effect on the live mycoplasma component when reconstituted. Experienced CBPP professionals often said there were very few problems when the broth vaccine was used in the 1970s and 1980s, though maintaining the cold chain was a challenge in the African heat (Windsor, personal communication).

Numerous new experimental vaccines have been produced over the last 30 years in an effort to improve the protection afforded by the T1/44, but none have so far succeeded in replacing it (Olorunshola *et al.*, 2017). The development of new vaccines for CBPP has been problematic. Two approaches were used initially, with the first concentrating on immunostimulating complexes (ISCOMs) as carriers for subunit vaccines. Whole detergent-solubilised cells of *M. m. mycoides* consisting mainly of membrane proteins have been used to obtain strong and long-lasting immunity in mice and vaccinated cattle. However, field trials were less successful with poor immune responses although some protection to challenge was seen in vaccinated animals.

Since then, work has been carried out using saponised whole cells and different purified proteins; however, these approaches have generally resulted in no protection and even exacerbation of disease (Nicholas *et al.*, 2005).

An understanding of the immunology associated with CBPP and the protective response may help in the formulation of a more effective vaccine. Scacchia *et al.* (2007) indicated that cyclosporine suppressed the immune response, which impacted on disease outcome. Information on the immune response can appear contradictory, with some indicating CD4 +T cells have a major contribution in animals that have recovered from infection whereas Sacchini *et al.* (2011) say CD4 +T lymphocytes have a minor role in the control of a primary infection of CBPP in cattle.

A new vaccine with none of the disadvantages of T1/44 would help but there would still be the problem of achieving the required 80% coverage required to have an impact on CBPP control. Work has been reported on the development of new vaccines that include sub-unit, attenuated and killed vaccines with variable reports of success. Using reverse vaccinology, the team at VIDO, Canada identified immunogenic recombinant proteins that provided similar protection to T1/44 in cattle using an improved aerosol challenge model. The vaccine is going through further trials in Kenya to achieve acceptance.

In a review of CBPP in Africa, Olorunshola *et al.* (2017) argued that the present tools for diagnosis and control are adequate for eradication and what is necessary are resources to improve vaccine coverage to levels of at least 80%, last seen in the 1970s when CBPP was restricted to very few countries of Africa. In addition, they note that a study in Namibia supported the concept that strategic and targeted antimicrobial treatment can play a critical part in the control alongside regular and comprehensive vaccination (Hűebschle *et al.*, 2006).

Historically, it has been believed that antibiotics have no role in the eradication of CBPP either at farm level or, more importantly, nationally and internationally. Antibiotics can, of course, alleviate clinical signs, enabling some improvement in condition. For the individual farmer, particularly the nomad, this prevents the loss of often their only form of income and livelihood; the fact that these treated animals may provide a constant source of infection to all those they come into contact with is not the farmer's primary concern. Strategically, it could be argued that any reduction in mycoplasma excretion inevitably leads to a reduction in disease incidence. However, this needs to be balanced against the damage caused by symptomless cattle spreading disease within and across international boundaries, which often results in explosive outbreaks among susceptible populations.

The reality is that, despite official condemnation, antibiotics *are* used, so advice is necessary on which are the most effective. Ayling *et al.* (2000) carried out an *in vitro* trial of the effects of five commonly used antibiotics on a number of strains of *M. m. mycoides* and concluded that tilmicosin and danofloxacin were effective both in terms of mycoplasmastatic and mycoplasmacidal activity; florfenicol and a tetracycline provide intermediate effectiveness while spectinomycin was ineffective against some strains. The use of fluoroquinolones, such as danofloxacin, is causing concern among regulatory authorities who feel these drugs should be restricted to human use because of rapid increases in microbial resistance.

More work needs to be done on the effectiveness of using antibiotics to control CBPP. Undoubtedly, treatment of single animals will not control the spread of disease among infected herds, so strategic treatment plans need to be investigated as stated by the FAO-OIE-AU/IBAR-IAEA Consultative Group Meeting on CBPP in Africa 2006 (FAO, 2007). Understandably, any recommendation to use antibiotics raises concerns about inducing antibiotic resistance in bacteria, and any possible subsequent effect on future disease treatment in animals and humans.

More recently, controlled *in vivo* experiments in Zambia and Kenya showed that the macrolide, tulathromycin, could achieve metaphylactic protection of up to 80% and prevent the spread of CBPP to untreated controls (Muuka *et al.*, 2019). Further studies are required to evaluate antibiotic strategies with and without vaccination.

Economic Impact

The economic effects of CBPP can be enormous, resulting in heavy losses in cattle populations. In Britain, 187,000 cattle died of CBPP in 1860 (Hutyra *et al.*, 1938). In the Netherlands, nearly 65,000 cattle died of CBPP between 1833 and 1850 (ter Laak, 1992). Over 100,000 cattle died within 2 years of the introduction of CBPP into South Africa (Trichard *et al.*, 1989). In the early 1860s when the disease spread rapidly throughout Australia, it behaved as a virulent epidemic, with losses of up to 75% of animals in an affected herd amounting to 1.4 million head. The Nigeria Animal Diseases Information System (NADIS) classified Nigeria as an endangered zone based on its CBPP status. The value of these losses was assessed nationally and across the four agro-ecological zones of Nigeria to be US$8.7 million (Olorunshola *et al.*, 2017). Economically, Nigeria suffers direct losses through infection and deaths of cattle, while indirect losses include exclusion from participation in international livestock and livestock product trade.

References

Ayling, R.D., Baker, S.E., Nicholas, R.A.J., Peek, M.L. and Simon, A.J. (2000) Comparison of in vitro activity of danofloxacin, florfenicol, oxytetracycline, spectinomycin and tilmicosin against *Mycoplasma mycoides* subspecies mycoides small colony type. *Veterinary Record* 146(9), 243–246.

Blancou, J. (2000) *History of the surveillance and control of transmissible diseases*. Office International Des Epizooties, Paris, France, pp. 133–160.

Bové, J.M. (1999) The 100th anniversary of the first culture of a mollicute. The contagious bovine pleuropneumonia microbe by Nocard and Roux with the collaboration of Borrel, Salimbeni and Dujardin-Baumetz. *Research in Microbiology* 150(4), 239–245.

Di Teodoro, G., Marruchella, G., Di Provvido, A., D'Angelo, A.R., Orsini, G. *et al.* (2020) Contagious bovine pleuropneumonia: A comprehensive overview. *Veterinary Pathology* 57(4), 476–489.

Done, S.H., Nicholas, R. and Palmer, N. (1995) Contagious bovine pleuropneumonia (CBPP). An emerging disease in Europe. *Cattle Practice* 3(1), 13–20.

Dupuy, V., Manso-Silván, L., Barbe, V., Thebault, P., Dordet-Frisoni, E. *et al.* (2012) Evolutionary history of contagious bovine pleuropneumonia using next generation sequencing of *Mycoplasma mycoides* subsp. mycoides 'Small colony'. *PLOS ONE* 7(10), e46821.

FAO (2007) CBPP control: Antibiotics to the rescue. Consultative Group Meeting of the FAO-OIE-OAU/IBAR-IAEA. FAO, Rome, Italy. Available at: https://www.fao.org/4/ah672e/ah672e00.htm (accessed November 2006).

Ferronha, M.H., Nunes Petisca, J.L., Sousa Ferreira, H., Machado, M. and Regalla, J. (1988) Localizacão de antigenios *Mycoplasma mycoides* subspecies mycoides nas lesoes do pulmao de bovinos com peripneumonia. In: *Nacional Repositorio de Trabalhos Do Laboratorio de Investigacao Veterinaria*. Numero Especial, pp. 25–36.

Firrao, G. and Brown, D.R. (2011) International committee on systematics of prokaryotes. Subcommittee on the taxonomy of *Mollicutes*. Minutes of the meetings, 11 and 16 July 2010, Chianciano Terme, Italy. *International Journal of Systematic and Evolutionary Microbiology* 61(3), 695–697.

Fischer, A., Shapiro, B., Muriuki, C., Heller, M., Schnee, C. *et al.* (2012) The origin of the '*Mycoplasma mycoides* cluster' coincides with domestication of ruminants. *PLOS ONE* 7(4), e36150.

Freundt, E.A. (1955) The classification of the pleuropneumonia group of organisms (*Borrelomycetales*). *International Bulletin of Bacteriological Nomenclature and Taxonomy* 5(2), 67–78.

Gonçalves, R., Ferreira-Dias, G., Belo, A., Correia, J., Ferreira, M.L. *et al.* (2002) Pathological and immunological characteristics of ewes experimentally infected with *Mycoplasma mycoides* subsp. mycoides SC strains isolated from cattle and sheep. *Small Ruminant Research* 46(1), 51–62.

Gosney, F., Corrò, M., Iob, L., McAuliffe, L. and Nicholas, R.A.J. (2011) Variable number tandem repeat (VNTR) typing of strains of *Mycoplasma mycoides* subspecies mycoides small colony isolated from the North-Eastern regions of Italy between 1990 and 1993. *Veterinary Microbiology* 147(1–2), 220–222.

Guadagnini, P.F., Simone, F. de, Panina, G.F., Gaffuri, A., Bugnetti, M. *et al.* (1991) Contagious bovine pleuropneumonia (CBPP). A review with field observations. *Selezione Veterinaria* 32(1), 3–31.

Houshaymi, B.M., Miles, R.J. and Nicholas, R.A. (1997) Oxidation of glycerol differentiates african from european isolates of *Mycoplasma mycoides* subsp. *mycoides* SC (small colony). *Veterinary Record* 140(7), 182–183.

Hudson, J.R. (1971) Contagious bovine pleuropneumonia. F.A.O. Agricultural Studies No 86, Food and Agricultural Organisation, Rome, 49 pp.

Huebschle, O.J.B., Ayling, R.D., Godinho, K., Lukhele, O., Tjipura-Zaire, G. *et al.* (2006) Danofloxacin (advocintm) reduces the spread of contagious bovine pleuropneumonia to healthy in-contact cattle. *Research in Veterinary Science* 81(3), 304–309.

Hutyra, F. and Marek, J. (1912) *Special Pathology and Therapeutics of the Diseases of Domestic Animals*, American edition. Bailliere Tindall, USA, pp. 389–391.

Hutyra, F., Marek, J. and Manninger, R. (1938) *Special pathology and therapeutics of the diseases of domestic animals*, 5th edition. Bailliere Tindall, USA, pp. 455–458.

Hyslop, N.St.G. (1958) The adaptation of *Asterococcus mycoides* to rodents. *Journal of Pathology and Bacteriology* 75, 189–199.

Jores, J., Baldwin, C., Blanchard, A., Browning, G.F., Colston, A. *et al.* (2020) Contagious bovine and caprine pleuropneumonia: A research community's recommendations for the development of better vaccines. *NPJ Vaccines* 5(1), 66.

March, J.B. (2004) Improved formulations for existing CBPP vaccines: Recommendations for change. In: Towards sustainable CBPP control programmes for Africa. *Proceedings FAO-OIE-AU/IBAR-IAEA Consultative Group on Contagious Bovine Pleuropneumonia, Food and Agriculture Organization of the United Nations (FAO)*, Third Meeting, Rome, Italy, pp. 102–109.

Masiga, M.N., Domenech, J. and Windsor, R.S. (1996) Manifestation and epidemiology of contagious bovine pleuropneumonia in Africa. *Revue Scientifique et Technique. Office International Des Epizooties* 15(4), 1283–1308.

Mbulu, R.S., Tjipura-Zaire, G., Lelli, R., Frey, J., Pilo, P. *et al.* (2004) Contagious bovine pleuropneumonia (CBPP) caused by vaccine strain T1/44 of *Mycoplasma mycoides* subsp. *mycoides* SC. *Veterinary Microbiology* 98(3–4), 229–234.

McAuliffe, L., Ellis, R.J., Miles, K., Ayling, R.D. and Nicholas, R.A.J. (2006) Biofilm formation by mycoplasma species and its role in environmental persistence and survival. *Microbiology* 152, 913–922.

McAuliffe, L., Ayling, R.D. and Nicholas, R.A.J. (2007) Identification and characterization of variable-number tandem-repeat markers for the molecular epidemiological analysis of *Mycoplasma mycoides* subspecies *mycoides* SC. *FEMS Microbiology Letters* 276(2), 181–188.

McAuliffe, L., Ayling, R.D., Ellis, R.J. and Nicholas, R.A.J. (2008) Biofilm-grown *Mycoplasma mycoides* subsp. *mycoides* SC exhibit both phenotypic and genotypic variation compared with planktonic cells. *Veterinary Microbiology* 129(3–4), 315–324.

Muuka, G., Otina, B., Wesonga, H., Bowa, B., Gicheru, N. *et al.* (2019) Evaluation of new generation macrolides for the treatment and metaphylaxis of contagious bovine pleuropneumonia (CBPP) in cattle experimentally infected with *Mycoplasma mycoides* subspecies *mycoides*. *BMC Veterinary Research* 15(451), 1–13.

Nicholas, R., Ayling, R. and McAuliffe, L. (2008) Contagious bovine pleuropneumonia. In: *Mycoplasma Diseases of Ruminants*. CABI Publishing, Oxford, UK, pp. 69–97.

Nicholas, R.A.J. and Palmer, N.M.A. (1994) Contagious bovine pleuropneumonia in Europe. *State Veterinary Journal* 4, 14–16.

Nicholas, R.A.J., Santini, F.G., Clark, K.M., Palmer, N.M.A., De Santis, P. *et al.* (1996) A comparison of serological tests and gross lung pathology for the detection of contagious bovine pleuropneumonia in two groups of Italian cattle. *Veterinary Record* 139, 89–93.

Nicholas, R.A.J., Tjipura-Zaire, G., Scacchia, M., Frey, J. and Hübschle, O.J.B. (2005) An inactivated vaccine against CBPP exacerbates disease in cattle. In: *Proceedings of FAO/OIE.OU Consultative Meeting on CBPP*, FAO, Rome, November 2004, pp. 91–97.

Nocard, E. and Roux, E. (1990) The microbe of pleuropneumonia. *Reviews of Infectious Diseases* 12(2), 354–358. Available at: https://www-jstor-org.er.lib.k-state.edu/stable/pdf/4455506.pdf?refreqid=fastly-default%3A2ba70aaea06d16af0c778db70b5041d6&ab_segments=&initiator=&acceptTC=1

Nunes Petisca, J.L., Duraco, J.F.C., Lage, M., Gonçalves, J.M.M., Ramos, M.J.A. *et al.* (1988) Pathogenesis and pathology of contagious bovine pleuropneumonia in Portugal. In: *Patogenia e*

Anatomia Atologica de Peripneumonia Contagiosa Dos Bovinos (PPCB) Em Portugal. Repositorio Des Trabalhos Do Laboratorio Nacional de Investigacão Veterinaria (Lisbon). Numero Special, pp. 1–10.

Nunes Petisca, J.L., Costa Durao, J.F., Lage, M., Goncalves, J.M., Azevedo Ramos, M.J. *et al.* (1990) Pathogenesis and pathological features of contagious bovine pleuropneumonia (CBPP). In: *Contagious bovine pleuropneumonia. A Seminar in the Community Programme for the Coordination of Agricultural Research*, Lisbon, 7-8 December 1988, pp. 2–6.

Olorunshola, I.D., Peters, A.R., Scacchia, M. and Nicholas, R.A.J. (2017) Contagious bovine pleuropneumonia – never out of Africa? *Veterinary Bulletin* 12(19), 1–7.

Privy Council (1874) Letter by Alexander Williams, 16 January.

Provost, A., Perreau, P., Bréard, A., Goff, C. le, Martel, J.L. *et al.* (1987) Contagious bovine pleuropneumonia. *Revue Scientifique et Technique, Office International Des Epizooties* 6(3), 565–679.

Regalla, J. (1984) Epidemiological aspects of the contagious bovine pleuropneumonia in Portugal. *Repositório de Trabalhos Do Laboratorio Nacional de Investigacao Veterinaria* 16(13), 15–18.

Regalla, J., Caporale, V., Giovannini, A., Santini, F., Martel, J.L. *et al.* (1996) Manifestation and epidemiology of contagious bovine pleuropneumonia in Europe. *Revue Scientifique et Technique. Office International Des Epizooties* 15(4), 1309–1329.

Sacchini, F., Naessens, J., Awino, E., Heller, M., Hlinak, A. *et al.* (2011) A minor role of CD4+ T lymphocytes in the control of a primary infection of cattle with *Mycoplasma mycoides* subsp. *mycoides*. *Veterinary Research* 42(1), 77.

Salmon, D.E. (1888–1889) Mediate contagion in pleuro-pneumonia. *American Veterinary Review* 12, 63–73.

Santini, F.G., D'Angelo, A.R., Scacchia, M., Giannatale, E. di, Visaggio, M.C. *et al.* (1992) A domestic buffalo with a pulmonary sequestrum caused by *Mycoplasma mycoides* subsp. *mycoides* SC: Isolation, pathology and immunohistochemistry. *Veterinaria Italiana* 28(4), 4–10.

Scacchia, M., Sacchini, F., Filipponi, G., Luciani, M., Lelli, R. *et al.* (2007) Clinical, humoral and ifngamma responses of cattle to infection with *Mycoplasma mycoides* var. *Mycoides* small colony and attempts to condition the pathogenesis of the infection. *Onderstepoort Journal of Veterinary Research* 74(3), 251–263.

Scanziani, E., Paltrinieri, S., Boldini, M., Grieco, V., Monaci, C. *et al.* (1997) Histological and immunohistochemical findings in thoracic lymph nodes of cattle with contagious bovine pleuropneumonia. *Journal of Comparative Pathology* 117(2), 127–136.

Shahram, M., Nicholas, R.A.J., Wood, A.P. and Kelly, D.P. (2010) Further evidence to justify reassignment of *Mycoplasma mycoides* subspecies *mycoides* Large Colony type to *Mycoplasma mycoides* subspecies *capri*. *Systematic and Applied Microbiology* 33(1), 20–24.

Shirlaw, J.F. and Iver, P.R.K. (1946) Studies on contagious bovine pleuropneumonia in Assam. *Indian Journal of Veterinary Science and Animal Husbandry* 16, 191–208.

ter Laak, E.A. (1992) Contagious bovine pleuropneumonia. *Veterinary Quarterly* 14(3), 104–110.

Trichard, C.J.V., Basson, P.A., Lugt, J.J. van der and Jacobsz, E.P. (1989) An outbreak of contagious bovine pleuropneumonia in the Owambo Mangetti area of South West Africa/Namibia: Microbiological, immunofluorescent, pathological and serological findings. *Onderstepoort Journal of Veterinary Research* 56(4), 277–284.

Tulasne, J.J., Litamoi, J.K., Morein, B., Dedieu, L., Palya, V.J. *et al.* (1996) Contagious bovine pleuropneumonia vaccines: The current situation and the need for improvement. *Revue Scientifique et Technique. Office International Des Epizooties* 15(4), 1373–1396.

Turner, A.W. and Campbell, A.D. (1937) A note on the application of the complement-fixation test to the control of bovine pleuro-pneumonia. *Australian Veterinary Journal* 13(5), 183–186.

Turner, A.W., Campbell, A.D. and Dick, A.T. (1935) Recent work on Pleuropneumonia contagiosa Boum in North Queensland. *Australian Veterinary Journal* 11(2), 63–71.

Windsor, R.S. and Masiga, W.N. (1977) Investigations into the role of carrier animals in the spread of contagious bovine pleuropneumonia. *Research in Veterinary Science* 23(2), 224–229.

Xin, J., Li, Y., Nicholas, R.A.J., Chen, C., Liu, Y. *et al.* (2012) A history of the prevalence and control of contagious bovine pleuropneumonia in China. *Veterinary Journal* 191(2), 166–170.

Yaya, A., Manso-Silván, L., Blanchard, A. and Thiaucourt, F. (2008) Genotyping of *Mycoplasma mycoides* subsp. *mycoides* SC by multilocus sequence analysis allows molecular epidemiology of contagious bovine pleuropneumonia. *Veterinary Research* 39(2), 14–21.

2 Europe: Birth of a Disease

Abstract

Beginning with the first crude descriptions (and supposed remedies) in the 16th century, European agriculturalists, veterinarians, microbiologists, and regulators have figured prominently in the global story of contagious bovine pleuropneumonia (CBPP). While often advocating bizarre remedies, late medieval texts consistently signal an understanding of the contagiousness of diseases, including sicknesses of the lungs. Due to continental Europe's critical mass of pioneering veterinary institutions (including the establishment of the first veterinary school, in France), CBPP's pathological characteristics became clearer in the 18th century. Concomitant with the disease's spread across nation state borders, additional scientific treatises on CBPP eventually appeared in all the major European languages. While practitioners and regulators alike grappled with CBPP, a relatively small group of science minded men – writing in English, Italian, French, German and other languages – have left today's scientists with a rich reservoir of information that, taken together, paints a picture of the circumstances that led to CBPP becoming a truly global challenge. Among Europe's contributions to the story of lung plague, the elaboration of its etiology, by French scientists at the close of the 19th century, stands out as most significant.

Introduction

Europe's first documented appreciation for the phenomenon of CBPP seems to appear half a millennium ago, in the year 1523. Authored by one of two brothers (John or Anthony Fitzherbert; as explained further on, most scholars have attributed authorship to John), the *Boke of Husbandrie* gives a description of 'longesaughte' (Fitzherbert, 1523, folio 25 recto). This ailment, which appears right after 'murrain' (presumably cattle plague or rinderpest) in a section on cattle diseases, is described as a long-lasting and contagious disorder (Smith, 1976, p. 133). While it remains unclear which of the Fitzherbert brothers authored the book (Gay, 1904), the *Boke of Husbandrie* enjoyed wide appeal, being published again a decade later (see Fig. 2.1 a,b).

The debate about the book's authorship is important for weighing the credibility of its scientific (albeit crude) clinical description and treatment of CBPP. One of the Fitzherbert brothers (Anthony) was a lawyer, but the other (John) was a bona fide agriculturalist; John's authorship would best explain the text's 'abundant indication of an exceptional knowledge of practical farming' (Gay, 1904, p. 591). A French chronicler of the history of veterinary medicine makes the following assessment of John as the author of the *Boke of Husbandrie*:

> Il n'a aucune connaissance de la medecine, mais il se revele comme un observateur attentif et avise [He has no knowledge of medicine, but he is an attentive and astute observer]. (Lechlainche, 1936, p. 147)

Synthesizing the original Old English prose with his own interpretive and explanatory comments, Walter Skeat's 1882 edited volume of the *Boke of Husbandrie* reveals that John Fitzherbert identified a beast with 'Long sought' as one that 'coughs 20 times an hour' (Skeat, 1882, p. 54). The *Boke of Husbandrie* emphasizes that the disease can persist for a long time, laments that 'fewe of them do mende [recover]' and, with some epidemiological foresight, advocates the separation of diseased and exposed animals (that is, 'as many as were in companye with that beast that fyrst fell sycke') from healthy ones. The most bizarre feature of the book's devotion to the disease is a proposed treatment involving bleeding, and inserting into the dewlap 'a rowel [circular slice] of 'seitergrasse' [setterwort, *Helleborus foetidus*, used in the primitive treatment method of settering]' (Skeat, 1882, p. 54; Lechlainche,

DOI: 10.1079/9781800627536.0002

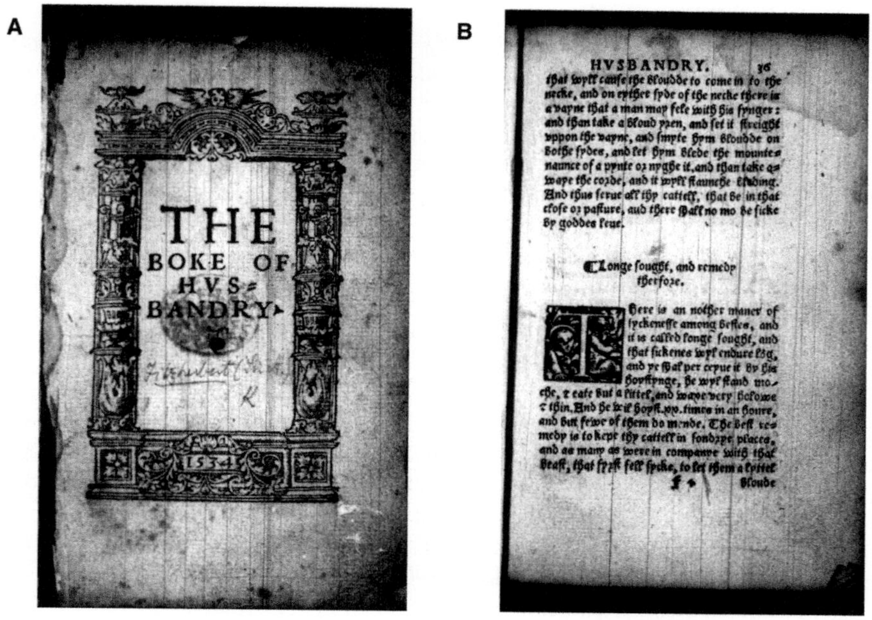

Fig. 2.1. The 1534 edition of Fitzherbert's *Boke of Husbandry*. First published in 1523, the author refers to CBPP as 'Longe sought'. (Cover (A) and 36 recto (B) from Fitzherbert, M., 1534, public domain via Internet Archive.)

1936, p. 148; Davidson, 1960; Smith, 1976, p. 133). The insights recorded in Fitzherbert's *Boke of Husbandrie* would be echoed in other agricultural publications, including those on the continent, during the late 16th and early 17th centuries.

In Germany, a 1570 treatise, authored in Latin by a humanist scholar (Conrad Heresbach, who fashioned himself as Conradus Heresbachius), argues that the presence of any and all livestock diseases should prompt owners to wisely 'segregandi incolumes a morbidis, ne contagio sanos corripiat, imprimisar cendi comunibus aquis, atq; stabulis [separate the healthy from the sick, lest the contagion overtake the healthy, to impose a ban on common water and stables]' (Heresbach, 1570). The 1601 English translation of this Latin text (*Foure Bookes of Husbandry*) goes beyond Heresbach's original text, adding Fitzherbert's dewlap-focused remedy for treating the 'sicknes of the loongs' (Heresbach, 1601). Further evidence that Fitzherbert was held in high esteem may be seen in the *Foure Bookes of Husbandry*'s impressive catalogue of 'names of such Authors, and Husbands, whole authorities' whose works were consulted; 'M. Fitzherbert' appears in the list – among 17 other Englishmen and 49 great names from classical antiquity (including Aristotle, Galen and Hippocrates) (Dannenfelt, 1982, p. 542; Heresbach and Barnaby Googe (translator), 1601, frontmatter folio iv verso). The 1601 translation also reveals a growing consensus among European agriculturalists to separate diseased and healthy animals; regarding all cattle ailments ('divers kindes'), the *Foure Bookes of Husbandry* emphasizes the essence of Heresbach's 1570 assertion: 'Every one of these kindes, are contagious and infective, and therefore as soone as you perceave them infected, you must presently put them a sunder for infecting the whole flock' (Heresbach and Barnaby Googe (translator), 1601, folios 124 verso and 125 recto).

In addition to a growing European consensus about the contagiousness of animal diseases, specific references to a lung disease (that we now assume to be CBPP) emerge during the second half of the 16th century in an array of agricultural writings on the European continent. Italy appears among the first. In 1552, not yet 20 years after Fitzherbert first wrote about 'long-sought' (one of several Old English spellings; see Table 2.1 further on) in England, Agostino Gallo – one of the most prolific agricultural writers of the Italian Renaissance – undertook authoring the first of a series of agricultural treatises that would contain an ever-growing number of chapters (ten chapters in the 1564 edition, 13 in 1566, and 20 in 1569). The first edition, titled *Le dieci giornate della vera agricoltura, e piaceri della villa* [Ten days of real agriculture, and pleasures of the villa], appeared in 1564 in Brescia and, following publication in Venice in 1565 (Cancrini, 2022), enjoyed widespread dissemination and acceptance (Smith, 1976, p. 141; Bifolco and Ronca, 2014). After Gallo died in 1570, his sequential editions of *Giornate della vera agricoltura* endured and were translated into multiple languages; Fig. 2.2 shows an excerpt of a 1584 copy of the 20 chapter treatise (Gallo, 1584). In a section focused on cattle, Gallo refers to CBPP as 'al male della polmonera [the disease of the lung]'. He declares the ailment to be a 'desperato [desperate]' condition, arguing that it is best 'cheseparar tutte le vacche sane subito dalle infette, & ponerle nell altre stalle, no ritornandoule per piu giorni [to separate all the healthy cows immediately from the infected, and place them in the other stables, not returning them for several days]' (Gallo, 1584, p. 233).

Gallo's term for CBPP would be embraced by other Italian writers, including Giuseppe Falcone of Piacenza. In a 1603 book focused on a range of animal diseases, he singles out 'polmonera', differentiating it from cattle plague (murrain, or rinderpest):

> La polmonera è mal pessimo. Presto separa la sane dalle ammalate, questo è mal contagioso, come peste fra l'animali bovini. [Polmonera is a very bad disease. Separate soon the healthy from the sick, this is badly contagious, like plague among cattle]. (Falcone, 1603, p. 17)

Building on the English 'longsoughte' and Italian 'male della polmonera', a Parisian medical scientist, printer and agriculture enthusiast – Charles Estienne – authored an agricultural treatise that also refers to CBPP. In 1564 (concurrent with Gallo's inaugural work), Estienne published in Latin his *Praedium Rusticum* (Estienne, 1564); Estienne died shortly thereafter, but a close colleague (Jean Liebault, also a medical man and student of agriculture) immediately translated it into French (Blancou, 2003; Smith, 1976, p. 177). A 1570 edition of Liebault's French translation, titled *L'Agriculture et maison rustique*, features a chapter on cattle and draws attention to 'au mal de poulmon [the disease of the lungs]' (Liebault, 1570). Liebault continued to build on Estienne's original work,

Table 2.1. First terms for CBPP to emerge in selected early-modern European languages.

Language	Term(s)	Author	Date of first mention
Old English	longe sought, longsought, longesaughte	John (or, less likely, Anthony) Fitzherbert	1523 (London) in *Boke of Husbandrie*
Italian	al male della polmonera, la polmonera, polmonite essudativa, pleuro-pneumonite essudativa[a]	Agostino Gallo	1564 (Brescia) and 1565 (Venice) in *Le dieci giornate della vera agricoltura, e piaceri della villa*
French	au mal de poulmon, péripneumonie contagieuse, maladie de poitrine du gros betail[a]	Charles Estienne, and Jean Liebault (translator)	1570 (Paris) in *L'agriculture et maison rustique*
German	Lungenseuche, lungenfaule[a]	Michael Bernhard	1695 (probably Geissen) in *Constitutio epidemica Hassiaca*
Other terms used in other languages[a]	Latin: peri-pneumonia exsudatoria contagiosa Belgian: pleuropneumonie typhoid exsudative Dutch: longziekte		

[a]Many CBPP names, appearing after early-modern history, come from Curasson (1936). *Traité de pathologie exotique vétérinaire et comparée,* Vigot, Paris.

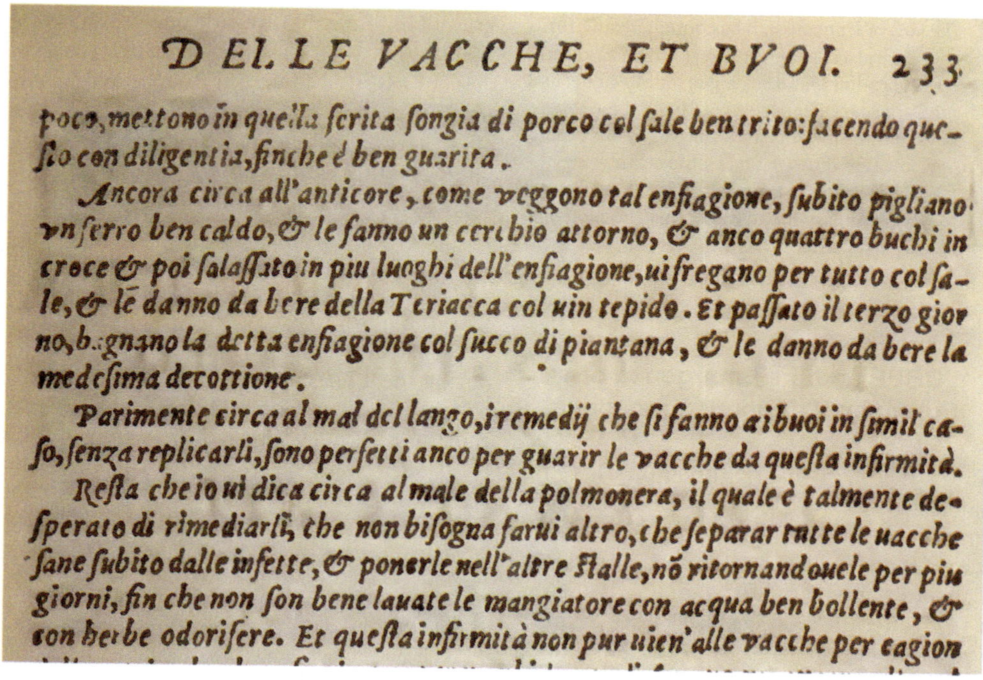

DELLE VACCHE, ET BVOI. 233

poco, mettono in quella ferita songia di porco col sale ben trito: facendo questo con diligentia, finche è ben guarita.

Ancora circa all'anticore, come veggono tal enfiagione, subito pigliano vn ferro ben caldo, & le fanno un cerchio attorno, & anco quattro buchi in croce & poi salassato in piu luoghi dell'enfiagione, ui fregano per tutto col sale, & lē danno da bere della Teriacca col uin tepido. Et passato il terzo giorno, bagnano la detta enfiagione col succo di piantana, & le danno da bere la medesima decottione.

Parimente circa al mal del lango, i remedij che si fanno ai buoi in simil caso, senza replicarli, sono perfetti anco per guarir le vacche da questa infirmità.

Resta che io ui dica circa al male della polmonera, il quale è talmente desperato di rimediarli, che non bisogna farui altro, che separar tutte le uacche sane subito dalle infette, & ponerle nell'altre stalle, nō ritornandouele per piu giorni, fin che non son bene lauate le mangiatore con acqua ben bollente, & con herbe odorifere. Et questa infirmità non pur uien' alle vacche per cagion

Fig. 2.2. One of the most widely read agricultural treatises of the Italian Renaissance features a section on 'vacche [cattle]' and 'buoi [oxen]'. The author, Agostino Gallo, terms CBPP as 'al male della polmonera [the disease of the lung]' and advises the separation of sick and healthy animals. (From Gallo, A., 1584, p. 233, public domain via Internet Archive.)

and an English translation of Estienne and Liebault's work (*Maison Rustique* or, *The Countrey Farme*) features a similar chapter structure and grammatically parallel language, referring to CBPP as 'the disease of the lungs' (Estienne and Liebault, 1616).

In addition to English, Italian and French monikers for CBPP, the German term 'Lungenseuche' emerges later (Table 2.1), as do other European linguistic terms for CBPP (Curasson, 1936). While the German writer Conrad Heresbach seems to demonstrate an appreciation for cattle diseases and their contagiousness, the most definitive first reference to CBPP in the German language occurs at the end of the 17th century. In 1695, a German medical doctor named Michael Bernhard (who styled himself as 'Valentini' despite not being Italian) superintended an investigation into an epidemic among cattle in his home region of Hesse. Bernhard's report focuses on 'eine *Seuche* des Viehs, welche von der *Lunge* auszugehen Schien [a *sickness* of cattle, which seemed to emanate from the *lungs*]' (Schrader and Hering, 1863, p. 437–438, italics added). Indeed, his report appears to lay a foundation for the German term '*Lungenseuche*, by which it [it would for many years be] known in Germany', according to James Law (Law, 1880). Law, who exercised leadership in both Britain and the USA (see Chapters 3, 4 and 5, this volume), demonstrated a wide understanding of the various terms used in Europe for CBPP. However, he expressed a preference for the German term, on which he built and derived his preferred English term for the disease: 'contagious lung-plague of cattle'. Illustrative of the power of words and cross-cultural awareness, Law's reasoning is noteworthy:

> Dr. Law has adopted that of *contagious lung-plague of cattle*, the new counterpart of the *Lungenseuche*, by which it has long been known in Germany. He regards the old term, *pulmonary murrain*, as equally good. The German *Lungenseuche* is especially apposite, the real meaning being *lung contagion*, which conveys

> the idea of transmission by contagion only. He therefore gives, as a definition of the malady, a specific contagious disease peculiar to cattle, and manifested by a long period of incubation (ten days to three months) by a slow, insidious onset, by a low type of fever, and by the occurrence of inflammation in the air passages, lungs, and their coverings, with an extensive exudation into lungs and pleurae. (Law, 1880)

CBPP and the Emergence of European Veterinary Education

During the 17th and 18th centuries, CBPP manifested itself in several locales in continental Europe, including Germany – where, as mentioned previously, medical doctors like Michael Bernhard rightly sounded the alarm in 1695 after the disease killed a large number of cattle in the region of Hesse (Blancou, 2003, p. 133). At the close of the 17th century, it was not uncommon to find CBPP in Switzerland and the Alpine regions of Germany and France (Hutyra *et al.*, 1938). By the beginning of the 1700s, discoveries of CBPP coincided with a wider and growing alarm regarding several livestock diseases – not just CBPP – spreading through an emerging livestock trade across nation-state borders. One husbandry guidebook, published in 1716 by an Englishman in London, and drawing on the 'Learned Van Helmount' (i.e. the pioneering Flemish physiologist Jan Baptista van Helmont), asserted that there were innumerable diseases facing livestock owners: 'There are several Epidemical and Destructive Diseases to Cattle, Fowl, &c. which sweep away a great part of the Husbandman's Stock before it ceaseth' (Worlidge, 1716, p. 353). This situation eventually prompted the establishment of Europe's – and, indeed, the world's – first veterinary educational institutions.

In 1711, and out of an aspiration to raise funds for the Russian treasury, Tsar Peter I (later, Peter the Great) sold cattle to Western European nations. Infected with cattle plague (the murrain, or rinderpest), this exchange facilitated the spread of the disease across Europe, prompting crude import controls that could not prevent innumerable livestock deaths (Blystone, 2001). In 1713, disease (including a respiratory ailment assumed to be CBPP) appeared in the Swabian region of Germany, several cantons of Switzerland, Italy, and Holland – where it killed 200,000 cattle within 10 years (Fleming, 1871, pp. 198–199). Three decades later, in 1743, another outbreak erupted in Zurich (New jersey office for the prevention of the spread, 1879, p. 5). Tragedy also soon struck France with the fresh arrival of rinderpest; there, the cattle plague 'eliminated half the national herd' during the 1740s and 1750s (Blystone, 2001, p. 8). Again, however, CBPP appeared alongside rinderpest throughout the 18th century and, in 1758, the widely respected Thomas Hale specifically addressed 'disorders of the lungs' in cattle (Hale, 1758, p. 448). Hale also provided the following recommendation for treatment:

> These are of various kinds [of lung disorders] in the cow...but one remedy will serve for them all. Sometimes the creature breathes with difficulty, sometimes coughs and wheezes. Bruise four heads of garlick, and press out the juice, mix this with a quart of new milk, and add a quarter of a pint of tar. This will serve for four doses. One is to be given every morning till the cure is compleated....If the disorder be obstinate, the creature should be blooded, and the medicine will then take effect. (Hale, 1758, pp. 448–449)

While Hale was regarded by the Royal Society for being an especially knowledgeable agriculturalist, such supposed treatments imply a lack of scientific sophistication (and even sound akin to the remedies advocated by the likes of John Fitzherbert 200 years prior). Fortunately, the 18th century witnessed a rapid maturation of scientific inquiry, with France demonstrating initial leadership in the European Enlightenment. As explained by scholars in the history of veterinary medicine, France had all the ingredients for leading the way in veterinary science: a robust printing culture, governmental sponsorship of education, an appreciation for the role of the human faculty of reason, and the study of nature (Jones and Koolmees, 2022, p. 88). In the 1760s, a veterinary education pioneer Claude Bourgelat (Fig. 2.3) was keen to establish a veterinary school. While he intended to establish one 'based on horse husbandry

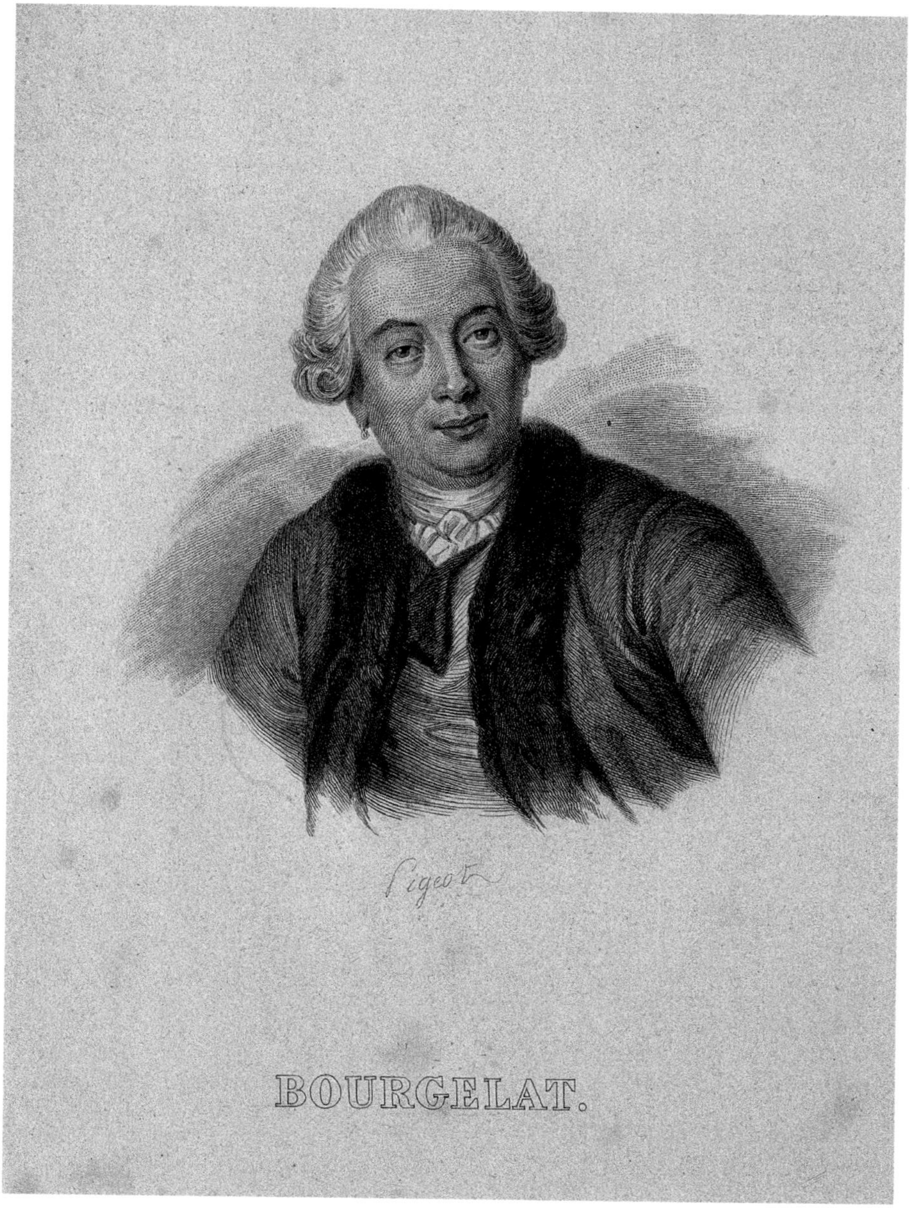

Fig. 2.3. Bourgelat founded the first veterinary school in Europe and, in 1769, authored one of the first, if not the first, comprehensive descriptions of CBPP. (From Pigeot, n.d., Claude Bourgelat (stipple engraving), Wellcome Library, London, CC-PD via Wikimedia Commons.)

and farriery', the head of the French treasury Henri-Léonard Bertin 'told Bourgelat that the French government would pay to establish a school if it included investigations into the diseases of cattle and other livestock' (Jones and Koolmees, 2022, p. 104). Bourgelat quickly acknowledged the need to train veterinarians to fight rinderpest, CBPP, and other diseases, and 1762 witnessed the establishment of the first modern era veterinary school, at Lyon (Blystone, 2001, p. 8). Bourgelat directed the École Vétérinaire de Lyon; in addition to emphasizing his passion for equine medicine, he was soon engaged with the livestock disease problem facing his country. In 1769, he was called upon to investigate a disease of cattle in the Franche-Comte region. The disease he discovered was initially referred to as 'murie' (likely a catch-all term for disease, akin to 'murrain'). Later scientists, reading the reports, concluded it was indeed CBPP, what Bourgelat's French predecessors had originally called 'au mal de poulmon' (see Table 2.1). By 1799, likely earlier, French veterinarians were routinely acknowledging that 'la péripneumonie' was 'une maladie contagieuse qui affecte les poumons [a contagious disease that affects the lungs]' (see Fig. 2.4) (Bonnaterre, 1799, p. 135). Soon thereafter, the combined term 'péripneumonie contagieuse' would be used (Salmon and Smith, 1896, p. 377).

Bourgelat's widely reported investigation of CBPP was foundational for European veterinary science; later veterinary textbooks would declare that CBPP 'was not definitely known until it was described by Bourgelat' (Walley, 1879, p. 5). Building on the momentum of Bourgelat and his school at Lyon, 22 more veterinary schools quickly sprouted up across Europe during the final decades of the 1700s (Lechlainche, 1936, p. 237). The new learning about the disease would spread to other countries – for example, Switzerland's Albrecht von Haller would join Bourgelat in 1766 in detailing the common symptoms of CBPP: fever, anorexia, sluggish rumination, coughing and foul-smelling breath (Blancou, 2003, p. 135). Growing European solidarity in the science of CBPP would prove fortunate, for a metaphorical 'army' of formally trained veterinarians would be needed in the coming years. Between 1790 and 1812, in particular during the Napoleonic Wars, CBPP would be spread across the European continent by cattle needed for the subsistence of marching soldiers (Salmon and Smith, 1896, p. 377). By the early 1800s, Italy, Switzerland, Belgium and Holland were commonly infected with CBPP; since Swiss and Dutch cattle were popular livestock imports (for breeding stock), CBPP would soon further fan its way across the continent (Hutyra *et al.*, 1938, p. 455).

LA PERIPNEUMONIE,

Ou affection gangréneuse du Poumon, qui règne ordinairement dans le printems, sur les bêtes à cornes.

La péripneumonie gangréneuse est une maladie contagieuse qui affecte les poumons ; elle est presque toujours épizootique dans les bêtes à cornes ; et c'est sous ce point de vue que nous la considérerons aujourd'hui.

Fig. 2.4. In the decades after Claude Bourgelat characterized CBPP, French scientists clearly understood the lung disease to be contagious, as illustrated in this excerpt from the 1799 textbook *Récueil de médecine vétérinaire*, and by the 19th century the term 'péripneumonie contagieuse' would become commonplace. (From Bonnaterre, P.J., 1799, *Récueil de médecine vétérinaire,* L.B., Carrere, Rodez, France, p. 135, public domain via Internet Archive.)

CBPP Spreads in 19th-Century Europe

With veterinary schools established in all the major European countries (including Great Britain, home to the London Veterinary College founded in 1792), a robust exchange of scientific insights ensued. Much insight continued to emanate from Lyon. In 1830, Professor Grognier of the École Vétérinaire de Lyon argued for the quarantining of CBPP-diseased cattle (Blancou, 1996, p. 1272). Three years later, an outbreak of CBPP in the French region of Avesnes caught the attention of yet another veterinary instructor at the École Vétérinaire de Lyon; Professor Lecoq's published report then caught the attention of other European veterinarians concerned about the disease (Dun, 1849, pp. 3–4). Among these was London's William Youatt, a pioneering educator and the editor of the *Veterinarian*. Youatt wanted veterinarians to embrace a more scientific approach to disease causation and treatment (Fisher, 1993, p. 288), and in his famous cattle textbook of 1833, he referenced Lecoq's account of CBPP (Dun, 1849, pp. 4). Youatt's index refers to Lecoq's account with 'Pleuro-pneumonia, interesting account of it' (Youatt, 1836). The Englishman then summarizes and comments on the French case:

> There is so instructive an account...in 'The Recueil de Médécine Vétérinaire,' for May, in the present year, (1833,) that the author is tempted to give it at considerable length. It is written by M. Lecoq, one of the teachers of the veterinary school of Lyons...He is speaking of Soire-le-Chateau, in the arrondissement of Avesnes, in which the farmers fatten more cattle than they breed, and therefore are obliged to purchase out of the neighbouring districts... The malady by which they are most frequently attacked, and which is particularly prevalent in some years, is one that is generally incurable, and the slaughter of the animal before he has perceptibly wasted, is the only means by which the farmer can avoid losing the whole value of the beast: this is *chronic pleura-pneumonia*... (Youatt, 1836, p. 407)

Youatt's focus on the *livestock economics* dimension (i.e. the need for purchasing cattle from other areas, thus spreading disease) of the emerging CBPP disease problem is significant. His observation reiterated what Switzerland's von Haller had previously noted – that CBPP's contagiousness was evidenced by the fact that new cases could almost always be traced to the *purchase* of an animal from another (infected) district (Nicholas and Kastner, 2024, p. 14). Youatt would continue to point to this economically rooted problem, fearing the almost inevitable spread of CBPP through international trade. One later memorialized Youatt for giving voice to the trade-related features of CBPP: 'Had his teaching been closely followed when the early outbreaks of the disease occurred in the United Kingdom, the waste of many millions of the nation's wealth would have been avoided, and the sorrows inflicted upon the owners of stock in seeing their animals swept away by disease, against which they were powerless to guard, would at the same time have been averted' (Duckham and Brown, 1893, p. 265).

Indeed, in the early 1840s, Great Britain would unwittingly import fresh cases of CBPP through livestock trading. As explained in Chapter 3 (this volume), there were likely previous instances of CBPP that spread into Britain from Holland in 1714 and 1745 (Horsburgh, 1859, pp. 278–279). However, the trade-associated cases of the 19th century would prove most impactful in Britain. Elsewhere across Europe, the story was the same; in concert with the growth of cattle trading in the middle of the 19th century, CBPP spread rapidly over large areas and in all directions. Economic historian Herbert Heaton documents the rapid liberalization of trade during this time in Europe. Britain repealed its tariffs in the 1840s (see Chapter 3, this volume), Belgium repealed its tariffs on agricultural imports in 1850, France and England signed a commercial treaty in 1860, Prussia signed a trade agreement with France in 1862, Holland too repealed tariffs between 1845 and 1877, and by 1870 Germany was effectively a free-trade market involving 40 million people connected by rivers, railroads, and roads (Heaton, 1948, pp. 640–643). Western and Central Europe soon formed a combined infected area that reached south to Spain and eastwards to Hungary and Russia (Hutyra *et al.*, 1938, p. 455). The disease truly prevailed from east to west. Between 1832 and 1840, reportedly 10,000 cattle died in Prussia, and, probably following a direct importation from this German kingdom in 1833, Holland was home to innumerable outbreaks of CBPP (Back, 2021, pp. 81–82). By 1863, nearly half of Holland's 14,000 farms had been affected by CBPP (Fisher, 2003). Fig. 2.5 illustrates one of the regions that would be implicated in spreading CBPP across to Britain and, as Chapters 4 and 5 (this volume) detail, even across the Atlantic Ocean.

Not surprisingly, those European areas most profoundly affected by the middle of the 19th century went to great lengths to come to grips with the disease, attempting various means by which to manage it. Belgium, for example, would give rise to scientists like Dr Louis Willems experimenting with new 'remedies' for the disease. Based at the Brussels veterinary school, Dr Willems pioneered a crude yet widely embraced inoculation method by which fluid from the lungs of a fatal CBPP case was injected into the skin of the tip of the tail (Pattison, 1990, p. 66). Not unlike the above account in which CBPP information was disseminated from France (Lecoq) to Britain (Youatt), Willems's innovation captured the attention of others across Europe. For example, council members of the Royal Agricultural Society of England expressed serious interest in the method, despite some British veterinarians remaining sceptical (Nicholas and Kastner, 2024, pp. 12–13). The discussion about inoculation was hotly debated across Europe, over a number of years. As the British veterinary authority J. Irvine Lupton remarked in 1882 to local leaders in Surrey, England: 'the inoculation of cattle as a preventive against the occurrence of pleuro-pneumonia has been often discussed during the past 25 years by more than one scientific Society in Europe' (Anonymous, 1882).

Almost every European government slowly (or reluctantly) instituted systematic slaughter campaigns targeting both infected and, importantly, suspect animals. By the close of the 19th century, these efforts came to fruition and had the practical consequence of ridding CBPP from such countries as Switzerland (1895), Great Britain (1898), Hungary (1902), and even Holland (1887). These efforts, however, came too late and could not prevent CBPP from spreading globally. Other European countries, notably Germany and Austria, initially enjoyed a measure of disease freedom in the early 20th century, only to see CBPP return during the First World War and the interwar period. Southern Europe, including Spain, would be home to an ongoing CBPP challenge (Hutyra *et al.*, 1938,

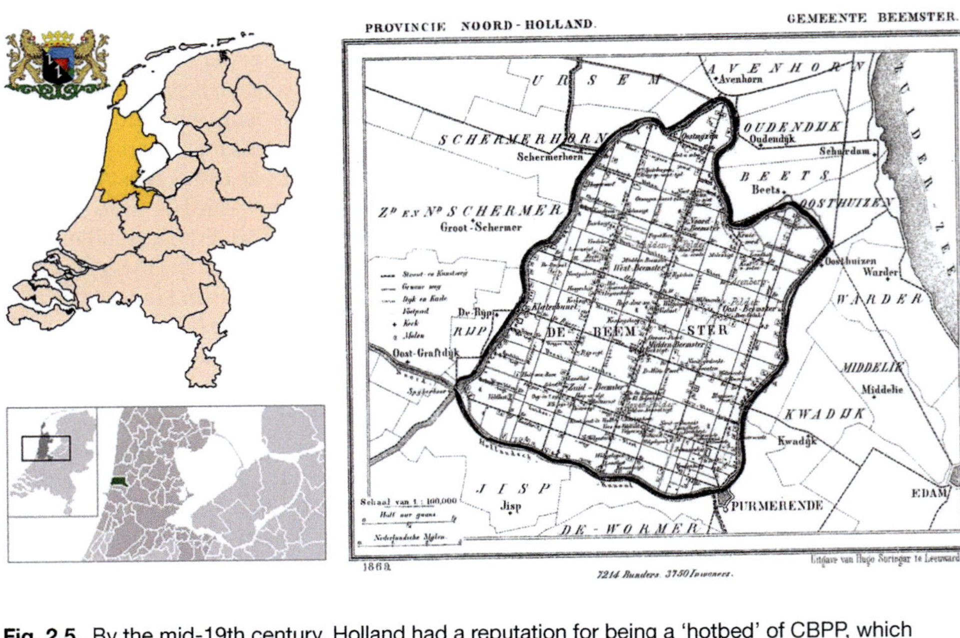

Fig. 2.5. By the mid-19th century, Holland had a reputation for being a 'hotbed' of CBPP, which had spread to Western Europe from Prussia in the east. (Image courtesy of Brian Altonen, https://brianaltonenmph.com/wp-content/uploads/2011/07/purmerend.jpg.)

p. 455). Italy, at first appearing to be rid of CBPP in the early 20th century, would later see the disease re-emerge (see Chapter 10, this volume).

Conclusion

Europe, while home to the 'beginnings' of the global challenge of CBPP, also boasted one of the most important scientific discoveries that would enable a worldwide response. In 1898, two French bacteriologists – Edmond Nocard and Émile Roux – published a groundbreaking article in the *Annales de l'Institut Pasteur* (Nocard *et al.*, 1990, p. 354). Their manuscript, titled *Le Microbe de la Péripneumonie*, marked the first scientific description of the mycoplasma organism responsible for CBPP. While the discovery was made just a few months after Britain's last case of CBPP (Pattison, 1990, pp. 67–68), these two scientists were duly honoured in the coming years (Anonymous, 2003). Their discovery had two consequences: First, it brought etiological explanation of a disease (see Chapter 1, this volume), a disease that had, since the 16th century, perplexed agriculturists, veterinarians, scientists and government regulators; second, it provided a foundation that would enable later diagnostic and disease-control tools for both the Northern and Southern Hemispheres.

References

Anonymous (1882) Minutes of 13 June 1882. In: *Minutes Book of the Executive Committee of the Justices of the Peace of the County of Surrey*. Surrey History Centre, Woking.

Anonymous (2003) Edmond nocard (1850–1903). *Historia Medicinae Veterinariae* 28(1), 11, cover.

Back, R. (2021) *Parlementaire Enquête omtrent de besmettelijke longziekte onder het rundvee in de negentiende eeuw* [Parliamentary Inquiry into the Contagious Lung Disease among Cattle in the Nineteenth Century]; *CAHIERS* [notebook series], *no. 8*. Veterinair Historisch Genootschap (Veterinary Historical Society), Utrecht, p. 8.

Bifolco, S. and Ronca, F. (2014) *Cartografia Rara Italiana: XVI Secolo L'italia e i Suoi Territori Catalogo Ragionato Delle Carte a Stampa*. Edizioni Antiquarius, Rome.

Blancou, J. (1996) Early methods of surveillance and control for contagious bovine pleuropneumonia. *Revue Scientifique et Technique (International Office of Epizootics)* 15(4), 1263–1282.

Blancou, J. (2003) *History of the Surveillance and Control of Transmissible Animal Diseases*. Office International des Epizooties, Paris.

Blystone, M. (2001) Rinderpest: One virus's impact on veterinary history. *Veterinary Heritage* 24(1), 8–12.

Bonnaterre, P.J. (1799) *Récueil de médecine vétérinaire: Ou collection de mémoires d'instructions et de recettes sur les maladies des animaux domestiques*. De L'imprimerie de L.B. Carrere, Rodez, France.

Cancrini, D. (2022) Agostino Gallo e la 'nobil'arte dell'agricoltura': Nuove acquisizioni dalle Raccolte Storiche. [Online]. Brescia, Italy: Università Cattolica del Sacro Cuore – Raccolte storiche [Historical collections]. Available at: https://brescia-raccoltestoriche.unicatt.it/storie/agostino-gallo-e-la-nobilarte-dellagricoltura/ (accessed 4 January 2024).

Curasson, G. (1936) *Traité de pathologie exotique vétérinaire et comparée*. Vigot, Paris.

Dannenfelt, K.H. (1982) The control of vertebrate pests in renaissance agriculture. *Agricultural History* 56(3), 542–559.

Davidson, T.D. (1960) A survey of some British veterinary folklore. *Bulletin of the History of Medicine* 34(3), 199–232.

Duckham, T. and Brown, G.T. (1893) The progress of legislation against contagious diseases of live stock. *Journal of the Royal Agricultural Society of England Third Series* IV, 262–286.

Dun, F. (1849) On the prevailing epizootic in cattle, called pleuro-pneumonia, prize essay published by the author.

Estienne, C. (1564) *Praedium Rusticum*. Apud Carolum Stephanum Typographu Regium, Lutetiae [Paris].

Estienne, C. and Liebault, J. (1616) Translated by R. Surflet. *Maison Rustique, or, The Countrey Farme... Now Newly Reviewed, Corrected, and Augmented*. Thomas Wight, London.

Falcone, G. (1603) *Rimedii*. Appresso Fabritio Zanetti, Treviso, Italy.

Fisher, J. (2003) To kill or not to kill: The eradication of contagious bovine pleuro-pneumonia in Western Europe. *Medical History* 47, 314–331.

Fisher, J.R. (1993) Not quite a profession: The aspirations of veterinary surgeons in England in the mid nineteenth century. *Historical Research* 66(161), 284–302.

Fitzherbert, M. (1523) *The Boke of Husbandrie*. Richard Pynson, London.

Fitzherbert, M. (1534) *The Boke of Husbandry*, 4th edition.

Fleming, G. (1871) *Animal Plagues: Their History, Nature, and Prevention*. Chapman and Hall, London.

Gallo, A. (1584) *Le vinti giornate dell'agricoltura, et de' piaceri della villa, Appresso Camillo Borgominerio al Segno di S*. Giorgio, Venice.

Gay, E.F. (1904) The authorship of the book of husbandry and the book of surveying. *The Quarterly Journal of Economics* 18(4), 588.

Hale, T. (1758) *A Compleat Body of Husbandry*. Thomas Osborne, London, 2nd edition.

Heaton, H. (1948) *Economic History of Europe*, Revised Edition. Harper & Row, New York.

Heresbach, C. (1570) *Rei rusticae libri quatuor*. Apud loannem Birckmannum, Cologne.

Heresbach, C. (1601) . Translated by B. Googe. *Foure Bookes of Husbandry*. Thomas Wight, London.

Horsburgh, J. (1859) On the contagious nature of pleuropneumonia in cattle. *Edinburgh Veterinary Review and Annals of Comparative Pathology* 278–285.

Hutyra, F., Marek, J. and Manninger, R. (1938) Contagious pleuropneumonia. In: Greig, J.R., Mohler, J.R. and Eichhorn, A. (eds) *Special Pathology and Therapeutics of the Diseases of Domestic Animals*, 4th English edition, ed. Alexander Eger, Chicago, Illinois, pp. 455–472.

Jones, S.D. and Koolmees, P.A. (2022) *A Concise History of Veterinary Medicine*. Cambridge University Press, Cambridge.

Law, J. (1880) Contagious pleuro-pneumonia or lung-plague of cattle. In: DUC, W.G.L. (ed.) *Report of the Commissioner of Agriculture for the Year 1879*. Government Printing Office Washington, DC, pp. 436–455.

Lechlainche, E. (1936) *Histoire de la Medecine Veterinaire*. Office du Livre, Toulouse, France.

Liebault, J. (1570) *L'Agriculture et maison rustique de M. Charles Estienne docteur en medecine*. Chez lacques Du-Puys, Paris.

New jersey office for the prevention of the spread (1879) *Report on Pleuro-Pneumonia among Cattle in the State of New Jersey*. Wm. S. Sharp, Trenton, New Jersey.

Nicholas, R.A.J. and Kastner, J. (2024) Contagious bovine pleuropneumonia: A tale of two countries. In: *Veterinary History* 22 new series, pp. 12–37.

Nocard, E., Roux, E., Borrel, M., Salimbeniet, M. and Dujardin-Beaumetz, M. (1990) The microbe of pleuropneumonia. *Reviews of Infectious Diseases* 12(2), 354–358.

Pattison, I. (1990) *A Great British Veterinarian Forgotten: James Beart Simonds 1810–1904*. J.A. Allen & Co, London.

Salmon, D.E. and Smith, T. (1896) Infectious diseases of cattle. In: Salmon, D.E. (ed.) *Special Report on Diseases of Cattle and on Cattle Feeding. U.S. Department of Agriculture Bureau of Animal Industry*. U.S. Department of Agriculture Bureau of Animal Industry, Washington, DC, pp. 371–438.

Schrader, G.W. and Hering, E. (1863) *Biographisch-literarisches Lexicon der Thierärzte aller Zeiten und Länder*. Ebner & Seubert, Stuttgart.

Skeat, W. (ed.) (1882) *The Book of Husbandry by Master Fitzherbert*. English Dialect Society, London.

Smith, F. (1976) *The Early History of Veterinary Literature and its British Development*. J.A. Allen & Co, London.

Walley, T. (1879) *The Four Bovine Scourges: Pleuro-Pneumonia, Foot-and-Mouth Disease, Cattle Plague, Tubercle (Scrofula) with an Appendix on the Inspection of Live Animals and Meat*. MacLachlan and Stewart, Edinburgh.

Worlidge, J. (1716) *A Compleat System of Husbandry and Gardening*. Printed for J, Pickard, London.

Youatt, W. (1836) *Cattle: Their Breeds, Management, and Diseases*. Grigg & Elliott, Philadelphia, Pennsylvania.

3 CBPP in Great Britain: The Problem of 'Flying Herds'

Abstract

Great Britain was affected by contagious bovine pleuropneumonia (CBPP) from continental Europe on at least one occasion in the 18th century. However, despite causing high mortality in cattle, it failed to establish – possibly because relatively little internal trade occurred, thereby inhibiting infected cattle from spreading the disease throughout the country. CBPP, nevertheless, became endemic both in Great Britain and Ireland in the 19th century following the liberalization of cattle trade in 1842. The Netherlands, which had become a 'hotbed of disease' and, unfortunately, an attractive market for dairy products and cattle by the British, was the source of many cattle imports and the fresh arrival of disease. Huge cattle losses resulted over the next 50 years, especially in the dairies of the big cities, notably in Edinburgh, Glasgow, Dublin, Manchester and Birmingham. Initially, there was little control over or even an understanding of the problem. However, slowly government and cattle owners were compelled to act, introducing legislation to control cattle movement, slaughter infected and in-contact animals and receive compensation, and, crucially, move responsibility for control from local to central government and enlist a robust corps of veterinary inspectors. While vaccination with crude lung extracts was used on a limited scale with mixed results, it was stamping out that finally led to the eradication of CBPP from the Great Britain in 1898.

Introduction: Origins on the Continent

Before its large-scale importation into the British Isles, CBPP was largely seen as a sporadic, enzootic disorder of the European continent – in the Pyrenees, Alps, Jura and Vosges mountains as well as the upland regions of Hesse, Swabia and Silesia in modern-day Germany. CBPP was also believed to be prevalent in the Prussian dominions (now eastern Germany and Poland) and Bavaria. Professor John Gamgee, the Italian-born British veterinarian and polymath who (as noted in Chapter 4, this volume) would exercise scientific leadership in more than one country, proposed that it existed in Europe in pockets, or 'stations' as he termed them. These 'stations' constantly infected cattle that passed by on established trade routes (Gamgee, 1863c). In one of his many voluminous reports, Gamgee paraphrased a scientific authority (Andreas Christian Gerlach, a pioneer of veterinary medicine in Germany) who reportedly believed, somewhat vaguely, 'that [probably] pleuropneumonia was not originally a European disorder' (Gamgee, 1863c, p. 633). Unfortunately, Gamgee does not provide a detailed citation for this claim attributed to Gerlach. Over a decade later, the ultimate origins of the disease were more specifically described at a parliamentary inquiry in 1877 in the Netherlands into the impact of 'longziekte' (Dutch for 'lung disease'; for other European names for CBPP, see Chapter 2, this volume). In the inquiry, a veterinarian named Gerardus Johannes Hengeveld argued:

> the lung disease originated in the Podolian and Kyrgyz steppes (Fig. 3.1), in the Crimea, between the Volga and the Don, and between the Urals and the Volga...These animals had [also] been the transmitters of the rinderpest. In conclusion: All breeds of cattle were susceptible to the lung disease. All infectious diseases, including those of humans, would come from the East. (Back, 2021, p. 21, original in Dutch, translated by Helen Steele)

As mentioned in Chapter 2 (this volume), there was an amplification of the number of outbreaks and, indeed, a worsening spread of CBPP, as a result of the countless wars erupting in Europe in the late 18th and early 19th centuries. These included, but were not limited

DOI: 10.1079/9781800627536.0003

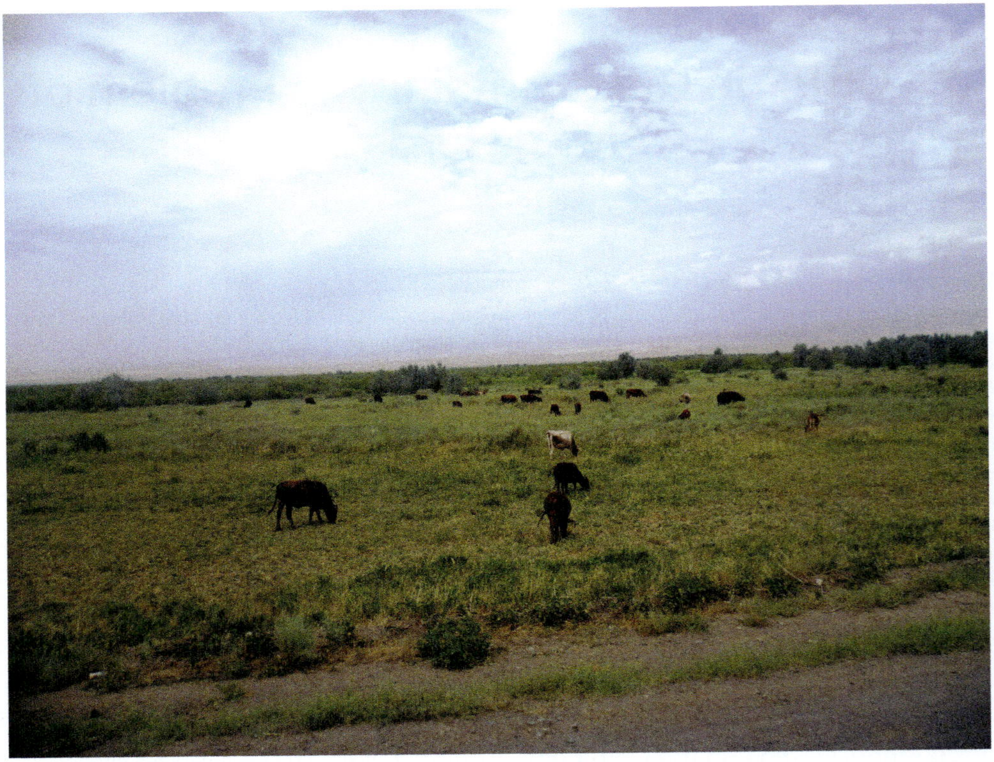

Fig. 3.1. The Kazakh steppe, part of the wider geographic region where Dutch and other European veterinary authorities believed CBPP likely originated (Back, 2021, p. 21). (From Botev, R., 2017, *Cattle on Kazakh Steppe*, CC BY 3.0 PL via Wikimedia Commons.)

to, the global Seven Years War (1756–1763), the Prussian invasion of Holland (1787), and the Russo–Swedish War (1788–1790). The north of Europe and Britain were largely uninvolved in large-scale cattle movements at this time. Furthermore, Britain was under a (largely unsuccessful) trade embargo with Europe, imposed by the French Emperor Napoleon; fortuitously (from a disease point of view), during this time Britain was prevented from trading livestock.

CBPP appeared all over the rest of Europe, even following Napoleon into Russia due to the need to feed and help transport the *Grand Armée* (Fig. 3.2; Gamgee, 1863c, p. 634). While there were likely other episodes of disease spread, one major outbreak of CBPP occurred in Russia in the year 1824 (Gamgee, 1871). The Scottish veterinarian James Horsburgh recounts contemporary reports of CBPP outbreaks (quite possibly of French origin) among the cattle accompanying the Russian army when they invaded Turkey (1828–1829):

> We learn that pleuro-pneumonia broke out among the cattle used by the Russian army when they invaded Turkey...their army being so reduced by disease among their...cattle that they could proceed no further, though Constantinople was almost in their grasp. (Horsburgh, 1859, p. 279)

Although otherwise militarily successful, Russia was obliged to sign a peace treaty because it could no longer support its soldiers; such was the impact of CBPP on its livestock (Horsburgh, 1859, p. 279).

The peace that followed the defeat of the French at the battle of Waterloo in 1815 brought a partial but short-lived reduction in CBPP-related losses as the disease retreated to its traditional home in central Europe (Gamgee, 1863c). However, new demographic and economic changes would soon perpetuate fresh patterns of CBPP transmission. The ensuing prosperity after the deprivations of war, coupled with increased industrialization, led to

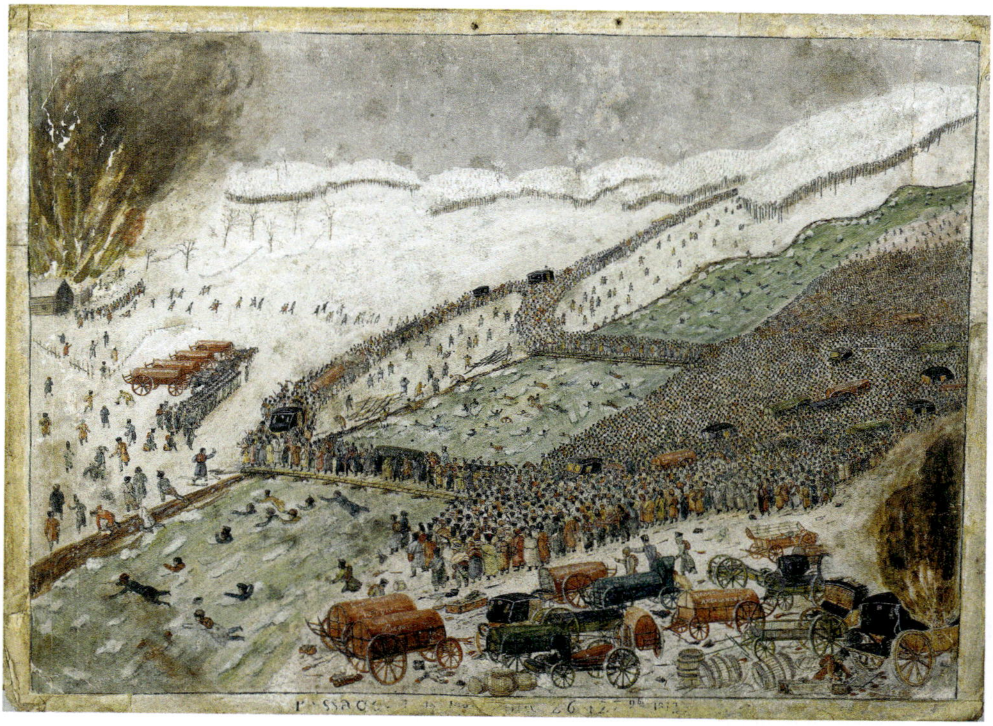

Fig. 3.2. The painting *The French Army Crossing the Berezina on 28 November 1812* depicts one of Napoleon's legendary marches, specifically the crossing of the Berezina River as part of a campaign into Russia in 1812. It required huge resources to maintain the *Grand Armée*, including cattle which spread CBPP across the continent into Russia (Horsburgh, 1859). (From Unknown artist, *c.*1812–1850, Musée de l'Armée, public domain via Wikimedia Commons.)

a population explosion that required greater resources, including cattle for beef and milk. This was met by Russian, Polish and Hungarian dealers, who moved large herds westwards. Due to these realities, CBPP re-emerged with renewed force through the German states. There were 'outbreaks of pleuropneumonia in the Rhine provinces of Prussia from 1830 to 1840', while 'lung plague prevailed severely in Hanover' and 'the malady appeared in Saxony in 1827' (Gamgee, 1871, p. 9).

CBPP noticeably appeared in the Netherlands in imported cattle through the border with Germany in 1835, a few years later than CBPP's arrival into Belgium and France. It was carried to Utrecht and then shortly afterwards to south Holland, where it infected the great cattle markets of Rotterdam and Schiedam – and, indeed, to the rest of the Netherlands. Gamgee was in no doubt of the origin of the British outbreaks in 1842, insisting 'we owe this disease *unquestionably* to our Dutch trade' (Gamgee, 1863c, p. 634, italics added). While he was certain about where CBPP ultimately came from, Gamgee believed it may have first been imported, along with cattle for breeding purposes, into County Cork, Ireland, as early as 1839 (or possibly in 1840 or 1841) by 'gentlemen related to a British Consul at one of the Dutch ports' (Gamgee, 1863c, p. 635). Writing 20 years after these events, Gamgee highlighted enduring genetic evidence of Dutch breeding stock being the source of CBPP's entrance into the British Isles: '[A]t the present day traces of these early importations are to be seen in county Cork, where they are numerous crosses, with a decided admixture of Dutch blood' (Gamgee, 1863c, p. 635).

At the time, and since the Act of Union of 1801, Ireland had been part of the UK and subject to the British government through its administration at Dublin Castle; any trade between Ireland and the rest of the UK was seen as internal and not subject to any additional legislation. To some extent, therefore, the precise port of CBPP's entry was largely academic because, once trade was liberalized in the 1840s, thousands of infected cattle poured into Britain from the Netherlands. Some estimates indicate that 0.04% of Dutch cattle exported to Britain was infected (Back, 2021); while this does not seem particularly high, immunologically naïve animals would be highly susceptible to disease and, with a reproductive (R) value calculated today of between 2 and 3, the mycoplasma organism (see Chapter 1, this volume) would spread rapidly through a herd.

CBPP's Early Impacts in Great Britain

While it is appropriate to focus on the mid-19th century introductions of CBPP into Britain from Holland (as the Netherlands was commonly known), the disease had, in previous centuries, exerted impacts on British herds and livestock raisers. As mentioned in Chapter 2 (this volume), knowledgeable agriculturalists in England recognized (and lamented and innovated supposed remedies for) an ailment called 'longesaught', presumed to be CBPP, as early as the 16th century. More conclusively, records suggest that CBPP was introduced into Britain from Holland on one or, perhaps, two occasions in the 18th century – that is, before the aforementioned circumstances that lead to CBPP becoming endemic in the mid-19th century. Little is known of CBPP's impact on its supposed arrival in 1714 from Holland. However, the impact must have been substantial, for the event prompted the British government to appoint an investigator into the 'distemper' at the livestock market in Islington, just north of London (Hall, 1976, p. 6). This 'distemper' may have actually been rinderpest (Hall, 1976, p. 6) and not CBPP – or, plausibly, a combination of the two (Horsburgh, 1859, p. 279). The 1714 cattle disease event in England would, in any case, later be referred to by some (including governments) as one involving CBPP (Butterfield, 1860).

The scientific investigator commissioned in 1714 was Thomas Bates – one of England's most pre-eminent scientists, a fellow of the Royal Society, and soon-to-be-appointed surgeon for the incoming King George I (Ministry of Agriculture, 1965, p. 3). His investigation led to a number of proposed measures for disease control. A remarkable document (Fig. 3.3) that testifies to Britain's growing participation in the early years of the scientific Enlightenment (which began in France; see Chapter 2, this volume), Bates's report is chock-full of analytical and ratiocinative sophistication, twinning observation with logic. His proposed measures to control the distemper included, but were not limited to, the following: (i) the purchase and destruction of diseased animals; (ii) the washing 'very clean' of all cow houses, followed by smoking them by burning pitch, tar and wormwood, and then waiting three months before bringing cows into the houses; (iii) waiting two months before grazing cattle on fields where diseased cattle had been; (iv) separation, from healthy cattle, of persons tending to sick animals; and (presumably to prevent further outbreaks) (v) that 'Cow-keepers be required to divide their Cows into small Parcels, not more than ten or twelve in a Field together' (Bates, 1718, p. 874).

In addition to the 1714 catastrophic disease event at Islington, another definitively CBPP-related event took place 30 years later, in Essex. Attributed by some to two infected calves imported in 1745 from Holland (Walley, 1879, p. 101), a lethal lung disease spread to the whole of Britain, ravaging herds for over a decade. At its height, 70,000 animals per month were dying or being killed. Attempts at control were, surprisingly, aided by financial support from the government. It had a devastating impact on the Midlands, where it killed over 100,000 cattle in 1747. Contemporary descriptions of the disease, such as the following, strongly implicate CBPP.

> The accounts given at that time [1747] show us that it began with a short, husky cough, which continued for eight or ten days, to which symptom little attention was paid; the cough increased, the breathing became difficult, the eyes heavy, and the coat staring. The secretion of milk ceased to be supplied in cows, and rumination was suspended; they mostly refused food and drink. This is exactly what takes place

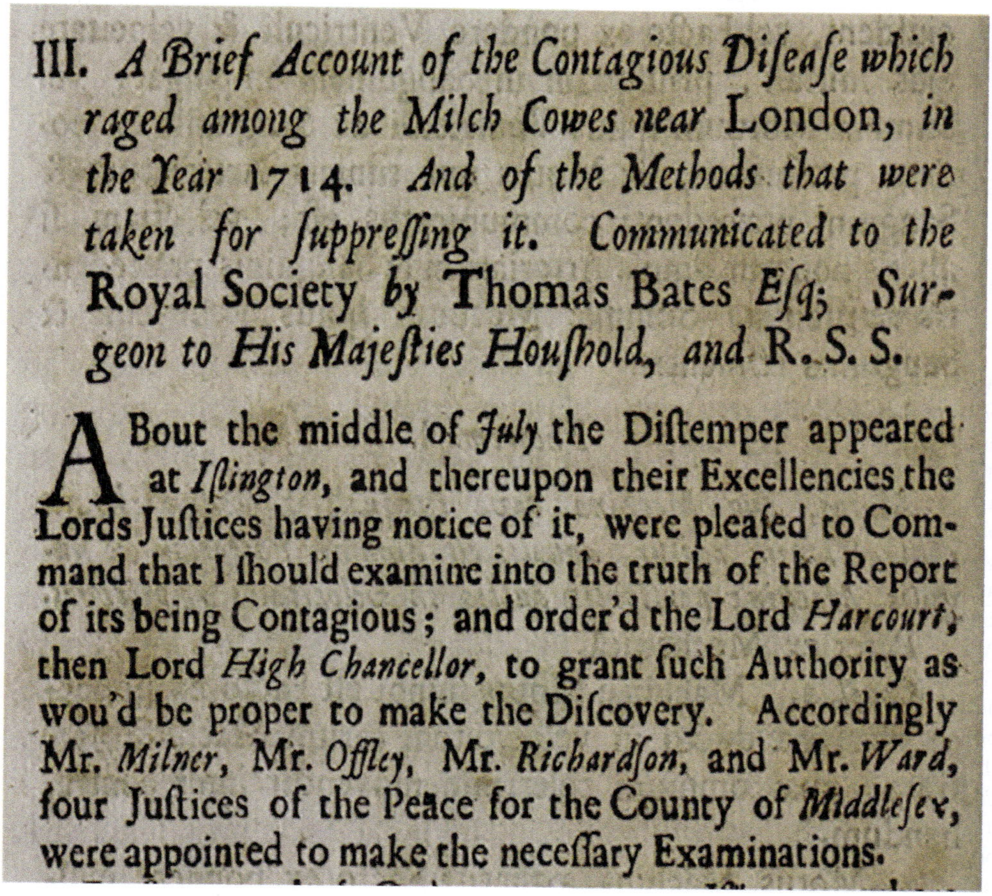

III. *A Brief Account of the Contagious Diſeaſe which raged among the Milch Cowes near* London, *in the Year* 1714. *And of the Methods that were taken for ſuppreſſing it. Communicated to the* Royal Society *by* Thomas Bates *Eſq;* *Surgeon to His Majeſties Houſhold, and* R. S. S.

ABout the middle of *July* the Diſtemper appeared at *Iſlington*, and thereupon their Excellencies the Lords Juſtices having notice of it, were pleaſed to Command that I ſhould examine into the truth of the Report of its being Contagious; and order'd the Lord *Harcourt*, then Lord *High Chancellor*, to grant ſuch Authority as wou'd be proper to make the Diſcovery. Accordingly Mr. *Milner*, Mr. *Offley*, Mr. *Richardſon*, and Mr. *Ward*, four Juſtices of the Peace for the County of *Middleſex*, were appointed to make the neceſſary Examinations.

Fig. 3.3. While it would be events in the mid-19th century that would cause more disease outbreaks, one possible early impact of CBPP in Britain took place in 1714, which Sir Thomas Bates, FRS, investigated at Islington. (From Bates, 1718, public domain via Internet Archive.)

> in the pleuro-pneumonia of our own times [1859]. No doubt it *was* the same disease. (Horsburgh, 1859, p. 279)

The disease(s) that impacted Britain in 1714 and 1745 were eventually eradicated, though it is not known exactly how. Eradication may have been due to government-aided culling and/or to a failure of the disease to establish because of insufficient cattle movements. During the second half of the 18th century, respiratory disease(s) continued to beleaguer British cattle raisers; this is evidenced by Thomas Hale's *A Compleat Body of Husbandry*, published in London in 1758. Hale's popular work enjoyed a wide readership that extended to the European continent and even overseas to pre-Revolutionary America. A copy may be found in the archives at Gunston Hall, the 18th century plantation of George Mason; and George Washington treasured a personal copy (Library of Congress, n.d.). Hale's practical resource, which was also translated into French, devotes an entire chapter to 'disorders of the lungs', acknowledging 'various kinds' but (perhaps simplistically) advocating 'but one remedy':

> Sometimes the creature breathes with difficulty, sometimes coughs and wheezes. Bruise four heads of garlick, and press out the juice, mix this with a quart of new milk, and add a quarter of a pint of tar. This will serve for four doses. One is to be given every morning till the cure is compleated...If the disorder be obstinate, the

creature should be blooded, and the medicine will then take effect. (Hale, 1758, pp. 448-49)

Such references and remedies to lung ailments persisted for the remainder of the 1700s; however, there were no more specific, substantial reports of CBPP until the mid-19th century.

CBPP in 19th-Century Britain: Devastation and Response

As mentioned, 19th-century Britain rapidly became a lucrative market for Dutch cattle and dairy products. Despite ongoing attempts by the Dutch authorities to eradicate CBPP, it was inevitable that Britain would become re-infected, particularly when the Conservative Prime Minister Sir Robert Peel liberalized the cattle markets in 1842 by removing import tariffs, causing a major upsurge in trade (North British Agriculturalist, 1860). For the rest of his career, Gamgee repeatedly indicted Peel's trade policy as the most determinative factor for CBPP's profound impact on Britain: 'British ports were thrown open to the cattle trade by Sir Robert Peel, and the demands of our markets caused a rush of stock through and from the northern provinces of Holland, which infected them' (Gamgee, 1871). Gamgee's lamentations about 'the legacy of Free-trade legislation' appeared not only in books. On 9 May 1877, Gamgee would speak at St James's Hall – a distinguished venue where noteworthy contemporaries like Charles Dickens also gave public addresses (Chappell & Company, 1869) – and point to 'the legacy of Free-trade legislation' as the culprit of CBPP (Gamgee, 1877, p. 5).

It was not that British livestock owners were unaware of what was happening in Holland, which had become widely reputed as a proverbial 'hotbed' of infection (Hutyra *et al.*, 1938, p. 455). English dealers and cattle owners knew that Dutch cattle 'contaminate English-bred stock more than any other foreign importations' (Anonymous, 1862a). Indeed, the Secretary of the Highland Society of Scotland had warned the Board of Trade of the dangers of allowing the importation of Dutch cattle (Horsburgh, 1859). With the trade doors now 'thrown open' (to use Gamgee's language), CBPP arrived in the south of England in 1842, taking but a year to reach the lowlands of Scotland, and another 12 months to bring infection to cattle in Inverness,

> by which time it was through all Britain, alike in the finest parks surrounded by lofty trees... in the clean-swept byres of the peer, or the single one built at the end of the solitary house of the shepherd, in the lonely glen among the mountains... (Horsburgh, 1859, pp. 279–80)

CBPP's impact across the British Isles was huge, and all the major towns with dairy herds were quickly affected. However, for the first 30 years following its introduction, there was little official data on the incidence of the disease or on attempts to control it – despite its impact on the national herd and an earlier governmental intervention in the previous century. This can perhaps best be explained as truly the time of *laissez-faire* politics – not only in Britain but also on Continental Europe. As one economic historian has detailed (and as described in Chapter 2, this volume), during these decades in Western Europe, it was increasingly *en vogue* to repeal trade restrictions on food imports. Indeed, 'up to 1870 there was a widespread trend toward freer trade' (Heaton, 1948, p. 641). Criticism of the inaction of the British government was voiced during these decades, and questions were posed as to why there was no ministry or minister of agriculture as there was in France or Canada (North British Agriculturalist, 1860).

In the autumn of 1863, Professor Gamgee (then living in Edinburgh, where he had recently established his own veterinary school) travelled 644 km (400 miles) south to speak to interested (indeed, concerned) dignitaries, some of whom were members of parliament (Gamgee, 1863a, p. 742). Delivered at the Marylebone Literary and Scientific Institution, then located in 'one of the richest, most fashionable parts of London' (Survey of London, 2019), Gamgee's lecture was published verbatim two months later in the *Edinburgh Veterinary Review and Annals of Comparative Pathology*. Gamgee was particularly withering in his characterization of the lack of proper preventative actions being taken against CBPP by the government:

> GENTLEMEN,—The subject on which I have the honour to address you this evening—the prevention of disease in town dairies—is one of great importance, not only to the people in large cities, but to the country generally...I have

> travelled 400 miles to address this audience... Twenty years ago we first knew what it was to see the much and justly abused cow-sheds swept clean of their inmates by the lung-disease, just as smallpox and scarlatina depopulate the human habitations they invade. Every one was taken by surprise...[and CBPP] has continued up to this time to kill twenty, thirty, and upwards of fifty per cent. per annum, without leading to the adoption of proper preventive measures; disgracing the professional men who have attempted to cure it, and ruining the wealthy stock-owners who, prior to 1842, were worth many thousand pounds, and owned many hundred cows as their stock in trade. (Gamgee, 1863a, p. 742)

It was not only governmental authorities who appeared apathetic in the face of this virulent disease; there were only occasional outcries from the farming communities which quickly died down after a few weeks. In 1862, an outbreak of 'smallpox' (known as sheep pox today) in sheep on a single farm in the Wiltshire Downs was causing *more* excitement because it transiently reduced the price of mutton throughout Britain. Gamgee stressed, however, that the damage caused by sheep pox was 'infinitesimal... as contrasted with the...destruction by pleuropneumonia' (Gamgee, 1863b, p. 402). Indeed, when considering other diseases, it was clear to not only Gamgee but other veterinarians that CBPP was having a greater impact than all other diseases combined. In Scotland J. Horsburgh remained alarmed (Horsburgh, 1859), and in England George Fleming decried 'contagious pleuro-pneumonia, to whose ravages at the present time we are so painfully accustomed' (Fleming, 1871, p. 461).

By the mid-1860s, a good number of scientifically and politically minded leaders believed that had the Government acted promptly on the first appearance of CBPP, its spread would have been greatly checked or wholly prevented. Dissatisfaction with the government over the inaction to the introduction of both CBPP and rinderpest (then especially devastating herds in Britain) led to the founding of both the Central and Associated Chambers of Agriculture. Formally created on 6 February 1866 at a meeting at the Salisbury Hotel on Fleet Street in London, the Central Chamber of Agriculture immediately gave voice to the need for regulation on behalf of livestock owners justifiably alarmed by the introduction of animal diseases of many kinds. Public letters from late 1865 (Fig. 3.4) and early 1866, reveal the principal hope attached to the organization's foundation: that it '*might eventually lead to the appointment of a Minister or Board of Agriculture*, which is much needed' (Matthews, 1915, p. 393).

Outspoken veterinarians like Gamgee, Horsburgh and Fleming, and the new collective voice of the Central and Associated Chambers of Agriculture, became increasingly influential in nudging the government to modify its free trade policies and adopt more robust animal disease regulations. In 1873, the Chambers of Agriculture, in partnership with the Royal Society of Agriculture, successfully pressed parliament to form a 'Select Committee of the House of Commons early in the session, to inquire into the operation of the Cattle Diseases Act and the constitution and working of the Veterinary Department of the Privy Council' (Matthews, 1915, p. 19). Five years later, and as the economic impact of animal diseases became clearer (see Table 3.1), their lobbying efforts led to a new Contagious Diseases (Animals) Act of 1878, which required the slaughter of all live cattle at the port of entry if they came from any country where CBPP was known to exist (for the trade impact, see Chapter 5, this volume).

Yet there were also voices of opposition that inhibited regulatory progress in the fight against CBPP. Somewhat ironically, one impediment to increasing controls was the influential first-ever state veterinary advisor, J.B. Simonds. He was appointed as the first Head of the Veterinary Department of the privy council, in October 1865 (Ministry of Agriculture, 1965, pp. ix, xviii), a position he held in addition to his other roles as Principal of the Royal Veterinary College, and editor of the journal *The Veterinarian*, which he held for 30 years. This busy man felt that, because CBPP was already endemic in Britain, further measures would be futile, delighting the liberal free traders (Fisher, 2003). Simonds's unfavourable views on 'inoculation' (Pattison, 1990, pp. 66–67) would also put paid to the demand for more widespread use of crude vaccination, for which many vets were clamouring.

A *The first of the following letters was copied by some of the London Agricultural papers in 1865, and proved the origin of the Central and Associated Chambers of Agriculture.*

Walton, near Wakefield, *December 5th*, 1865.

PROPOSAL FOR A FARMERS' LEAGUE, OR CENTRAL CHAMBER OF AGRICULTURE.

Sir,—The idea of a general meeting in London of deputations from all the Farmers' Clubs and Agricultural Societies in the Kingdom, to consider the questions arising out of the Cattle Plague—which I had the pleasure of suggesting and proposing to the members of the Wakefield and West Riding Farmers' Club—having been so well received throughout the country, induces me (after mentioning it to a few friends) to venture upon another subject which has for some years appeared to my mind to be a great want, and which (if properly carried out) would tend greatly towards the efficient management of agricultural affairs. My present suggestion is embraced in the title of "A Farmers' League." The means of forming such an Association are so ready to hand that I almost wonder it has not been carried out long ago. I would adopt the same plan as suggested for the Cattle Plague Meeting, viz., forming the Chairman and Secretaries, for the time being, of every Farmers' Club and Society—with such other members as it may be found desirable to enrol—into one central "Farmers' League or Association," each Club paying, say, £5 5s. to the funds of the League annually, which (as there are some 400) would give at once about £2000 per annum. With such pecuniary means and such extensive influence capable of being exerted at any moment over the whole country, and brought to bear with all its force upon any and every measure affecting the farmer, it cannot but be evident, I think, that the agricultural interest would thereby have a power ready at command which it does not possess at present, simply because there is no organisation; each Club exhausts its influence locally—

B The special object of the League would be to undertake duties now much neglected and beyond the rules of all existing societies; viz., the charge of measures in the Houses of Parliament and before the Government, calculated to benefit agriculture, as well as to oppose or modify any movement detrimental to that important interest. It cannot be denied that more attention to such matters would result in some improvement, and might *eventually lead to the appointment of a Minister or Board of Agriculture*, which is much needed; for although the present House of Commons contains many members who are friendly to the farmer, yet the prominence with which his younger but more energetic brother, "The Manufacturer," has contrived to push forward his own measures seems to be obliterating the fact that there is such an interest in agriculture—which equally requires and fully deserves the application of those free trade and progressive principles which have been of so much benefit to commercial enterprise.

Fig. 3.4. In a public letter that appeared in the press in December 1865 at the height of alarm and anxiety over rinderpest (and other animal diseases, including CBPP), the writer (Charles Clay) advocates for the establishment of an organization or 'league', which was officially established as the Central Chamber of Agriculture. The italicized text expresses an aspiration for the eventual establishment of a proper governmental ministry of agriculture. (From Matthews, 1915, public domain via HathiTrust.)

Table 3.1. Estimates of losses to cattle disease in Great Britain prior to the Contagious Diseases (Animals) Act of 1878. (Adapted from Fisher, 1980, p. 294.)

Disease	Years	Cattle attacked	Value (£)
Rinderpest	1865–1867	278,943	5,000,000
	1872	72	5000
	1877	248	22,000
CBPP	1855–1860	1,000,000	12,000,000
	1860–1865	960,000	No estimate
	1869–1887 (includes some outbreaks after 1878)	74,552	670,790
Foot and Mouth Disease	1867–1871	1,344,525	No estimate
	1871	519,523	No estimate
	1872	No estimate	13,071,392

The Role of 'Flying Herds' in the Spread of CBPP

As in other countries, CBPP was having its biggest effect on Britain's town dairies, housing so-called 'flying herds', which were kept purely for milk production with replacements, often freshly calved cows, brought in continuously from other sources. The continuous movement (and spread of disease) extended to open pastures and other herds, too, as Gamgee explained:

> A cow yielding milk thrives best when she is left quiet...To run the animals about, to travel them on roads, and turn them into fields where cattle of all kinds are permitted to graze, only tend to favour the spread of contagious diseases... (Gamgee, 1863a, p. 743)

Once unhealthy or unproductive, the cows would be slaughtered for their meat. Long before rapid and/or refrigerated transport, the town dairies were seen as essential for providing milk close to the largely populated communities that consumed it; however, these dairies were also seen as a public health hazard. Between 1841 and 1848, at the beginning of Britain's widespread CBPP outbreaks, London had at least 1.25 million cattle distributed among the many town dairies living cheek by jowl with the human population. Edinburgh was singled out for having the dirtiest dairies and for being one of the most heavily infected cities in Britain: in a one-year period just over 55% of 1800 cattle from 88 dairies were sent to slaughter because of CBPP (Hall, 1976), and livestock owners were strongly advised not to buy their cattle. Fattening premises where cattle were fed on cheap waste from food processing became especially susceptible to CBPP. Writing in the early 20th century, Hutyra and Marek estimated losses of 187,000 cattle in Britain in 1860 alone (Hutyra *et al.*, 1938). This same statistic, mentioned by an historian in the context of the wider animal disease devastation of the 1860s and 1870s, persuaded the government to act:

> During the 1860s and 1870s Britain was swept by a number of epidemics of animal diseases which decimated the cattle and sheep population. Cattle plague, foot and mouth and contagious bovine pleuro-pneumonia swept the country. The contagious bovine pleuro-pneumonia outbreak of 1860 alone left 187,000 cattle dead in Britain and the government eventually realised that the only way to control these appalling diseases was to slaughter infected herds to try to eliminate the disease and to impose restrictions on the import of foreign animals to prevent the diseases reintroduction. (McCarron, 1991, p. 19)

Meanwhile, other health-minded leaders were concerned for what this all meant for British agriculture. A report in the *British Medical Journal* in 1870, at the height of the CBPP epidemic, stated, 'Probably no fatal disease of stock is so constantly present in the minds of agriculturalists and cow owners as that known under the name of "pleuro-pneumonia", "pleuro", and lung sickness"

(Anonymous, 1870, p. 604). For its part, the government did deploy a growing number of inspectors – including, notably, travelling inspectors serving on behalf of the Veterinary Department of the Privy Council. One such travelling inspector was Henry Sleeman, who was in charge of an expansive area of England, extending from Lancaster to Bristol as well as the whole of Wales. During 1876, Inspector Sleeman 'paid 459 visits to Railway Stations', conducted '31 visits of inspection to cattle-carrying ships', helped execute 'one conviction against a Railway Company', and assisted with 'investigations affecting Port Inspectors' as well as 'negotiations with Shipping Companies' (Williams, 1876, pp. 3–4). As Fig. 3.5 shows, he routinely visited areas in Birkenhead, a critical livestock port area near Liverpool, one that figured prominently in trade-related matters between the USA and Great Britain (see Chapter 5, this volume).

The 1870s was an important decade in the governing of Great Britain. Powers delegated by the Privy Council enabled local authorities to take concrete action in the battle against CBPP. In the county of Surrey, decisive action was taken at the local level in areas of compensation and staffing. The following excerpt in the deliberations of the local authority illustrates how personal local government of CBPP had become:

> [I]t is ordered that the sum of £9.10.0 be awarded to W. Edwin Jay of Headley for One Cow, and the sum of £18.7.10 to W. Edward Hilder of Woking for two Cows so slaughtered, the said sums not exceeding One half of the value of the above Animals... (Anonymous, 1872)

Indeed, in order to make progress in the fight against CBPP, decision making was often in the hands of such local authorities. This was not an easy task, as judgement calls had to be made about a host of matters, including the right pay level to retain local inspectors: '[The] Chertsey Sub Committee notify that they have increased the Salary of the Inspector of their Division, from 7/- to 15/- for every day he shall be actually employed' (Anonymous, 1872).

As explained later, inspection and condemnation efforts accelerated in the late 1870s and 1880s, raising critical challenges about funding the national goal of CBPP eradication.

While there were no official records of losses until later that century, statistical reports of various cattle insurance societies are telling. Over half of insurance claims came from losses due to CBPP and, indeed, this was the cause of many firms' financial collapse when they underestimated the problem. The original corporate documents for one company, the Alcester Cattle Plague and Pleuro Pneumonia Prevention Company, illustrate the economic trepidation with which many livestock raisers were consumed when considering both rinderpest and CBPP. The firm was organized 'for the prevention of the Cattle Plague and Pleuro Pneumonia ... and to make compensation to persons who may issue in the Company for any loss which they may sustain in consequence of such diseases or either of them and exceeding two thirds in value of the amount for which animals are insured' (Anonymous, 1865, p. 1). The company's directors clearly appreciated the nature of the risk against they were hedging, engaging local veterinary inspectors for their expertise and insisting on its members taking 'precautions against infection', and stipulating that subscribers 'purchasing fresh Cattle...shall keep the newly purchased animal or animals separate, and at as great a distance as practicable, from the rest of his Cattle for 21 days' (Anonymous, 1865, p. 5). It was not uncommon for insurance firms to closely monitor the mortality rate of CBPP infection; one in England reported that during 1863–1866, CBPP annually killed 'fifty to sixty-three per cent' of infected animals that it had insured (McEachran, 1879, p. 212). CBPP was clearly a costly disease.

The always-prolific John Gamgee estimated at least 1 million cattle deaths, attributable to CBPP, occurred during the six-year period 1855–1860, which 'represented a value of about twelve millions [£12 million] sterling' (Gamgee, 1866, p. 487); these figures correspond to the data summarized in Table 3.1. Gamgee was also one of the first to raise concerns about the effects of human consumption of beef from CBPP-affected cattle (Gamgee, 1857). Gamgee was not alone in exploring this issue. While food safety-related worries later proved unfounded, they signal an early awareness of potential zoonotic diseases. Not surprisingly, given these uncertain times, advice on what to do with the meat from CBPP-affected

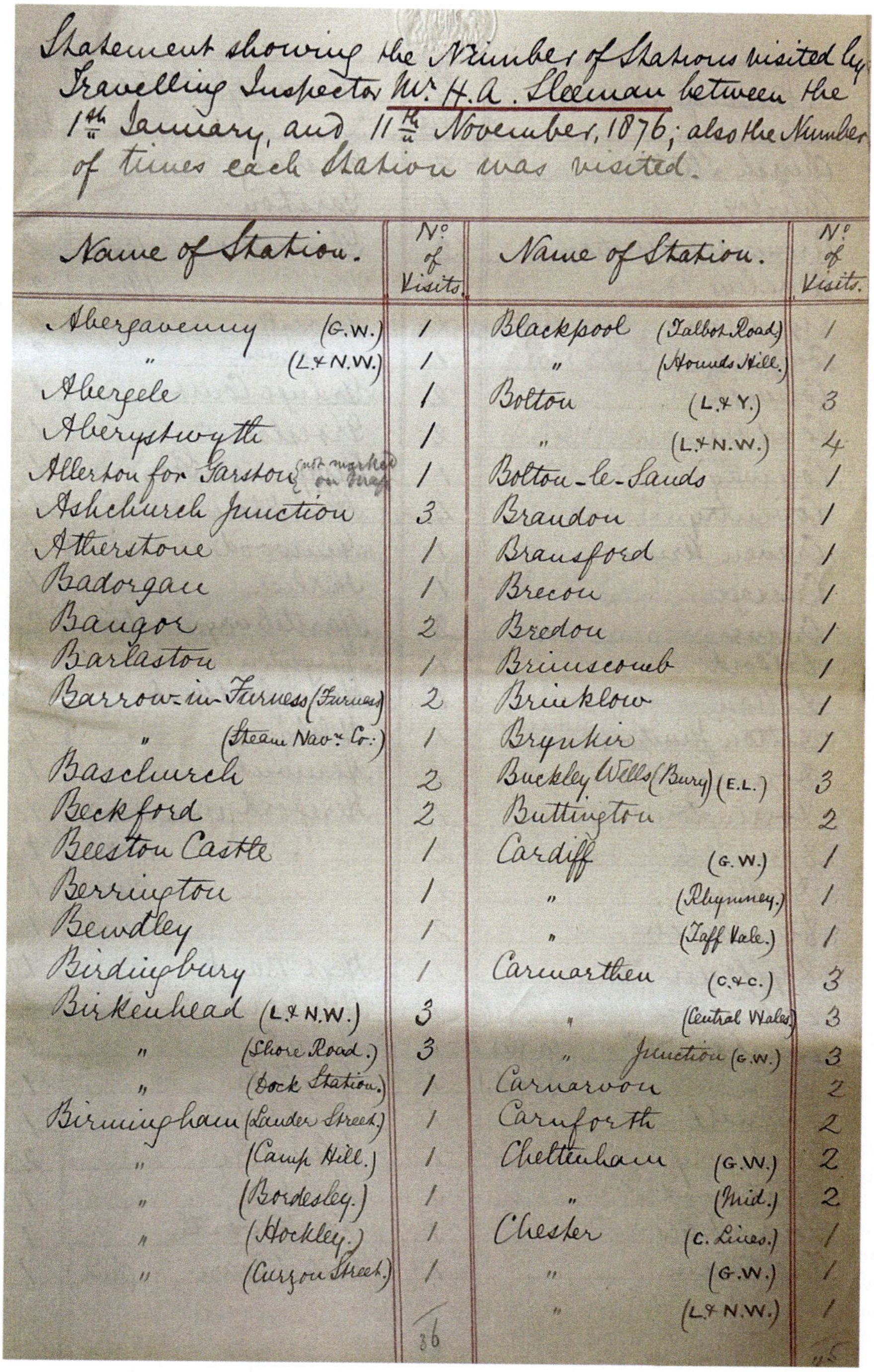

Statement showing the Number of Stations visited by Travelling Inspector Mr. H.A. Sleeman between the 1st January, and 11th November, 1876; also the Number of times each Station was visited.

Name of Station.	No. of Visits.	Name of Station.	No. of Visits.
Abergavenny (G.W.)	1	Blackpool (Talbot Road)	1
" (L.& N.W.)	1	" (Hounds Hill.)	1
Abergele	1	Bolton (L.& Y.)	3
Aberystwyth	1	" (L.& N.W.)	4
Allerton for Garston (not marked on map)	1	Bolton-le-Sands	1
Ashchurch Junction	3	Brandon	1
Atherstone	1	Bransford	1
Bodorgan	1	Brecon	1
Bangor	2	Bredon	1
Barlaston	1	Brimscomb	1
Barrow-in-Furness (Furness)	2	Brinklow	1
" (Steam Navn. Co.)	1	Brynkir	1
Baschurch	2	Buckley Wells (Bury) (E.L.)	3
Beckford	2	Buttington	2
Beeston Castle	1	Cardiff (G.W.)	1
Berrington	1	" (Rhymney.)	1
Bewdley	1	" (Taff Vale.)	1
Birdingbury	1	Carmarthen (C.& C.)	3
Birkenhead (L.& N.W.)	3	" (Central Wales)	3
" (Shore Road.)	3	" Junction (G.W.)	3
" (Dock Station.)	1	Carnarvon	2
Birmingham (Lawley Street.)	1	Carnforth	2
" (Camp Hill.)	1	Cheltenham (G.W.)	2
" (Bordesley.)	1	" (Mid.)	2
" (Hockley.)	1	Chester (C. Lines.)	1
" (Curzon Street.)	1	" (G.W.)	1
		" (L.& N.W.)	1
	36		45

Fig. 3.5. Statement showing the activities of travelling inspector Henry A. Sleeman. During 1876, Sleeman served as one of five travelling inspectors for the Veterinary Department of the Privy Council; he conducted inspections in locales that included Birkenhead (column 1), the Liverpool-area port through which ever increasing numbers of cattle were then imported. (From Williams, C., 1876, public domain via National Archives (Kew) PC 8/223.)

cattle varied internationally. In the USA during its eradication efforts, all beef was condemned; meanwhile, in France, the decision was left to the discretion of the veterinary inspector, presumably to gauge the degree of spoilage. In Britain, the rule was to pass the meat as marketable with diseased portions removed where possible. Thomas Walley, the distinguished professor, and for many years principal of the renowned Dick Veterinary School in Edinburgh, stated that he was not aware of any instance where the disease had been transmitted to humans through CBPP-affected meat (Shelley, 1892). A respected medical officer of health, Francis Vacher, noticed 'when pleuropneumonic beef was openly sold in London' and that, despite 'thousands of tons of such meat' having been eaten, 'it has never been alleged that one single case of rinderpest or pleuropneumonia has been communicated to a consumer' (Vacher, 1882, p. 3). Other studies involved feeding 'pleuro-pneumonic meat' to a host of carnivorous animals in London's Zoological Gardens, with none of the caged animals suffering ill effects (Vacher, 1881, p. 9).

Global and Local Impacts

The UK writ large was affected by CBPP. As the centre of the British empire, it was inevitable that it would also serve as a source of global infection. Indeed, Gamgee was sorrowful about how Britain's failure to control CBPP impacted other dominions, which then became seeds of global re-transmission:

> I should emphasize the lesson that our injury is the injury of all – the non-suppression of international disease means international mischief – and this is...illustrated by the way in which we have, since the days of free trade in cattle plagues, shipped pleuro-pneumonia to America, Australia, the Cape of Good Hope, and also to Holland, Germany, Denmark, and even Sweden. ...We may still suffer for having shipped lung disease to the United States, and I am very sorry to see constant attempts to land live cattle in Liverpool from the New World. (Gamgee, 1877, pp. 16–17)

Indeed, and as explored elsewhere in this volume – especially in Chapters 4 and 5 (on USA), 6 (on Africa), 7 (on Australia) and 9 (on India) – the UK's colonial and trade connections helped fuel a diaspora of CBPP. Meanwhile, *local*, county-level impacts, as well as trade within the British Isles, continued to consume the British Government and, eventually, compelled it to take more regulatory action.

As previously mentioned, the first outbreak in Ireland occurred in Cork sometime between 1839 and 1841, just before the British cases, and spread into county Limerick and then Carlow, Kilkenny, Tipperary, Galway and the rest of Ireland, inflicting enormous losses exceeding those of England and Scotland combined. Insurance companies could not cope, and many were obliged to relinquish protection to save themselves from bankruptcy. The north was initially spared but imports of cattle from Glasgow in 1844 provoked large outbreaks which continued for a decade, with Derry being particularly impacted. In 1885, official returns recorded 384 outbreaks in Leinster Province alone, with 314 occurring in the Dublin dairies that included 600 cowsheds in the city (Anonymous, 1887).

Ireland also became a major source of infection for the rest of the British Isles, particularly in Scotland where Irish store cattle were in great demand. Over 200,000 cattle were annually exported to Great Britain; 75% went to Scottish ports, and more than half of these were fat cattle fit for slaughter. The rest were store cattle – that is, cattle imported and brought inland for further fattening and subsequent slaughter. Concerns were raised by the Privy Council that the poor conditions of transport and inadequate inspection exacerbated the disease in the Irish cattle, leading to severe outbreaks in Scotland (Anonymous, 1887). In 1886, the Council proposed that the importation of cattle should be banned from infected regions of Ireland and inspections increased. This was considered too punitive by the Royal Agricultural Society of Ireland, who argued that it would adversely affect Irish livestock owners. They called for a Royal Commission to identify the exact distribution of CBPP as they maintained that at least 80% of Ireland was free of the disease. The inquiry, led by the Chief Veterinary Inspector Alex Cope, confirmed the society's opinion that the disease was largely restricted to Dublin and adjoining counties and that reports in other provinces were often misdiagnosed, mostly as tuberculosis. However, due to an increase in cases in Scotland between 1885 and 1886 that were blamed on Irish imports, some local authorities were severely restricting the introduction of all Irish cattle, much to the annoyance of Irish farmers, cattle dealers, and shipping companies, including the largest cattle carrier, A. Laird and Company of Glasgow (Anonymous, 1887). These local authorities required the animals to be kept in quarantine outside their districts for nearly two months at a time. These steamboat owners certainly had a point as many of their consignments came from Belfast, located in the CBPP-free province of Ulster. Consequently, pressure was brought to bear on the Government to lift these restrictions. Perhaps cunningly, the Privy Council rejected the protestations of the Irish lobby by stating:

> it would be impossible to take away from local authorities the power to protect their districts in the present state of disease in Scotland, and where they have prohibited or regulated the entry of cattle from all districts there can be no special grievance as regards Irish cattle, which does not equally apply to cattle from healthy districts in England or Scotland. (Anonymous, 1887, p. 51)

This tricky issue resolved itself shortly, as some of the Scottish local authorities voluntarily modified their regulations to allow some imports – but mainly because of the progress of the eradication programme during the next decade, which saw the beginning of the end of CBPP's prevalence throughout the British Isles.

Livestock owners, agriculturalists, veterinarians, insurance companies and government regulators were not the only ones to express opinions about CBPP's spread to and from Ireland. During the 1890s, animal welfare activists, including the Humanitarian League, loudly decried how Irish cattle shipped to Great Britain suffered atrocious conditions. 'One of the most objectionable features of the Irish trade is the length of time which the animals are kept without food and water', they argued (Greg and Towers, 1894, p. 10). The Humanitarian League – including one of its most notable female spokespersons, Isabel Greg – successfully lobbied the government for the gradual improvement of shipping regulations to both prevent the spread of diseases and minimize the discomfort of animals (Anonymous, 1897).

On the island of Great Britain, local impacts appeared everywhere. CBPP spread quickly from London to Manchester and Birmingham to Liverpool, Leeds, Sheffield and Newcastle. The large towns were the first to be affected by CBPP but soon farms in the countryside witnessed outbreaks. Between 1844 and 1845, the counties of Norfolk, Lincolnshire, Derbyshire, Lancashire, Yorkshire and Northumberland were all affected. Shortly after, the breeding districts in the west of England 'lost early and much' (Gamgee, 1863c, p. 636). English cattle then took the disease into Scotland, with Glasgow, Edinburgh, Perth and Aberdeen feeling its full force. In an 1882 commentary in *The London Times*, the varying local impacts of CBPP in England, Scotland and Wales are detailed; many communities had been distressed by the 'frequent years of disease' (Anonymous, 1882a, p. 6).

As explored in the next section, observation of local disease dynamics helped scientists better understand CBPP. Many farms in sparsely populated regions escaped the disease completely, providing helpful evidence of how CBPP was spread. In one illustrious example recounted by Gamgee, the parish of St Martin's in Perth was first infected in 1845 and then spread to ten farms, all of which could be linked to direct contact with diseased cattle. In contrast, 19 farms in the same area 'enjoyed perfect immunity' as they were all closed breeding premises with no introduction of replacement animals (Gamgee, 1863c, p. 639).

Contagion and Environmental Spread

Gamgee, Horsburgh, and many others including James Law, who referred to the propagated pathogen as a 'poison' (Law, 1876, p. 15), were convinced of the contagiousness of CBPP though they were not the first. In the previous century, the French veterinary giants Bourgelat in 1765, Haller in 1773, and Chaberts in 1794, had all argued that pleuropneumonia clearly spread from animal to animal. The introduction of the disease into countries previously free of the disease was convincing evidence enough for many. To emphasize the fact even more, in the 'Fifth Report of the Medical Officer of the Privy

Council' Gamgee had provided 26 examples nationwide where farms that had previously been CBPP-free became infected following the purchase of cows at local markets that were in contact with infected cattle, usually belonging to neighbours. Owners who raised their own stock, particularly breeders, were rarely affected and for those that were, the source could be traced to exposure to passing infected carriers on public roads or to diseased cattle that had been moved surreptitiously (Gamgee, 1863c).

Despite this overwhelming evidence going back nearly a century, some British veterinarians, the so-called 'non-contagionists' as they were known, were still not persuaded; this situation undoubtedly influenced government action or inaction. In true British style, a kind of disease-explanation compromise was reached in 1860:

> Those who have bestowed the most attention on the disease [i.e., CBPP], are generally of the opinion that the disease is contagious, but that it also occurs spontaneously... (North British Agriculturalist, 1860, p. 214)

To some extent, the doubts expressed by a few veterinarians and cattle owners about contagiousness could be understood with hindsight as, generally, not all cattle that came into contact with affected animals went down noticeably with CBPP. Moreover, it was still widely believed the causes of diseases like CBPP arose from miasmas ('bad air', defined as unhealthy fogs or vapours) brought on by damp and cold weather, wind direction, or conversely no wind at all. Miasmatic blame was often aimed at the cowsheds with their dirt, bad ventilation, improper food and blocked drains. One of the earliest summaries of the debate was authored in a prize student essay by Finlay Dun, then a junior at the Edinburgh Veterinary College; upon graduation, he was made a lecturer. His comments are illustrative of how veterinary scientists in mid-19th-century Britain were coming to grips with the disease.

> Many persons refuse to admit the contagion of pleuro-pneumonia, because, in some instances, the communication of the sick animals with the healthy cannot be proved to have taken place... [W]e hold that, although contagion may not be the sole exciting cause of all cases of pleuro-pneumonia, IT IS UNDOUBTEDLY the principal and the most fertile cause...Although contagion is admitted as producing many cases of pleuro-pneumonia, still it is very generally asserted that there must be other...causes at work capable of generating it independently of contagion. But if this be so, none of the many theories adduced to account for its exciting causes seem fully to explain its phenomena...Miasmata issuing from the earth have long been supposed to possess the power of producing epidemic and epizootic diseases. Endemics occurring partially, and varying at different times in intensity, may be referable to that cause; but were pleuro-pneumonia...dependent upon miasmata, their attacks would be local, and more or less intermittent, their diffusion more rapid, the type of disease more liable to change with the season of the year, the weather, or the locality, and its appearance and progress would be affected by the physical and geological character of the country; none of which circumstances are in any great degree observable in pleuro-pneumonia, as it appears in this island. (Dun, 1849, pp. 6–7, 10–11, 16)

Dun's prescient essay was written in 1849. By the 1850s and 1860s, transmission of contagion was more broadly accepted. The British Board of Trade received a report in May 1856 from the north of Germany of 'a *contagious* pulmonary disease having broken out among the horned cattle in Mecklenburgh' (Blackwell, 1856b, p. 2). Two weeks later, the British consular agent based at Lübeck confirmed it was 'Lungenseuche – the equivalent of "pulmonary murrain" in England – and, while distinct from rinderpest "equally contagious and almost equally fatal" (Blackwell, 1856a, pp. 3–4). As discussed in Chapter 4, this volume, contagion theory was vindicated in 1859 in the undeniable 'importation of pleuro-pneumonia into the United States from Holland' (Gamgee, 1864, p. 596).

In Britain, Gamgee pointed to evidence that showed that the disease 'was no less destructive in the fields of our best cattle-rearing counties or on the hills on which it may accidentally be carried...while mortality was often twice as high in summer than winter' (Gamgee, 1863a, p. 743). In the 1870s, the Privy Council began to explicitly acknowledge CBPP to be a transmissible disease; the 'attention of the Lords of the Council has been drawn to the continued prevalence of *contagious* pleuro-pneumonia among cattle', the Council secretary wrote in February 1874 (Williams, 1874, italics added). Later that summer, local authorities were assuming CBPP to be contagious as well as infectious, as illustrated in the county of Surrey:

> Animals affected with Pleuro-Pneumonia should be slaughtered at once, and buried as directed by the Order in Council. All persons engaged in looking after or slaughtering and burying Diseased Animals, should be disinfected by washing their hands in a solution of Condy's Fluid in Water (an ounce to the quart). The clothes should be carefully cleaned, and the boots washed with a solution of Carbolic Acid in Lime Water or Oil...The Dung and all Litter which has been on Contact with infected Animals should be burnt as far as practicable, an if wet, dug into arable land upon which Cattle are not likely to be pastured, until a crop has been grown upon it. (Anonymous, 1874)

Such statements illustrate a growing consensus among veterinarians and government officials that CBPP ought to be treated as a contagious disease capable of being transmitted through the environment. Yet, until the the establishment of the germ theory two years later (in 1876, when German bacteriologist Robert Koch discovered *Bacillus anthracis*, clearly linking a disease – anthrax – to a specific organism for the first time), scientific debate between and among contagionists and non-contagionists persisted.

Contrary to other European countries, where slaughtering all clinically affected animals with whole or partial compensation was recommended, Britain's confused opinion set back disease control for several decades. Fear of legislative interference by cattle owners was also a factor in the decision not to control the disease, even if it meant the continual introduction of infected cattle from the European mainland. By the time government surveillance finally began in 1870, at least 1500 outbreaks were reported annually, doubling five years later. Elsewhere in the British Empire, CBPP was about to wreak havoc. A report written by the Pleuro-pneumonia Commissioners for Victoria, three years after the introduction of CBPP into Australia in 1858, pleaded the following: 'Our best sheet-anchor is prevention. The time now is approaching when men must act vigorously, or else lose their cattle – if they wish to save the country, *unite*' (Anonymous, 1862b, p. 65).

Surprisingly, perhaps, this remains the best advice for preventing the spread of this and many other mycoplasma diseases. Sadly, and as explored in Chapter 7, this volume, the Australian authorities did not heed this impassioned warning, and CBPP spread throughout the continent and was not eliminated for another 110 years.

Within a few decades, the contagiousness of CBPP was all but accepted. Yet, as late as 1890, some instructors still felt the need to assert the point. On 22 October of that year, Professor Robert Wallace told an incoming class of agriculture students to abandon miasmatic or other non-contagionist theories: "It should not be forgotten that there is no such thing as spontaneous generation of such diseases as Foot-and-Mouth and Pleuro-pneumonia; they must be directly passed on from one animal to another' (Wallace, 1890, pp. 21–22).

Treatment

With cattle dying of CBPP while veterinarians and cattle owners stood around helplessly, it was natural for them to seek a quick cure, but surprisingly most authoritative advice was not to treat but to isolate and even slaughter without delay. However, a few seemingly sensible practitioners and, of course, the ubiquitous 'snake oil salesmen' were only too willing to advocate a range of treatments from powdered woodlice to honeyed barley (Blancou, 2000). In the absence of controlled experiments, it can only be inferred that most failed or the cattle improved naturally. James Moore, a recent convert to homeopathy, advocated originally by the German physician Samuel Hahnemann in 1796, was sure his homeopathic approach was the answer. Moore noted in the 9th edition of his slim book that despite 'diseased cows [being] assiduously purged, violently blistered and setoned...they still died...the only known method of cure is that called the Homoeopathic system of treatment' (Moore, 1871, pp. 5–6).

While believing the disease was caused by the gases from decomposing vegetation, he also believed (rightly) it was contagious and exacerbated by over-production and intensification and that early diagnosis and isolation was essential. The medication he recommended was based on definite stages of the disease and varied from the grandly termed ammonium causticum (more commonly known as ammonia water), which would be greatly diluted and given every few hours depending on the severity of the clinical signs or dilutions of the poisonous plant monkshood. Sulphur and phosphorus were to be used for the most severe cases. Some dietary advice was also offered, such as giving livestock mashes of boiled turnips and carrots which, unlike some of the homeopathic recipes, were unlikely to do much harm. Descriptions of cases of successful treatment are appended in his book (Moore, 1871). Whether his medications were truly homeopathic whereby 'healing' substances are diluted beyond detection is not clear.

In contrast, James Law (1887) was set against any form of treatment unless isolation could be guaranteed and 'where no strange men or animals can get access' (Law, 1887, p. 93). Where it was possible, he advocated a variety of treatments including warm water mild laxatives and blisters applied to the sides of chests, sulphur fumes and carbolic acid vapours. Finally, he recommended covering the cattle in water-soaked rugs, but this required: 'intelligence, enthusiasm and activity on the part of the attendants' (Law, 1887, p. 94).

Later, on a more scientific level, an organoarsenic compound called neosalvarsan, which had successfully treated cases of syphilis, was reported to improve the disease course and reduce mortality to 5–6% but did not appear to catch on (Salmon, 1896). Repeated injections of immune serum had some therapeutic effects if given shortly after fever developed but were expensive, time-consuming and ultimately of little value at this period of our knowledge of immunology (Hutyra *et al.*, 1938).

Legislation

As mentioned, the 1840s – which inaugurated three decades of 'laissez-faire' policy – begged questions about how to curtail the introduction of animal diseases, including CBPP. British historian of science Michael Worboys summarizes well the national reluctance of early legislative responses:

> [T]he repeal of protectionist legislation and improvements in transportation times...allowed animals carrying disease to be more readily imported. In 1848 outbreaks [of a number of animal diseases] demonstrated what many had feared, namely, that free trade in livestock had brought with it free trade in livestock disease. The proposed introduction of veterinary policing was very controversial, since it was seen by supporters of laissez-faire as a means of re-introducing protection. (Worboys, 1991, pp. 309–10)

The 1848 outbreaks mentioned by Worboys were actually primarily of sheep-pox (which had begun in 1847), yet CBPP would soon again be on the rise. In response, bills were introduced and, in September 1848, 'two acts were passed which sought to regulate imports in the interests of controlling disease' (Fisher, 1980, p. 279). Taken together, the two laws 'gave powers to the Queen in Council to prohibit the importation of sheep, cattle, and other animals, or to admit them after quarantine, for the prevention of contagious diseases...[and] to prohibit or regulate the movement of animals, including horses; also of meat, hides, fodder, and other things likely to spread contagion' (Duckham and Brown, 1893, p. 282). Significantly, the 1848 laws failed for a number of reasons. First, the contagiousness of CBPP (as well as other animal diseases) was still being debated. Second, the 1848 Order did not name specific diseases; therefore, 'which diseases were covered and whether they were contagious or "foreign" or both had to be decided case by case' (Worboys, 1991, p. 310). Third, and as mentioned earlier in this chapter, veterinary leaders like J.B. Simonds were reluctant to take action on imports; he continued to feel that 'the dangers of foreign cattle diseases had been exaggerated' and that CBPP was one of several 'native diseases which flared up under certain conditions' (Worboys, 1991, p. 310). Fourth, while general powers had been conferred on the Privy Council, the 1848 laws provided no special powers to the Privy Council regarding specifically CBPP; such powers would not come until two decades later in 1868 (Duckham and Brown, 1893, p. 264). These factors contributed to 'the association of imports and disease' being generally, but not entirely, 'forgotten for two decades' (Fisher, 1980, p. 279).

It should be acknowledged that the two 1848 laws were periodically invoked in new Orders of Council. One such example occurred in July 1856 while the Queen was on the Isle of Wight. Receiving news of fresh animal disease outbreaks on the continent, the Privy Council saw fit to require veterinary inspections when 'any sheep, lambs, cattle, or pigs imported or brought into this country shall appear at the time of their importation to be infected with, or labouring under, any contagious or infectious disorder' (Bathurst, 1856, p. 2). Nevertheless, the 1848 laws were largely inconsequential in preventing disease. The ever-vigilant John Gamgee recognized this and, in 1864, proposed two bills to replace the impotent 1848 legislation. Gamgee's proposed measures were opposed – indeed 'by most agricultural and livestock interests, as well as by leading veterinarians' – and were not adopted by Parliament (Worboys, 1991, p. 311).

In the late 1860s and early 1870s, Great Britain was fast losing control of CBPP but had passed a series of Acts – most notably, the Contagious Diseases (Animals) Acts of 1869 and 1878 – that made the disease notifiable and imposed movement controls on cattle (see Table 3.2). Local authorities were now forced to act more decisively. Official figures were to be collected and, in 1875, just over 3000 outbreaks were recorded in 68 counties across the country (Anonymous, 1887). While the intention was to slaughter all infected and contact cattle with compensation, this was applied inconsistently and hampered by the fact that a local authority could only deal with its own area whereas the trade in cattle involved extensive movements across counties. Nevertheless, and despite these imperfect control measures, the number of outbreaks fell in the late 1870s when full compensation (up to £40 per animal) was paid – a significant indemnification policy that accompanied the trade-related policies enshrined in the 1878 Animals Order (see Table 3.2). More regulatory progress followed, and an Act of 1884 (Animals Order) recognized, farsightedly, that clinical examination would not identify all infected animals; therefore, clearance of all cattle from an infected holding was now required. Outbreaks slowly declined thereafter. By 1887, while the disease stubbornly persisted in London and the large cities of Yorkshire and mid-Scotland (see Fig. 3.6, this volume), most areas of Wales and the West Country were probably CBPP-free given the limited methods of detection available at the time (Agriculture Department, 1888, map facing p. 292).

As late as 1889 – by which year Holland, Norway, Switzerland, Sweden and Denmark had eradicated CBPP – Professor Thomas Walley, Principal of the Dick Veterinary School in Edinburgh, was leading a debate on whether the wholesale cattle slaughter would ever eliminate the disease, or it would always be a scourge to British herds (Walley, 1889). He must have vacillated between frustration and hopefulness. In Edinburgh, if a dairyman observed a cow showing symptoms of CBPP, he could summon Principal Walley (or another local inspector) to slaughter the animal. If a post-mortem examination turned up CBPP, then three-fourths of the value of the animal was paid to the dairyman (Walley, 1888, p. 143). As indicated in Table 3.2, this practice of compensation (up to 75% of the value up to £30) began in 1875, yet more authority (and more funds) were needed. The funding pressures were acutely felt at the local authority level, where delegated powers from the Privy Council were being enacted. In some instances, differing degrees of expertise and scrutiny among inspectors raised eyebrows and prompted surprising comments, as evidenced in the county of Surrey in 1882. There, the competent J. Irvine Lupton (who had been hired to serve as veterinary inspector for two divisions in Surrey, namely Wandsworth and Richmond) was singled out by the Justices of the Peace for the high cost of what Lupton likely considered prudent disease-control decisions:

> The Committee observing the very large amount awarded in the Wandsworth Division for compensation in respect of Cattle slaughtered in consequence of having been in contact with others affected with Pleuro Pneumonia Resolve that a Communication be sent to the Inspector for that Division [i.e., Mr. Lupton] requesting him before directing in future the slaughter of healthy animals to fully consider the effect

of inoculation as a preventive against Disease. (Anonymous, 1882b)

For his part, Lupton rejected their suggestion and remained undeterred in aggressively stamping out CBPP. By the end of the 1880s, he remained aggressive in his work, consistently notching some of the highest numbers of inspections, condemnations and recommended reimbursements for the entire county (Anonymous, 1888a).

National thought leaders like Thomas Walley must have been heartened by the Act of

Table 3.2. Legislation introduced to control CBPP. (From Robin Nicholas and Justin Kastner.)

Date	Name	Function
1848	An Act to prohibit the Importation of Sheep, Cattle, or other Animals, for the Purpose of preventing the Introduction of contagious or infectious Disorders An Act to prevent, until the First Day of September One thousand eight hundred and fifty, and to the End of the then Session of Parliament, the spreading of contagious or infectious Disorders among Sheep, Cattle, and other Animals	Conferred general (but not CBPP-specific) powers upon the Privy Council
1856	Order of Council making further provision for the prevention of the importation of diseased Cattle, Sheep, &c.	Provided for the seizure and inspection of ships carrying cattle that were suspected of carrying disease
1867	Contagious Diseases (Animals) Act	Offence to expose an affected animal at a market or fair
1869	Contagious Diseases (Animals) Act	Local authorities' power to stop the movement of cattle for slaughter from farms with CBPP; restrictions withdrawn after 30 days
1869	Animals Order	CBPP made notifiable
1875	Animals Order	Slaughter with compensation of 75% with value up to £30; restrictions on rest of herd for 2 months; local authorities to enforce
1878	Contagious Diseases (Animals) Act	Slaughter of in-contacts with 100% compensation up to £40
1884	Animals Order	Movement of cattle onto a farm with CBPP to be stopped until all resident cattle are removed
1888	Pleuropneumonia Slaughter Order	Slaughter of all animals exposed or in contact with CBPP within 10 days; after slaughter, farm to be disinfected
1888	Pleuropneumonia (Infected Circles) Order	All movements prohibited within half-mile of outbreak
1890	Contagious Diseases (Animals) (Pleuropneumonia) Act	Responsibility for control transferred from local authority to veterinary department
1891	Pleuropneumonia Order	Prescribed scheduled districts in place of infected areas
1896	Cowshed Pleuropneumonia Order	Prohibited movement of cows out of any shed in East London except under licence for local slaughter

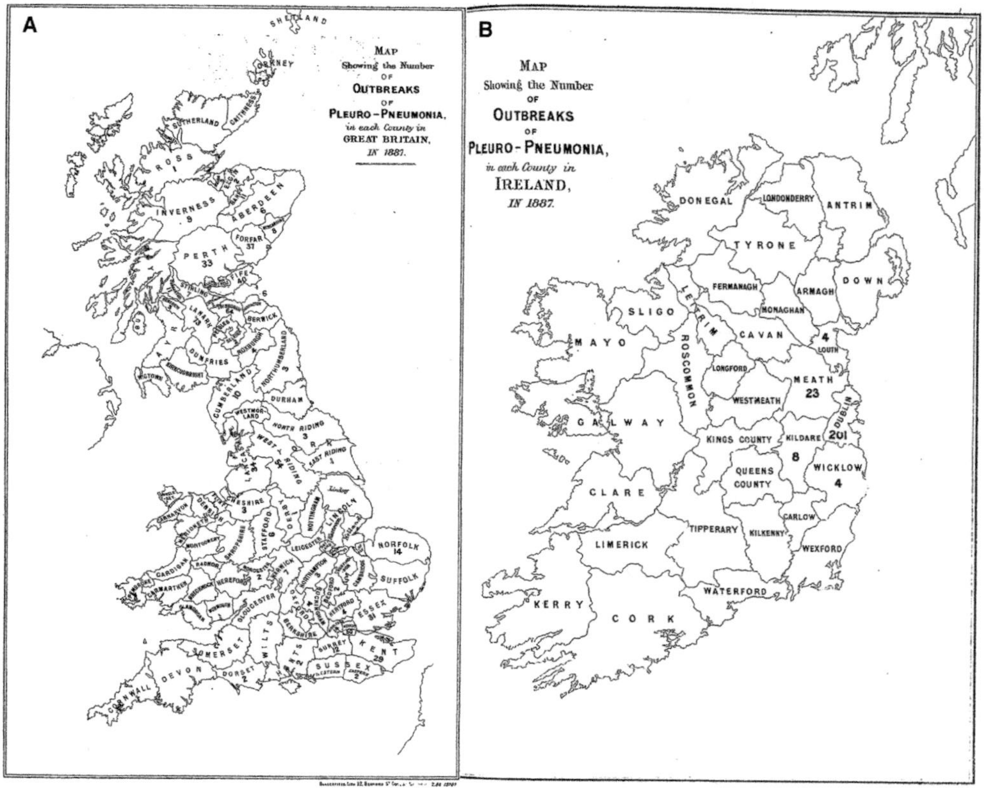

Fig. 3.6. Two maps depicting the prevalence of CBPP in 1887, in Britain (A) and Ireland (B). (From Agriculture Department, 1888, Her Majesty's Stationery Office, London, public domain.)

1890 (see Table 3.2), which transferred responsibility to the central government, providing a final impetus for the complete eradication of the disease from Britain. Essentially, this provided £140,000 (worth nearly £5 million in 2025) for CBPP control, while also enabling official inspection and post-mortem examination of cattle on suspected farms. Moreover, tracing and slaughter of affected contacts were ordered to be carried out; this had the positive effect of drastically reducing the number of outbreaks from just over 2000 in 1890 to a single case five years later. A scattering of outbreaks followed over the next few years with one outbreak near London in 1897 attracting the attention of parliament. Dr Farquharson, an MP for Aberdeen, asked whether this case may have arisen spontaneously. Walter Long, MP for Liverpool West and President of the Board of Agriculture, gave the following reply: 'The hon. Gentleman knows perfectly well that the opinion of our expert advisers is that the disease cannot have a spontaneous origin. But it may be lying dormant for a long time' (Commons Sitting, 1897, column 1545).

It seems that not everyone had got the message of contagion even after living with the disease for nearly 50 years. The very last case was recorded in East London in January 1898 and, as if to finally lay the ghost of spontaneous generation, Nocard and Roux in France isolated 'a strange causal organism' in the very same year (see Chapter 1, this volume).

The Deptford Ox

By 1892 the term contagious bovine pleuropneumonia (CBPP) was being used widely in Britain, particularly by the leading figures of the day such as Professor John McFadyean (McFadyean, 1892). Referring to the difficulty some veterinarians were having in diagnosing CBPP at post-mortem, McFadyean argued that lesions were pathognomonic and outlined those features which were essential in order to confirm a case of CBPP. The key features he outlined included the following: different animal ages; variety of colour and appearance of the hepatized areas (marbling); the prominent participation of the inter-lymphatic apparatus shown by extreme inflammation of the interstitial lymphatics, with the formation of thrombi inside the vessels and marked inflammatory infiltration of the interstitial connective tissue leading to a broadening of the latter; and an exudative fibrinous pleurisy (McFadyean, 1892, p. 355). However, there was a great divergence of opinion, even among experts, particularly in response to several cattle imported from the USA into the London port of Deptford in April 1891. An American government veterinarian, Mr Wray, thought the lesions were a non-infectious bronchopneumonia, a diagnosis supported by Professor William Williams (of the New Veterinary College in Edinburgh) using microscopic evidence; as explored in Chapter 5, this volume, this was not the first time Williams had voiced such a claim, for he had weighed in similarly over a decade earlier in an equally debatable CBPP-diagnosis case at the port of Liverpool (Kastner *et al.*, 2005). Williams recalled the event in these terms:

> [A] lung of an ox was found at Deptford in April 1891, and said by Professors Brown and Duguid and Mr. Cope, and confirmed by Professors Walley and M'Fadyean, to have *pleuro-pneumonia contagiosa*, and in further support of the correctness of the diagnosis Mr. Chaplin, the Minister of Agriculture, said it was pleuro, for he had seen the lungs. But Dr. Wray, the American veterinary inspector, disputed this opinion, and on 18th April brought a portion of the lungs to me. I, along with my son, examined this portion of lung, and we both came to the conclusion that it was not pleuro-pneumonia. I was again in the minority... (Williams, 1893, p. 187)

Indeed, in April 1891, Professors McFadyean and Walley disagreed with Williams; they were sure that these cattle had true CBPP, a view finally accepted by other experts including six European pathologists who all examined a piece of the lung (presumably fixed in formalin) from the 'Deptford ox'. To placate Williams, experts at a meeting at the Lancashire Veterinary Medical Association meeting where McFadyean spoke accepted the possibility that the affected lung may have also contained a 'small lesion' of bronchopneumonia (McFadyean, 1892, p. 358).

Stamping Out Versus Inoculation

The successful eradication of CBPP from Great Britain, and indeed the USA, was achieved solely by slaughtering affected herds without any real insight into the nature of the cause but informed eventually by the overwhelming knowledge that the disease was contagious. Pressure on the British authorities to experiment with crude vaccines being developed in Europe, particularly Belgium, over this period was not just resisted but actively scorned. A review in the *British Medical Journal* mixed patronization with sarcasm at the attempts by Dr Louis Willems to vaccinate cattle with 'lung matter' from an animal that had died of CBPP: 'In 1850 Dr Willems having failed to arrest the disease...tried inoculation as an experiment and convinced himself of its success' (Anonymous, 1870, p. 604).

Describing the adverse reactions of death and severe ulceration produced by tail inoculation, the *BMJ* quotes Willems as saying that the cattle do not suffer. The journal's response was scathing: 'If experience proves this to be true, it must be regarded as a new fact in medicine' (Anonymous, 1870, p. 604).

Despite growing evidence from the private veterinary sector especially in the Netherlands that inoculation in certain situations could bring about good results in a short time with little loss of animal life and crucially at little cost, the government, including the privy council, were very single-minded, influenced by Simonds and the *BMJ*, in their pursuit of 'stamping out' which became official policy in 1888 (Slateford, 1888). It must be said, however, that this decision was not made without consideration but was based on a thorough two-week-long review by a departmental committee, of evidence from 44 witnesses comprising veterinarians, physicians and stock owners, which produced a report of over 300 pages (Anonymous, 1888b).

One witness had testified that inoculation had been used with excellent results in Edinburgh, but his evidence had come unstuck when he stated that the amount of compensation paid was less than the salary of the state inspector; eventually, under questioning, he had to admit that he was unaware of the costs of either. In fact, official figures showed that compensation was still exceeding the costs of inspection.

The issue of inoculation versus stamping out was thoroughly explored. The following excerpt from the report is also telling:

> [W]e have found very conflicting opinions as to the necessity or practical value of experiments on inoculation as a remedy for pleuro-pneumonia. Many of the advocates of inoculation on the one hand declared that their faith in its efficacy required no confirmation, whilst its opponents maintained that, the only object being to get rid of pleuro-pneumonia as quickly as possible, it is undesirable and illogical to perpetuate the disease in order to carry out experiments, which after all could be valuable only on the most abstract scientific grounds... Most of the witnesses, however, were decidedly averse to any experiments being carried out if the policy of compulsory slaughter as at present being pursued were to be in any way weakened or impeded thereby. (Privy Council Office, 1888, p. 17)

On completion of the inquiry, the committee concluded that it could not be rigidly proved that inoculation practised on a healthy animal protects it against subsequent infection, but promised to search the committee's minutes for evidence of any proof that inoculation exerted a curative effect. In the words of the editor of the influential *Journal of Comparative Pathology and Therapeutics*, who studied the report, 'No loophole of escape is left from the conclusion that the only known method that could reasonably be expected to eradicate the disease is that which is familiarly known as stamping out' (Anonymous, 1888b).

But to cover themselves perhaps, the government appointed another departmental committee to investigate the merits of inoculation. Its findings would be purely academic as, by the middle of the 1890s, outbreaks of CBPP had declined to single figures. On balance, stamping out was a brave decision leading to the total eradication of the disease from Great Britain – and would remain policy to this day both in Great Britain and Europe. Furthermore, it is a fact that vaccination has never been shown to eradicate CBPP without other measures being applied, anywhere in the world.

While vaccination would not, knowingly, play any role in CBPP's control in Europe for the next 100 years, vaccines based on Willems's work would participate in CBPP control alongside movement control and test and slaughter in China (see Chapter 8, this volume), in Australia and New Zealand (very successfully; see Chapter 7, this volume), and (still today) in sub-Saharan Africa where CBPP remains a major livestock problem (see Chapter 6, this volume).

Costs of Eradicating CBPP From Great Britain

The total costs of the eradication of CBPP have never been fully costed, but Sir John McFadyean, eminent professor at the Royal Veterinary College, writing a quarter of a century after the last case of CBPP, provided an approximation. He estimated the losses inflicted by the disease during its 49-year presence in Britain could not have been less than £3 million (Windsor, n.d.). It was estimated that, in the 25 years ending 1894, 79,000 and 24,000 cattle in Great Britain and Ireland, respectively, were recorded as afflicted with CBPP. The Government eventually voted £1.25 million over nine years for the eradication campaign. McFadyean believed it was worth it; since the cost of eradication was less than the effects of the disease during one year, it was money well spent.

Although later than planned, CBPP was finally eradicated in 1898, 13 years later than the Netherlands which had adopted a combined policy of stamping out and inoculation of contacts. Ironically, it was partly the ban by Britain on imports from the Netherlands that reduced the risk of infection caused by the movement of cattle across the Dutch countryside.

Postscript

While, today, many will think the term 'fake news' is a relatively new phenomenon, a look at the 16 January 1892 issue of *The Veterinary Record* will find an article entitled 'Why Pleuro Prevails', which reports on an item from *The New York Herald* suggesting that the number of reported cases of CBPP in England was greatly exaggerated and simply a means for owners to fraudulently obtain compensation at 'double the value' of their slaughtered cattle (Anonymous, 1892, p. 383). *Plus ça change!*

References

Agriculture Department (1888) *Report of the Departmental Committee Appointed to Inquire into Pleuro-Pneumonia and Tuberculosis in the United Kingdom (Part II: Minutes of evidence and appendix)*. Eyre and Spottiswoode for Her Majesty's Stationery Office, London.

Anonymous (1862a) Pleuro-pneumonia in Holland. *Edinburgh Veterinary Review and Annals of Comparative Pathology* 4, 225–235.

Anonymous (1862b) Report on pleuro-pneumonia in cattle. *Edinburgh Veterinary Review and Annals of Comparative Pathology* 4(11), 61–67.

Anonymous (1865) *Memorandum of Association of the Alcester Cattle Plague and Pleuro Pneumonia Prevention Company, Limited.* Alfred Doubble, Law and Public Companies' Stationer, London.

Anonymous (1870) Infectious pleuropneumonia. *British Medical Journal* 1(493), 604–606.

Anonymous (1872) Minutes of 4 October 1872. In: *Minutes Book of Executive Committee of the Justices of the Peace of the Country of Surrey*. Surrey History Centre, Woking.

Anonymous (1874) Minutes of 25 July 1874. In: *Minutes Book of Executive Committee of the Justices of the Peace of the Country of Surrey*. Surrey History Centre, Woking.

Anonymous (1882a) Agricultural decline. *The Times*, 19 April p. 6.

Anonymous (1882b) Minutes of 20 March 1882. In: *Minutes Book of Executive Committee of the Justices of the Peace of the Country of Surrey*. Surrey History Center, Woking.

Anonymous (1887) *Correspondence Relating to Pleuro-Pneumonia in Ireland. Presented to both Houses of Parliament*. HMSO, London.

Anonymous (1888a) *Minutes Book of the Executive Committee of the Justices of the Peace of the County of Surrey*. Surrey History Centre, Woking.

Anonymous (1888b) The report of the departmental committee on pleuro-pneumonia and tuberculosis. *Journal of Comparative Pathology and Therapeutics* 1, 234–237.

Anonymous (1892) Why pleuro prevails. *The Veterinary Record* 4(184), 383–384.

Anonymous (1897) The cattle trade. *The Londonderry Sentinel* 2 December, p. 3.

Back, R. (2021) *Parlementaire enquête omtrent de besmettelijke longziekte onder het rundvee in de negentiende eeuw* [parliamentary inquiry into the contagious lung disease among cattle in the nineteenth century]; *CAHIERS* [notebook series], no.8. Veterinair Historisch Genootschap (Veterinair Historisch Genootschap), Utrecht.

Bates, T. (1718) A brief account of the contagious disease which raged among the milch cowes near London, in the year 1714. and of the methods that were taken for suppressing it. *Philosophical Transactions of the Royal Society of London* 30(358), 872–885.

Bathurst, W.L. (1856) *General Order no.74/1856: Order of Her Majesty in Council*. Isle of Wight.

Blackwell, J.A. (1856a) *Dispatch Relative to Cattle Diseases, Including Lungenseuche*. Board of Trade, Germany Lubeck.

Blackwell, J.A. (1856b) *General Order no.52/1856: Reports from Lubeck and Hamburg Regarding a Contagious Pulmonary Disease in Mecklenburgh and Response of the Lubeck Government*. Board of Trade (Office of Committee of Privy Council for Trade), London.

Blancou, J. (2000) Contagious bovine pleuropneumonia. In: *History of the Surveillance and Control of Transmissible Animal Diseases*. OIE, Paris, pp. 133–160.

Butterfield, M. (ed.) (1860) *House Report 651: House Agriculture Committee Report on Cattle Disease*. Government Printing Office, Washington, DC.

Chappell & Company (1869) *St. James's Hall: Mr. Charles Dickens's Farewell Readings, Tuesdays, October 6 and 20, November 3 and 17, and December 1*. The New York Public Library, Berg Collection of English and American Literature, New York.

Common Sitting (1897) Pleuropneumonia. *Hansard's Parliamentary Debates Series* 4, 47.

Duckham, T. and Brown, G.T. (1893) The progress of legislation against contagious diseases of live stock. *Journal of the Royal Agricultural Society of England IV* 262–286.

Dun, F. (1849) On the prevailing epizootic in cattle called pleuro-pneumonia. Prize essay published by the author, Edinburgh.

Fisher, J. (2003) To kill or not to kill: The eradication of contagious bovine pleuro-pneumonia in Western Europe. *Medical History* 47(3), 314–331.

Fisher, J.R. (1980) The economic effects of cattle disease in Britain and its containment, 1850-1900. *Agricultural History* 54(2), 278–294.

Fleming, G. (1871) *Animal Plagues: Their History, Nature, and Prevention*. Chapman and Hall, London.

Gamgee, J. (1857) *Diseased Meat Sold in Edinburgh, and Meat Inspection in Connection with The Public Health and with the Interests of Agriculture: A Letter to the Right Hon*. The Lord Provost of Edinburgh, Southerland Knox, Edinburgh.

Gamgee, J. (1863a) Disease in town dairies, and its prevention. *Edinburgh Veterinary Review and Annals of Comparative Pathology* 5(44), 742–758.

Gamgee, J. (1863b) The health of stock in the United Kingdom during the year 1862. *Edinburgh Veterinary Review and Annals of Comparative Pathology* 5(39), 401–418.

Gamgee, J. (1863c) Pleuro-pneumonia in cattle. *Edinburgh Veterinary Review and Annals of Comparative Pathology* 5(42), 632–643.

Gamgee, J. (1864) *Our Domestic Animals in Health and Disease: Organs of Circulation and Respiration*. MacLachlan & Stewart, Edinburgh.

Gamgee, J. (1866) *The Cattle Plague; with official reports of the International Veterinary Congresses, held in Hamburg, 1863, and in VIenna, 1865*. Robert Hardwicke, London.

Gamgee, J. (1871) Report of Professor Gamgee on the lung plague. In: Capron, H. (ed.) *Report of the Commissioner of Agriculture on Diseases of Cattle in the United States*. Government Printing Office, Washington, DC, pp. 3–63.

Gamgee, J. (1877) *The Meat Question: Free and Food Taxes, being an address delivered on the 9th of May 1877 at the St. James's Hall*. T.W. Hannaford, London.

Greg, I. and Towers, S.H. (1894) Cattle ships and our meat supply. *The Humanitarian League's Publications* 15.

Hale, T. (1758) *A Compleat Body of Husbandry*, 2nd edn. Thomas Osborne, London.

Hall, S.A. (1976) The stimulus for the statutory control of animal diseases in Great Britain in the 19th century. *Veterinary History* 6, 3–12.

Heaton, H. (1948) *Economic History of Europe*, Revised edition. Harper & Row, New York.

Horsburgh, J. (1859) On the contagious nature of pleuropneumonia in cattle. *Edinburgh Veterinary Review and Annals of Comparative Pathology* 1(3), 278–285.

Hutyra, F., Marek, J. and Manninger, R. (1938) Contagious pleuropneumonia. In: Greig, J.R., Mohler, J.R. and Eichhorn, A. (eds) *Special Pathology and Therapeutics of the Diseases of Domestic Animals*, 4th English edition. Alexander Eger, Chicago, Illinois, pp. 455–472.

Kastner, J., Powell, D., Crowley, T. and Huff, K. (2005) Scientific conviction amidst scientific controversy in the transatlantic livestock and meat trade. *Endeavour* 29(2), 78–83.

Law, J. (1876) The lung-fever of cattle. Contagious pleuro-pneumonia. In: *The Farmer's Veterinary Adviser: A Guide to the Prevention and Treatment of Disease in Domestic Animals*. Published by the author, Ithaca, New York, pp. 14–17.

Law, J. (1887) *The Farmer's Veterinary Adviser, A Guide to the Prevention and Treatment of Disease in Domestic Animals*. Published by the author, Ithaca, New York.

Library of Congress (n.d.) Washington and the New Agriculture. Online. Library of Congress, Washington, DC. Available at: https://www.loc.gov/collections/george-washington-papers/articles-and-essays/introduction-to-the-diaries-of-george-washington/washington-and-the-new-agriculture/ (accessed 22nd January, 2025)

Matthews, A.H.H. (1915) *Fifty Years of Agricultural Politics, Being the History of the Central Chamber of Agriculture, 1865–1915*. P.S. King & Son, Ltd, London.

McCarron, K. (1991) *Meat at Woodside: The Birkenhead livestock trade 1878–1981*. Merseyside Port Folios and the National Museums and Galleries on Merseyside Birkenhead.

McEachran, D. (1879) Report of special investigation into existence of cattle disease in the United States (extract report). In: Walley, T. (ed.) *The Four Bovine Scourges: Pleuro-Pneumonia, Foot-and-Mouth Disease, Cattle Plague, Tubercle (Scrofula)*. MacLachlan & Stewart, Edinburgh, pp. 206–212.

McFadyean, J. (1892) Pleuro-pneumonia: A paper read before the Lancashire Veterinary Medical Association. *The Veterinary Record* 4(182), 351–358.

Ministry of Agriculture, F.a.F (1965) *Animal Health: A Centenary 1865–1965*. Her Majesty's Stationery Office, London.

Moore, J. (1871) *The Lung Disease of Cattle, or Pleuro-pneumonia, Curable by Homeopathy*. Henry Turner and Co., London.

North British Agriculturalist (1860) Pleuro-pneumonia. *Edinburgh Veterinary Review and Annals of Comparative Pathology* 2(6), 214–216.

Pattison, I. (1990) *A Great British Veterinarian Forgotten: James Beart Simonds 1810–1904*. J.A. Allen & Co., London.

Privy Council Office (1888) *Departmental Report to the Lord President of the Privy Council (on Pleuro-Pneumonia and Tuberculosis)*. Privy Council Office, London.

Salmon, D.E. (1896) *Diseases of Cattle and on Cattle Feeding*. Government Printing Office, Washington, DC.

Shelley, C.E. (1892) The relations of the diseases of animals to those of man. In: *Transactions of the 7th International Congress of Hygiene and Demography*, Eyre and Spottiswoode, London, p. 174.

Slateford, C.C. (1888) Proceedings of the Scottish Metropolitan Veterinary Medical Society. *The Veterinary Record* 1, 7–8.

Survey of London (2019) Marylebone Literary and Scientific Institution. Online. Available at: https://blogs.ucl.ac.uk/survey-of-london/2019/11/01/marylebone-literary-and-scientific-institution/ (accessed 21 January 2025).

Vacher, F. (1881) *What Diseases Are Communicable to Man from Diseased Animals Used as Food?* T. Richards, London.

Vacher, F. (1882) *The transmission of disease by food (reprint of article published in the British Medical Journal, September 16, 1882)*. The author, Birkenhead.

Wallace, R. (1890) Edinburgh university, session 1890–91. In: *Introductory Lecture to the Agriculture Class on American Cattle and the American Export Trade in Beef and Live Cattle to Great Britain, Wednesday*. Oliver and Boyd, Edinburgh.

Walley, T. (1879) *The Four Bovine Scourges: Pleuro-Pneumonia, Foot-and-Mouth Disease, Cattle Plague, Tubercle (Scrofula) With An Appendix on the Inspection of Live Animals and Meat*. MacLachlan and Stewart, Edinburgh.

Walley, T. (1889) Pleuro-pneumonia. Proceedings of the Royal Scottish Veterinary Society. *The Veterinarian* 62, 812–825.

Walley, T. (1888) Animal tuberculosis in relation to consumption in man. In: Craig, W. (ed.) *The Transactions of the Medico-Chirurgical Society of Edinburgh: Session 1887–88*. Oliver and Boyd, Edinburgh, pp. 110–153.

Williams, A. (1874) Copy of order from the veterinary department of the privy council. In: *Minutes Book of the Executive Committee of the Justices of the Peace of the County of Surrey*. Surrey History Centre, Woking.

Williams, C. (1876) *Statement of Work Done by the 5 Travelling Inspectors of the Privy Council Veterinary Department*. Veterinary Department of the Privy Council, London.

Williams, W. (1893) *The Principles and Practice of Veterinary Medicine*. William R. Jenkins, New York.

Windsor, R. (n.d.) Personal communication to Robin Nicholas regarding the costs of CBPP eradication efforts.

Worboys, M. (1991) Germ theories of disease and British veterinary medicine, 1860–1890. *Medical History* 35(3), 308–327.

4 Going Westwards: The Arrival of CBPP in the USA

Abstract

Beginning in the mid-19th century with the first documented instances of arrival of contagious bovine pleuropneumonia (CBPP) in the USA, this chapter explores how CBPP spread to multiple locales along the eastern seaboard of North America. The USA's initial decades of grappling with the disease included a noteworthy watershed outbreak event (1859–1860), initially affecting herds in the state of Massachusetts; the outbreak was attributed to the importation of a small number of cattle from Holland, illustrating the contagiousness of the disease. The Massachusetts outbreak spread to other states, prompting a series of state-by-state regulatory actions and, ultimately, measured federal-government intervention. Meanwhile, important collaborations emerged as American livestock raisers, veterinarians, microbiologists and regulators learned from the scientific and policy responses of Great Britain and continental Europe. As the spread of CBPP sparked alarm and anxiety in the USA, these agriculturalists and professionals embarked on disease-management and regulatory schemes that aimed at ensuring the continued export of American cattle, an important economic priority for the rapidly expanding country. These schemes ultimately helped achieve in 1892 the eradication of CBPP from American shores.

Introduction

James Law (Fig. 4.1), a Scottish veterinarian who, in 1868, emigrated to New York to become the first veterinary professor in the USA (Warwick and Macdonald, 2003, p. 380), authored, in 1879, a self-published book, *The Lung Plague of Cattle, Contagious Pleuro-Pneumonia*. Law's treatise sketched out some of the epidemiological history of CBPP in the USA (Law, 1879, p. 14). This was not the first time that Professor Law had sounded the alarm regarding the presence of this disease in the USA. Two years earlier, in an extract cited by both the US President Rutherford B. Hayes and the US Commissioner of Agriculture, William G. Le Duc, Law had asserted the presence of 'lung fever' in herds in the US states of New York, New Jersey, Pennsylvania, Maryland, Delaware and Virginia, as well as the environs in and around Washington DC. Law lamented what he viewed as complacency regarding the disease, adding a warning in colourful, metaphorical terms: 'At present it creates little apprehension, but we are asleep over a smouldering volcano, which only wants a little more time to gather strength, when the general infection of the country will be imminent' (Le Duc, 1878, p. 144). Law was but one of many US-based veterinarians who, during the second half of the 19th century, slowly but surely came to grips with the reality of the lung plague's presence in the USA.

'Clearly Contagious': Emerging Scientific Understanding and Regulatory Response

Law's views on CBPP were largely influenced by the concerns voiced by his long-time mentor, Dr John Gamgee, from whom Law had learned much in both Edinburgh and London. As one historian would later put it, 'As Gamgee's disciple, Law [would eventually become] America's leading livestock sanitarian, and his comprehension of the causes of disease... was the fountainhead from which the scientific eradication of diseases of animals in the United States' would eventually come (Eby, 1959, p. 48). Gamgee's and Law's collaborations dated back to as early as 1857 when the two of them superintended over half of the lectures and anatomical demonstrations for Gamgee's newly founded veterinary college (Macdonald and

DOI: 10.1079/9781800627536.0004

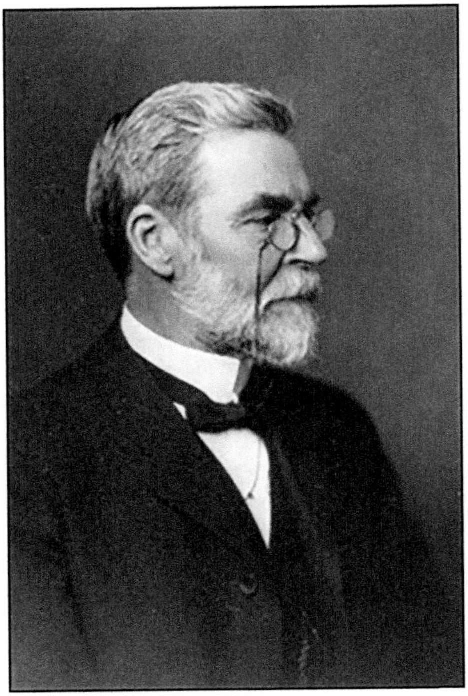

Fig. 4.1. James Law, born and educated in Scotland, was the first veterinary professor in the USA, helping to found Cornell University's veterinary college in Ithaca, New York. He devoted much of his career to highlighting the presence of CBPP in the USA. (From Anonymous, c. 1890, public domain via Wikimedia Commons.)

Warwick, 2023, pp. 50–52), and in 1861 the two veterinarians co-authored a book (Gamgee and Law, 1861), which was noted for being a substantial work consisting of two volumes and several illustrations (Thompson, 1974, p. 102). The illustrations include drawings from Law and Gamgee as well as such pre-eminent scientists as Rudolf Virchow (1821–1902), the founder of cellular pathology (Meachen, 1936, p. 11).

The year 1861 was still 15 years short of Robert Koch's establishment of the germ theory of disease, and Gamgee and Law asserted that '[a] sound knowledge of General and Descriptive Anatomy is required, to be proficient in Pathological Science' (Gamgee and Law, 1861, p. ix). At the same time, Gamgee seems to be an early adopter of the view that CBPP was indeed *contagious*. In fact, as early as 1864, Gamgee made the distinction between 'sporadic pleuro-pneumonia' and 'contagious pleuro-pneumonia in cattle', and pointed to its spread between countries as evidence of this reality: 'The outbreak of pleuro-pneumonia in different countries beyond the centres of spontaneous origin...is wholly due to contagion, and the contagious nature of this virulent malady is incontestably proved by an overwhelming amount of evidence' (Gamgee, 1864, pp. 595–596).

One of Gamgee's most persuasive pieces of evidence for a kind of CBPP contagion theory included 'the recent importation of pleuro-pneumonia into the United States from Holland' (Gamgee, 1864, p. 596), which had taken place 5 years earlier, on 23 May 1859, in the state of Massachusetts (Butterfield, 1860, p. 7). Gamgee referred to a US report that the disease could be traceable to one of two, or three, possible sources, all of which were ultimately connected to four milk cows imported from Holland by a well-known agriculturalist, Winthrop W. Chenery, who brought the cows to his dairy farm in the town of Belmont, on the outskirts of Boston (Butterfield, 1860, p. 7). In public testimony for the legislature of a neighbouring state (Connecticut), a Massachusetts commissioner (one of several appointed to investigate the disease and stop its spread) offered a detailed account of the recent events:

> [T]his disease was imported into the country [last year, in 1859] by Mr. [Winthrop W.] Chenery, of Boston, from Holland...Mr. Chenery imported several animals from Holland, which, on their arrival here, were found to be in a very bad condition, but this was supposed to be the result of the treatment they had received while on their way from Holland to this country—indeed, such was their miserable condition that one of them was conveyed home on a truck, being so much reduced that it was unable to go without aid. This matter, however, occasioned no alarm for some time. But in the month of June, 1859, Mr. Chenery sold three calves which had been kept with the stock he had imported—half Dutch, half Ayreshire. Mr. Chenery at that time had not the slightest idea that his herd contained the disease. They were brought by a Mr. Stoddard to North Brookfield, and in the month of October [1859] one of these calves was taken very sick....Very soon the herd...was taken sick, but this fact created no sensation for a time, until the month of January [1860], and then few people knew anything about it; but in the month of February [1860], the public

began to be alarmed, for it was found that the cattle belonging to a Mr. Neeham, at whose stable these diseased cattle had been put up, were attacked in the same way as the others had been. The cattle of another neighbor, Mr. Woodruff, were taken in the same manner, and began to die. A Mr. Oldstead, who had purchased some of the infected cattle, began to lose his stock, as did his neighbors in the month of January. All these facts taught the people that the disease was contagious, and that it was a dangerous one.' (Connecticut Legislature, 1860, p. 3)

Contemporary reports (for example, see Fig. 4.2, this volume) illustrate detailed, local-community awareness of CBPP's spread in the towns of Massachusetts.

While there were indeed previous introductions of CBPP into the USA (as explained later in this chapter, as early as 1843) (Gamgee, 1871, p. 12), Chenery's importation of the implicated Dutch cattle and the ensuing events of 1859–1860 in Massachusetts and New England mark the most substantial awareness and response. In fact, the 1859–1860 events prompted many of the first instances of actual biosecurity legislation in the USA. As indicated above, the neighbouring state of Connecticut was concerned about the CBPP situation in Massachusetts, with its governor, William Buckingham, on 2 May 1860 calling 'attention to the cattle-disease in Massachusetts' (Vincent, 1860).

The Massachusetts commissioners appointed to investigate the disease especially recognized the gravity of CBPP's spiralling spread from Chenery's originally imported Dutch cattle and, therefore, on 18 May 1860 urged an extra special session of the Massachusetts legislature. Illustrating the simultaneous nature of unrelated events in a dynamic period of US westward expansion, that same day and 1000 miles west of Boston, a restless politician named Abraham Lincoln awaited the outcome of his unlikely bid for the Republican Party's nomination as its candidate for president. During the morning of 18 May, Lincoln was running various errands, going to and from his law office and various stately buildings, and, curiously, passing the notable *Chenery* House (5Goodwin, 2006, p. 5). The 130-room hotel, 'at the time the finest in the entire state' (Lowe, n.d.), was owned by a William Chenery (Abraham Lincoln Presidential Library, 2018), a farmer who had come from Massachusetts a few decades before (Lowe, n.d.). (It is unclear if this Chenery was of relation to the Dutch cattle importer Winthrop W. Chenery of Belmont, Massachusetts, but one wonders.) In a book authored by the veterinary activist George Dadd, Chenery's farm is illustrated as the source of a family-tree-like spread of CBPP (Fig. 4.3).

The Massachusetts commissioners' request for the special session 'was supported by... the State Board of Agriculture...and by many influential and honorable citizens', and the Massachusetts state government's leaders re-assembled 12 days later, on 30 May (9Butterfield, 1860, p. 9). At the noon-time opening of the special session, Governor Nathaniel Banks

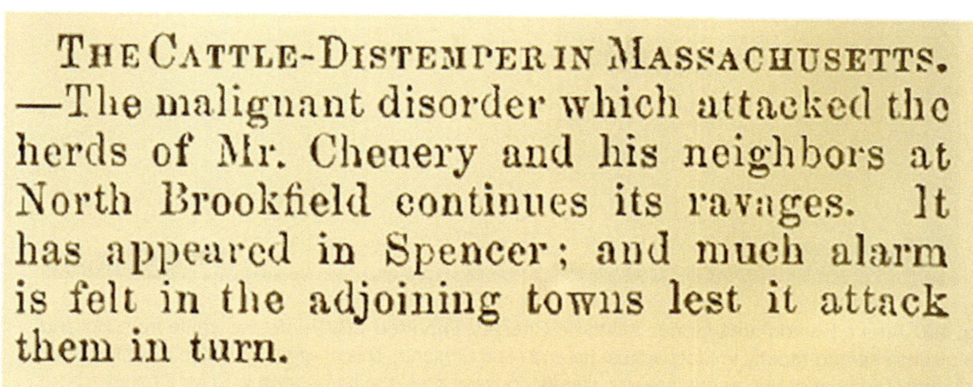

THE CATTLE-DISTEMPER IN MASSACHUSETTS.—The malignant disorder which attacked the herds of Mr. Chenery and his neighbors at North Brookfield continues its ravages. It has appeared in Spencer; and much alarm is felt in the adjoining towns lest it attack them in turn.

Fig. 4.2. A March 1860 account of CBPP spreading to the town of Spencer, Massachusetts. (From Vincent, F. (ed.), 1860, Library of Congress, public domain.)

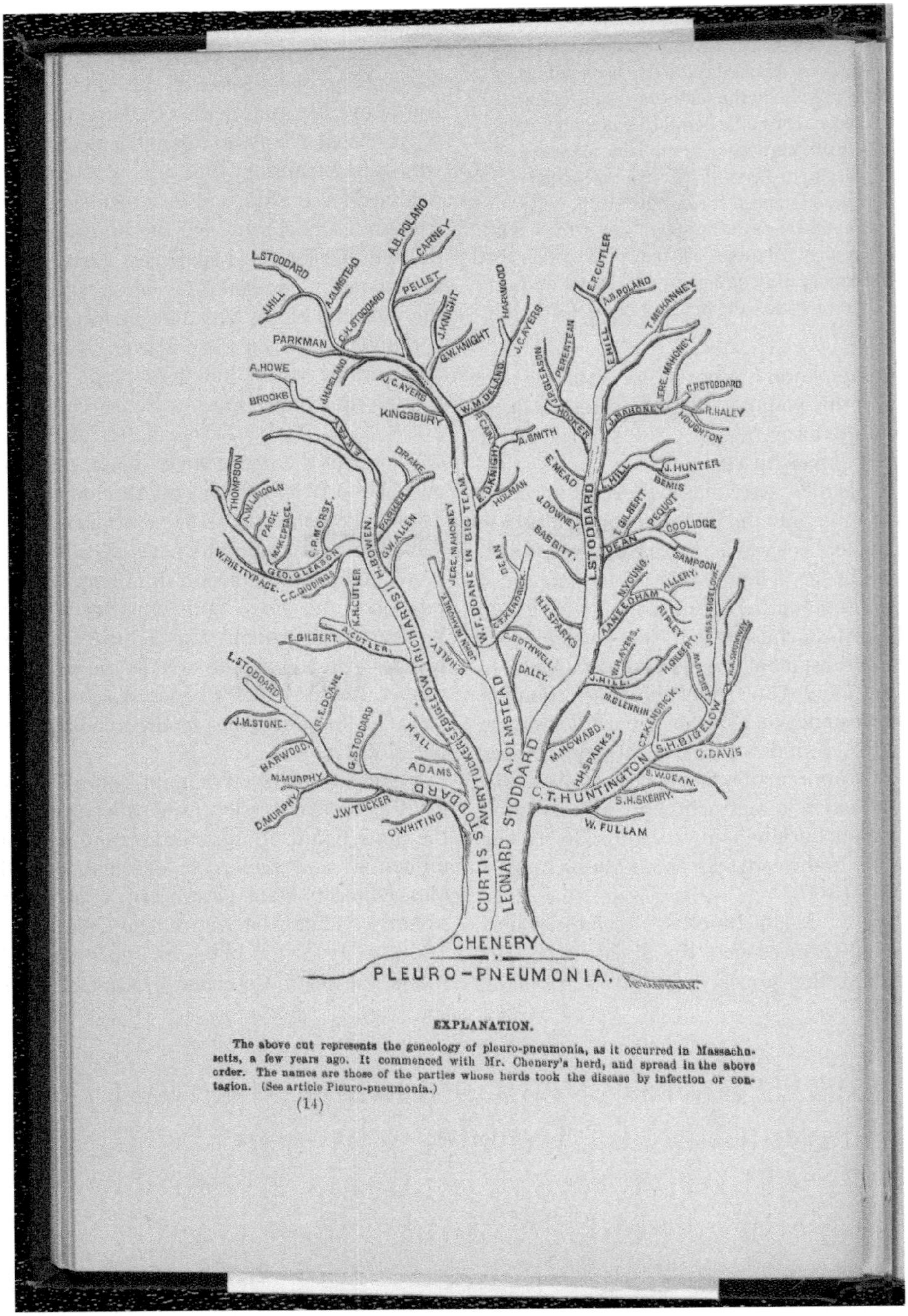

Fig. 4.3. After a Boston-area farmer, Winthrop Chenery, imported CBPP-infected cattle from Holland, the disease spread rapidly in Massachusetts and New England. This engraving, which identifies the sequential farms affected by the disease, clearly conveys how it 'commenced with Mr Cheney's herd'. (From Dadd, G.H., 1869, Orange Judd Company, New York, public domain. Image scan courtesy of the Richard L. D. & Marjorie J. Morse Department of Archives and Special Collections, Kansas State University.)

(a skilled politician who Lincoln would later consider for a cabinet post) emphasized 'the importance of checking the contagion [and] a thorough investigation of the character of the disease', while acknowledging 'that the transit of cattle through the several towns may require additional legislation' (Vincent, 1860, p. 460). Two bills were proposed. The first sought to empower local authorities (including, but not limited to, the mayors of towns) 'to adopt measures, pass and enforce regulations to prevent the spread of any contagious disease among cattle by isolation of suspected herds, and killing diseased animals, when necessary', and to 'regulate or prevent the transit of cattle in and through their respective towns and cities' (Nash, 1860, p. 2). Importantly, a second bill called for the state commissioners to be further empowered to appraise, slaughter and bury diseased cattle, setting aside US$10,000 in state funds for the commissioners to compensate the owners of condemned cattle (one-fifth of the value paid for by the town to which the cattle belonged, and four-fifths paid for by the state) (Nash, 1860, pp. 2–3). Both bills passed, but the US$10,000 in appropriated funds was soon exhausted as 842 animals valued at US$20,432.82 were slaughtered. To help sustain the disease response, private citizens raised an additional US$20,000 for the effort (Gamgee, 1871, p. 13). A detailed breakdown of the 842 pre-emptively slaughtered animals later appeared in an extracted summary of agriculture data originally gathered for the 1860 US Census; Table 4.1 presents these statistics, along with an approximate number (500) of cattle that naturally died from the disease.

The deaths and pre-emptive slaughter of hundreds of infected animals in Massachusetts contributed to American scientific understandings of the disease and a crude refinement of the disease's epidemiology. The officially designated commissioners involved in the Massachusetts disease-control response were assisted by bona fide medically skilled personnel – notably, Drs E.F. Thayer (a veterinary surgeon) and George Bates (a physician) – and their testimonies featured a characterization of the disease, including a detailed list of the signs and symptoms that they witnessed (see Table 4.2). Other interested agriculturalists, including members of the New York State Agricultural Society, held hearings in which they marvelled at the profound challenges of diagnosing CBPP, a disease with an unclear period of incubation (see Table 4.3).

One of the more medically qualified Massachusetts commissioners, physician George B. Loring, provided testimony on both the pathology and the risk of transmission. His insights included a colourful description of the infected lungs:

> Dr. Loring, of Salem, one of the commissioners, said that that he had known of no cattle being killed that were getting better; so far as external appearances were concerned, some were getting better; one ox killed had imparted the disease to twenty-three yoke of cattle; he looked well when he was killed, apparently in good condition for beef, but had a slightly 'pinched' appearance: he was killed because it was known he had been exposed, and believed that he had imparted the disease to the others; the general appearance of the lungs was that of fair health; in the left lung was found a bunch about the size of a fowl's gizzard, and of the same color; it resembled decayed cheese, and was a little harder...
> (Vincent, 1860, p. 488)

Referring to a unit of measure ('rod') equivalent to 16.5 ft, Dr Loring also explained that while 'Mr Chenery's herd has been very much isolated', CBPP had 'been carried two or three rods in the air, with the wind blowing', adding that 'he would be willing to have cattle

Table 4.1. CBPP-related deaths in Massachusetts during the 1859–1860 outbreak. (From Kennedy, 1864.)

Disease Status	Number of Cattle
Casualties of CBPP (not pre-emptively slaughtered, and found to be diseased)	~500
Pre-emptively slaughtered and found to be healthy ('exposed to contagion... killed...on post-mortem examination found to be sound')	657
Pre-emptively slaughtered and found to be infected ('killed [and] proved to be diseased')	185

Table 4.2. Distinctives for the diagnosis of contagious bovine pleuropneumonia (CBPP), elaborated by Drs E.F. Thayer and George Bates in 1860. (From Butterfield, 1860, pp. 9–11)

Pre-mortem Signs and Symptoms	Post-mortem Pathology
Separation from the herd	Lungs showing red hepatization, dark spots, and effusion of serum
Arched back	Rupture or distension of capillaries
Refusal to eat in the morning, improved health during the day	Increased weight and solidity of the lungs
Initial slight, husky cough	Blocking of air-cells, vessels, etc. in the lungs
Diminished milk production	Collections of pus and other morbid products
With disease progression, more frequent and more husky cough, increasingly laborious	
Humid respiration	
Diminished appetite, suspension of rumination	
Constipation	
Cold body surface and limbs	
Rigidity of skin over the ribs	
Flinching upon pressure being applied to the spine	
Discomfort upon percussion of the sides of the chest and costal regions	
Frequent lying down (when standing, head protruded)	
Frothy saliva	
'Dull or dead sound' or 'crepitating sound or rattle', when percussing the affected side of the animal	

Table 4.3. The challenges of diagnosing CBPP in Massachusetts during June 1860, as explained to the New York State Agricultural Society. (From Johnson, 1860, p. 779.)

Insidious	'*Insidious*, inasmuch as it often creeps upon an animal so stealthily that it is difficult and impossible to fix, with any accuracy, the date of the attack.'
Deceptive	'*Deceptive*, in that, in animals which have had the disease, and may be fairly presumed, from appearances, to have recovered, one or both lungs have been found, on slaughtering them, to be little else than a mass of disease.'
Unclear incubation period	'Term of incubation' – 'In some cases the disease is apparent within ten days after exposure; in others, twenty, thirty, sixty, ninety days, or even more, are supposed to elapse. One case is reported where the exposure was seven months previous'.

of his own within half a mile of a diseased herd' (Vincent, 1860, p. 489). As a Harvard-trained physician who was also a state leader in agriculture, Dr Loring was seen as a credible voice in discussions about CBPP. He provided additional scientific commentary regarding CBPP, compared and contrasted it with human respiratory ailments that he had seen as a physician, and demonstrated an impressive knowledge of European CBPP quarantine and isolation strategies. At the time of his testimony, Loring would have likely been mindful of Massachusetts's neighbouring states' anxieties about the disease; a few weeks after his testimony, farmers in northern Connecticut would take decisive action to seize a small number of animals, on the basis of one 'having a slight cough', that had been brought to their town (Vincent, 1860, p. 627) (see Fig. 4.4).

Some 19th-century agriculturalists were sceptical of governmental intervention, whether state-based or national. This is most clearly evidenced by a Chicago-based farming weekly, the *Prairie Farmer*, which emphasized a lack of scientific consensus on the disease's contagiousness. One of its correspondents, covering the Massachusetts legislature's special session, reported: 'It is...asserted that it is contagious; and with equal confidence that it is not contagious! How do doctors disagree!' (Anonymous, 1860a, p. 340).

Such sarcastic comments admittedly reveal some popular resistance to governmental intervention; however, the report is likely more telling of the practical realities of the then still-maturing scientific understanding of CBPP. The *Prairie Farmer* would go on to be one of the most important publishing voices for an important American agriculture lobbying group – the 'Patrons of Husbandry', also known as the national Grange (Hurt, 1994) – yet still encouraged its constituents to 'have a care about their purchases' in light of the advice of 'some of the older English Veterinarians' warning of CBPP's contagiousness (Anonymous, 1860a, p. 340).

In the end, the intentional effort by the state of Massachusetts to financially indemnify livestock owners for their condemned animals was celebrated by many as a costly but prudent approach in light of the strategy's success in disease containment in continental Europe. Writers for the *North British Agriculturalist* noted that by slaughtering all animals labouring under the disease, and indemnifying their owners in whole or in part...certain States, as Belgium ...[have] almost wholly eradicated pleuropneumonia (North British Agriculturalist, 1860, p. 214). According to a US Census report, the Massachusetts disease-response approach included marking sick, suspect, and exposed animals with a 'P' brand: 'All cattle that are diseased or have been exposed to the infection,

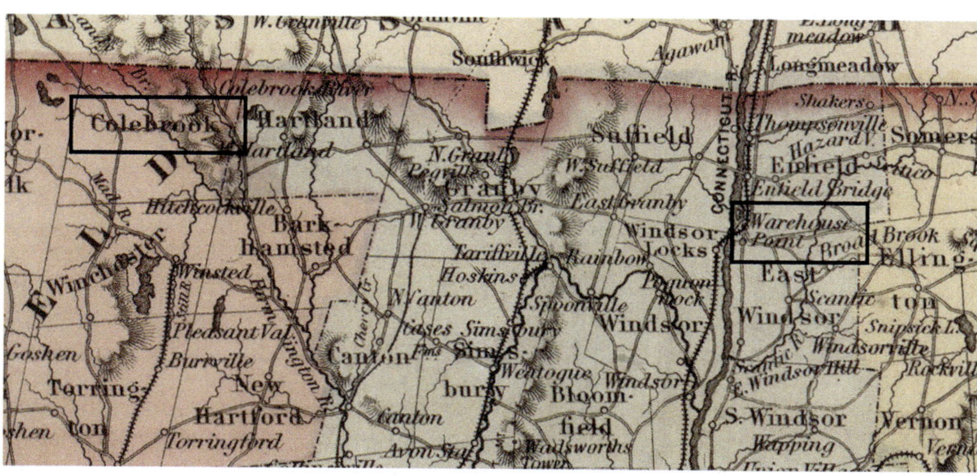

Fig. 4.4. Northern Connecticut agriculturalists (situated close to Massachusetts, the origin of the 1859–1860 outbreak) were wary of potentially diseased animals infecting their herds. In June 1860, one 'Mr Abiel Pease, of Warehouse Point [right], drove a pair of cattle (healthy, but one of the animals having a slight cough) over the river to find pasturage; and...he kept on west till he reached Colebrook [left], where the people seized the cattle and compelled their immediate return' (627Vincent, 1860, p. 627). (From J.H. Colton & Co, and Millard Fillmore, 1859, Library of Congress, public domain.)

to be marked on the rump with the letter P; and no animal so branded shall be sold or disposed of without the consent of the authorities' (Kennedy, 1864).

Key advocates of this approach included, of course, Dr George Loring and the other Massachusetts commissioners. In the coming decades, Loring would go on to serve as the US Commissioner of Agriculture and eventually be eulogized in *The New York Times* for 'his efforts... in 1860 [by which] the spread of pleuro-pneumonia in New-England was checked' (Anonymous, 1891, p. 5). Eventually, other US officials would recognize that the US would have to adopt the same CBPP approach as that adopted by European governments – 'many of them have found it necessary to expend millions of dollars in its suppression' (Bierer, 2019, p. 68). However, progress in the US effort would prove slow, in part because of the country being a *union* of individual *states*.

National Action Needed: Initial, State-by-State Action

While the Massachusetts regulatory response was largely successful, it was clear that, in the US, *national* (not merely individual state) action would be essential for CBPP control, as at least two states expressed concern about the situation. On 31 May 1860, just one day after the Massachusetts legislature convened its special session, the state of New Jersey reported a case of CBPP 'in the neighborhood of Newark', with authorities reporting four out of seven cattle dying and post-mortem exams showing 'the disease to be the same as that in Massachusetts' (Vincent, 1860, p. 465). Concerns continued to be expressed in neighbouring Connecticut (Connecticut Legislature, 1860), and that state's cattle commissioners 'caused notices to be posted in every Connecticut town on the Massachusetts line, east of the Connecticut River, forbidding the driving or bringing into the State from Massachusetts, sick or well, on penalty of five hundred dollars fine and six months' imprisonment' (Vincent, 1860, p. 627). On Wednesday, 6 June, the New Hampshire house of representatives appointed 'a committee to consider what legislation is necessary to prevent the spread of the cattle-disease' (Vincent, 1860, p. 508), and that same month local authorities (so-called selectmen) in Bellow's Falls, Vermont, enacted their own embargo of sorts, disseminating 'posters forbidding the driving or carrying of cattle across the State line in that town' (Vincent, 1860, p. 628). In the previously cited hearings of the New York State Agricultural Society, similar sentiment had been expressed: 'The cattle disease prevailing in Massachusetts has excited much interest in our own State' (Johnson, 1860, p. 777). In July 1860, *Scientific American* reported CBPP-related deaths of two oxen in New York's central park (Anonymous, 1860b).

Revealing growing conviction for the need for inter-state (i.e. national) regulation, cattle commissioners or veterinary surgeons from at least six states (New York, Connecticut, Rhode Island, Ohio, Kentucky and Illinois) paid visits to Massachusetts to investigate the matter (Johnson, 1860, pp. 781–782). With forward thinking, both chambers of the Massachusetts legislature adopted a joint resolution calling for truly federal (national) regulatory action: 'That our senators and representatives in Congress be requested to use their influence to procure the passage of such quarantine laws as shall prevent the importation into this country of animals affected with any contagious or infectious disease, and of laws to extirpate the disease called pleuro-pneumonia now existing in this country' (Banks and Warner, 1860, p. 1).

The Massachusetts legislature's call for congressional action was met with mixed results. On 18 June 1860, the US House of Representatives Committee on Agriculture acknowledged CBPP was 'already of sufficient importance to receive the attention of the legislatures of several States [including] that of Massachusetts' (Butterfield, 1860, p. 1). The committee applauded Massachusetts's and the other states' 'praiseworthy exertions to restrain its ravages, and, if possible, to extirpate it', while expressing worry that CBPP 'may sweep over the entire country, unless timely precautions are taken to arrest its progress' (Butterfield, 1860, p. 1) . However, contrary to the wishes expressed by the original Massachusetts resolution, the House Committee on Agriculture was reluctant to recommend any federal action. 'The committee do not as yet feel authorized to advise legislation on the part of the government', they reported, adding, 'Some believe that the disease is less terrible than has been represented' (Butterfield, 1860, p. 3). Nevertheless, the House Committee adopted two important resolutions, one urging the US Secretary of State to reach out to US diplomats in Europe to ascertain from those CBPP-infected countries 'what sanitary measures have been adopted, and with what success' and another encouraging the US Secretary of the Interior to gather statistics on the prevalence of the disease and report such data back to the House (Butterfield, 1860, p. 13).

The next year, 1861, featured the start of the US Civil War, and American accounts of CBPP decreased in number. Nevertheless, 1862 did witness the establishment of a department of agriculture by America's wartime President, Abraham Lincoln. President Lincoln appointed Isaac Newton, the agriculturalist, as the nation's first commissioner of agriculture (Hurt, 1994). While not a truly cabinet-level department, the new federal agency took on important *national* work in the area of animal diseases and, for the remainder of the decade, annual reports by commissioner Newton and his successors would make mention of CBPP. Having a federal agriculture department seems to have advanced a more comprehensive approach to managing such threats as animal diseases. Commissioner Newton's first such report, for the year 1862, included a section authored by an Illinois-based reporter familiar with the western cattle sector. The report explained that the original Massachusetts outbreak of 1859–1860 had caught his state's attention, prompting the governor to convince all 'railroad, canal, and steamboat lines [to] prohibit the introduction of all cattle from the east' (Corbett, 1863, p. 335). This temporary embargo, the report explained, was soon lifted after the New England outbreaks came under control. The 1862 report revealed how the American west was an integral part of the US livestock and meat trade; the next year's (1863) report included an analysis highlighting the economic importance of being able to move cattle from the west to eastern markets and overseas export (Loomis, 1863). While fewer in number than during 1859–1860, periodic reports of CBPP continued to haunt the New England states, and the Boston Board of Trade called the attention of the Massachusetts legislature to its threat: '[S]hould the disease increase, the commerce of the State cannot but be impaired' (Converse and Sabine, 1864, p. 2).

As the Civil War drew to an end (in 1865), a growing number of animal diseases caught the attention of the department of agriculture. These included CBPP, rinderpest, and the so-called Texas Cattle Fever (bovine babesiosis). In the report for 1864, commissioner Newton mixed troubling news with optimism: 'The pleuro-pneumonia has again shown itself in New England, but strenuous efforts are being made to prevent its spread, which it is hoped will prove successful' (Newton, 1865, p. 5). During the summer and autumn of 1865, reports of the supremely dreaded rinderpest (or cattle plague) in Great Britain excited comparative commentaries, with a government statistician reminding commissioner Newton that it was 'worse than the pleuro-pneumonia' (Dodge, 1866, p. 569). Commissioner Newton added a call for action in his 1865 report: 'The importance of the subject seems to demand the immediate action of Congress, prohibiting the importation of farm-stock during the prevalence of the disease' (Newton, 1866, p. 4). Newton's report, along with diplomatic and news reports of the rinderpest disaster unfolding in Britain, prompted Congress to act; on 18 December 1865, the Congress passed and President Andrew Johnson (who had succeeded Abraham Lincoln, assassinated 8 months earlier) signed into law *An Act to prevent the Spread of foreign Diseases among the Cattle of the United States* that (i) temporarily prohibited any and all cattle imports; and (ii) granted the President powers to resume importation 'when [he] shall give...notice that no further danger is to be apprehended from the spread of foreign infectious or contagious diseases among cattle', allowing cattle to 'be imported in the same way as before its passage' (39th Congress, 1st Session, 1865, p. 2). Three months later, in March 1866, Congress amended the law (39th Congress, 1st Session, 1866) to address perceived risks posed by the importation of cattle hides. Throughout 1866, US diplomats stationed abroad wrote home to the US Secretary of State with reports of how Great Britain, as well as continental European countries (most notably, Belgium, whose response was seen as a successful exemplar), were responding to the rinderpest crisis. As an indicator of an increasing openness to regulatory action to fight animal diseases, one Belgium-based diplomat reported the following:

> The wisdom of radical measures enforced by this government at the outset, for the prevention and eradication of the cattle plague, in causing the immediate slaughter of animals infected by the disease, isolating localities where it appeared, and forbidding the entry or transit of sheep, cattle, hides, &c., has been vindicated by the result. While the disease [rinderpest] has extended to an alarming extent in England and Holland, it has been smothered here [in Belgium]... (Sanford, 1866, pp. 191–92.)

In late 1866, Commissioner Newton reported his satisfaction that Congress had acted to keep rinderpest out, but expressed worry that the US lacked truly national laws to quickly respond to stamp out such a disease if it did nevertheless reach the US (Newton, 1867, p. 8). During the third quarter of the 19th century, US regulatory responses would happen primarily in piecemeal, state-by-state action against animal diseases generally, and CBPP particularly.

For its part, the state of Massachusetts remained vigilant during the 1860s in combatting subsequent outbreaks of CBPP. In December 1866, Dr Thayer and the Massachusetts commissioners were able to cautiously declare 'the *probable* extinction of the disease' from their state, noting that in 1865 'but three herds were found affected with the disease' and that 'no cases of the diseases' had come to their attention during the last year (Thayer *et al.*, 1867, p. 1). However, if Massachusetts was successful in containing CBPP, many other farms and dairies in the region remained beset with the disease. The US government statistician, Jacob Dodge, reported in 1866 a number of CBPP cases and outbreaks across five states – Rhode Island, New York, New Jersey, Pennsylvania and Maryland. Dodge's report was not entirely dire, though, as he cited a department correspondent based in Newport, Rhode Island, describing the semblance of a containment strategy: 'To prevent the spread of the disease, we have kept isolated all cattle known to have been exposed to it until danger of contagion was past, by which means it has been kept within narrow limits' (Dodge, 1867, p. 72). In June 1867, commissioner Newton died, and his successors – first John Stokes (acting commissioner) and then Horace Capron (commissioner beginning in 1868) – continued to convey statistical insights, courtesy of Dodge, on the CBPP situation. For Stokes's and Capron's joint Agriculture Commissioner report for 1867, Dodge cited a Baltimore-based department correspondent who found several stables infected by a disease that was 'probably pleuro-pneumonia' (Dodge, 1868, p. 97); given the attack rates reported by the correspondent, they were most likely right (for this crudely reported data, see Table 4.4).

Thus, by 1867, the US regulatory approach to CBPP and other animal diseases was still in its infancy. While a decent disease-data collection effort was being superintended by the department of agriculture, the meagre federal laws adopted in 1865 and 1866 (to restrict imports of cattle and cattle hides, in response to the rinderpest threat) were generally inconsequential; the laws granted the Secretary of the Treasury the authority to lift the prohibitions on a country-by-country basis (39th Congress, 1st Session, 1865), and the US President retained permission to suspend the entire prohibition (39th Congress, 1st Session, 1866), which was not uncommon. While some states (i.e. Massachusetts) appeared to be competently responding to animal disease threats, other 'younger' states in the American West were less equipped. Kansas, the 34th state to be admitted

Table 4.4. Cases and mortalities from selected stables in Baltimore, Maryland in 1867. (From Dodge, 1868, p. 97.)

County and Stable Designation	Number of Animals in Stable	Number of Mortalities (Mortality Rate)
Baltimore county stable A	14	14 (100%)
Baltimore county stable B	20	20 (100%)
Baltimore county stable C	38	35 (92%)
Baltimore county stable D	70	30 (43%)
All stables	142	99 (70%)

to the union, illustrates this quite well. Faced with the threat of bovine babesiosis (then referred to as splenic fever, Spanish Fever, or, most commonly, Texas Cattle Fever in reference to the Texas longhorn cattle being driven northwards, trampling crops and spreading the mysterious ailment), the Kansas legislature adopted, in February 1865, a law restricting cattle movement into the state (Kansas Legislature, 1865). One year later, this law was repealed (Kansas Legislature, 1866), but in 1867 the legislature adopted a resolution explicitly requesting the US department of agriculture to appropriate funds for a scientific investigation of the perplexing tick-borne protozoan disease (Morton *et al.*, 1867). That resolution, adopted by the legislature of Kansas in January 1867, was followed by a summer in which 'Spanish fever [was] less severe than for many years past' (Dodge, 1868, p. 97); however, the plea for help would eventually catch the attention of Commissioner Capron who, after several additional outbreaks of Texas Fever during the summer of 1868, hired the world-renowned John Gamgee to conduct an investigation of this disease (Capron, 1869, pp. 4–5) . As explained in the next section, Capron's decision to hire Gamgee would ultimately lead to profoundly disturbing insights into not only Texas Fever but also CBPP.

Clarifying the USA's CBPP Situation: Gamgee's Contribution

As previously mentioned, in both Edinburgh and London, the highly influential John Gamgee had served as a colleague and mentor to James Law, the eventual patriarch of US veterinary medicine who would give due attention to the USA's CBPP problems. Gamgee's early career included serving as an anatomy lecturer on the staff at what was initially the sole veterinary school in Edinburgh. The Edinburgh Veterinary College – the antecedent institution to now world-renowned Royal (Dick) School of Veterinary Studies – was established in 1823 through the persistence of the pioneering William Dick and a partnership with the Highland and Agricultural Society of Scotland (Warwick and Macdonald, 2003, p. 380). Dick, who had ascended in Edinburgh society from a family of farriers, diligently laboured to establish his school, eventually negotiating with the Royal College of Veterinary Surgeons (RCVS) to allow its graduates to sit for the RCVS licensing exam alongside those completing studies at the London Veterinary College, where Dick himself earned a diploma following 3 months of study in 1817 (Macdonald and Warwick, 2023, p. 26).

While Gamgee initially lectured at Dick's school, and while Gamgee had met Law there, it seems that Gamgee's prescient insights into contagion theory in general, and CBPP's seriousness in particular, would compel the two to abandon Dick's original Edinburgh Veterinary College. Gamgee views on CBPP were publicly declared as early as 1857, when Gamgee authored a report decrying a range of public health and animal disease matters, including the 'fact that great numbers of the cattle labouring under the fever of pleuropneumonia were slaughtered, and that the meat was sold in [Edinburgh] and other large towns for human food' (Gamgee, 1857, p. 31). Shortly after writing this report, Gamgee and Dick appeared to have a falling out:

> There is...one...occurrence to record as disturbing the even and steady evolution of the Edinburgh veterinary school during the lifetime of the Founder [Dick]. In 1857, John Gamgee, who had been engaged by Dick as his assistant for one year, and whose engagement was not renewed at the end of that time, determined to establish a veterinary school in Edinburgh in opposition to [the Edinburgh Veterinary College]. (Bradley, 1923, p. 42)

Gamgee brought Law with him to his new rival institution, and named it the New Veterinary College, which opened on 4 November 1857 (Macdonald and Warwick, 2023, p. 50). Within 2 years, Gamgee secured royal recognition of his institution, but in 1865 he was persuaded by some enterprising businessmen to move its operations to London (Bradley, 1923, p. 43). There he established the short-lived Albert Veterinary College. Not surprisingly, he brought with him James Law, who was made a professor of Veterinary Anatomy and curator of the Anatomical Museum (Thompson, 1974, p. 106). From this base in London, Gamgee would actively speak out regarding the unfolding rinderpest (Cattle Plague) disaster of 1865–1867; this, in turn, cemented Gamgee's national (see

Chapter 3, this volume) and international reputation as an authority on communicable diseases in animals, including CBPP.

As mentioned previously, the US government hired Gamgee to investigate the issue of Texas Fever. Conducted during the last 2 years of the 1860s, his investigation uncovered the prevalence of both Texas tick fever and CBPP, resulting in a published report on pleuropneumonia. During the 2 years he was in America, Gamgee lectured widely on contagion theory and the still-being-established theory of diseases being transmitted by micro-organisms. Consulted by the leaders of upstate New York's Cornell University, Gamgee also recommended his mentee James Law for a professorship there in 1868 (Anonymous, 2019, p. 74).

Professor Law, distinguished as the first faculty member of veterinary medicine in the USA, would use his influence to highlight the realities that the USA had a major CBPP problem. During the 1870s, Law would frequently cite his mentor's (that is, Gamgee's) published report from 1869 – that CBPP widely prevailed along the eastern seaboard (specifically, in eastern New York, New Jersey, Pennsylvania Maryland, Delaware, Virginia and the District of Columbia) (Gamgee, 1869). As a protégé of Gamgee, Law would have also understood that CBPP had been lurking in the USA for several decades – indeed, since the 1840s (the same decade in which Great Britain was embattled with fresh CBPP incursions from Holland by way of Ireland; see Chapter 3, this volume). This was Gamgee's understanding:

> [During the early 1840s] while the lung disease was ...lighting up in different parts of Ireland, it was committing great ravages in England. All the large towns containing dairy cows suffered... It was in...1843, that English cattle carried the disease into Scotland...*From England and Holland the disease has been propagated far and wide...* (Gamgee, 1871, italics added)

According to Gamgee, the 'far and wide' places to which CBPP was exported included Sweden, Denmark, Germany, Norway and overseas – into both Australia (see Chapter 7, this volume) and, in the year 1843, Brooklyn, New York (Gamgee, 1871, p. 12). James Law, in multiple writings from the mid-1870s onwards, would repeatedly reference and provide additional detail on these and other early introductions of CBPP into America. In 1876 he authored the first edition of his soon-to-be-famous book *The Farmer's Veterinary Adviser*; in it, Law elaborates on Gamgee's insights, repeating again how England and Holland were both sources of infection:

> It invaded Ireland in 1839-40 by Dutch cattle, England in 1842 by Irish and Dutch cattle, Sweden and Denmark in 1847 by English stock, and later again by English and Dutch, Norway in 1860 by infected Ayrshires, Oldenburg in 1858, and Schleswig in 1859, in each case by Ayrshires, the Cape of Good Hope in 1854, Australia in 1858 by an English cow, Brooklyn, L.I. [Long Island, New York], in 1843 by a Dutch cow, and again in 1850 by an English one, New Jersey in 1847 by English stock, and Boston, Mass., by Dutch cattle in 1859. (Law, 1876, p. 14)

Law was writing in 1876 from his veterinary college in upstate New York. While based in Ithaca, he spent much of the 1870s venturing downstate (to today's boroughs of Manhattan and Brooklyn), the very environs where Dutch and English cow imports had first brought the disease to the USA. As he communicated with local veterinarians and dairy farmers, Law likely heard stories about how CBPP had made its way into the USA. At some point, he came to the conclusion (which he later declared in a speech before the New York State Agricultural Society) that CBPP had been 'landed in Brooklyn in 1843...from an English ship' (Law, 1880). Further explanation of what happened comes from scholar Calvin Schwabe, who argues the following:

> [A] dairyman named Peter Dunn from near South Ferry in New York City purchased a cow from the captain of the British ship *S. S. Washington*. Mr. Dunn's herd became infected and, from this focus, pleuropneumonia quickly spread throughout dairy farms in New York City and Brooklyn. (Schwabe, 1984, p. 23)

Interestingly, the 1843 arrival of CBPP may have very well been via a Dutch cow, and an English ship captain was definitely involved. Primary source shipping documents confirm the arrival, on 24 April 1843 into New York, of a *Ship George Washington*, which had sailed from Liverpool (U.S. Bureau of Customs, 1957, pp. 630–631). The master of the ship, A. Burrows, is the likely agent who sold the cow to Mr Dunn (Fig. 4.5).

The purchaser of the cow, Mr Peter Dunn, is said to have been a dairyman. While Schwabe had referred to this person as a dairyman from South Ferry (i.e. the southern port area of lower Manhattan), it seems that in fact the purchaser was from the Brooklyn area (the very area that Law noted as the place of importation). Indeed, a directory for the Williamsburg neighbourhood of Brooklyn indicates the following person, occupation and address in the late 1840s: 'Dunn, Peter, milkman, 54 North 4th' (Payson, 1850, p. 39). Since most shipments into the New York port arrived at south Manhattan, it seems most likely that Dunn met Burrows there, purchased the cow, and then took it back to Williamsburg, which in 1843 was still its own town but in 1855 was incorporated into Brooklyn. The Williamsburg area – and even the street address for Mr Dunn – featured in the 1840s stables, hay and feed vendors, and other agricultural businesses (Bowers, 2025). Perhaps it was here that the Dutch cow (imported from England aboard the *Ship George Washington*, sold by Captain Burrows, and bought by Peter Dunn)

A

B

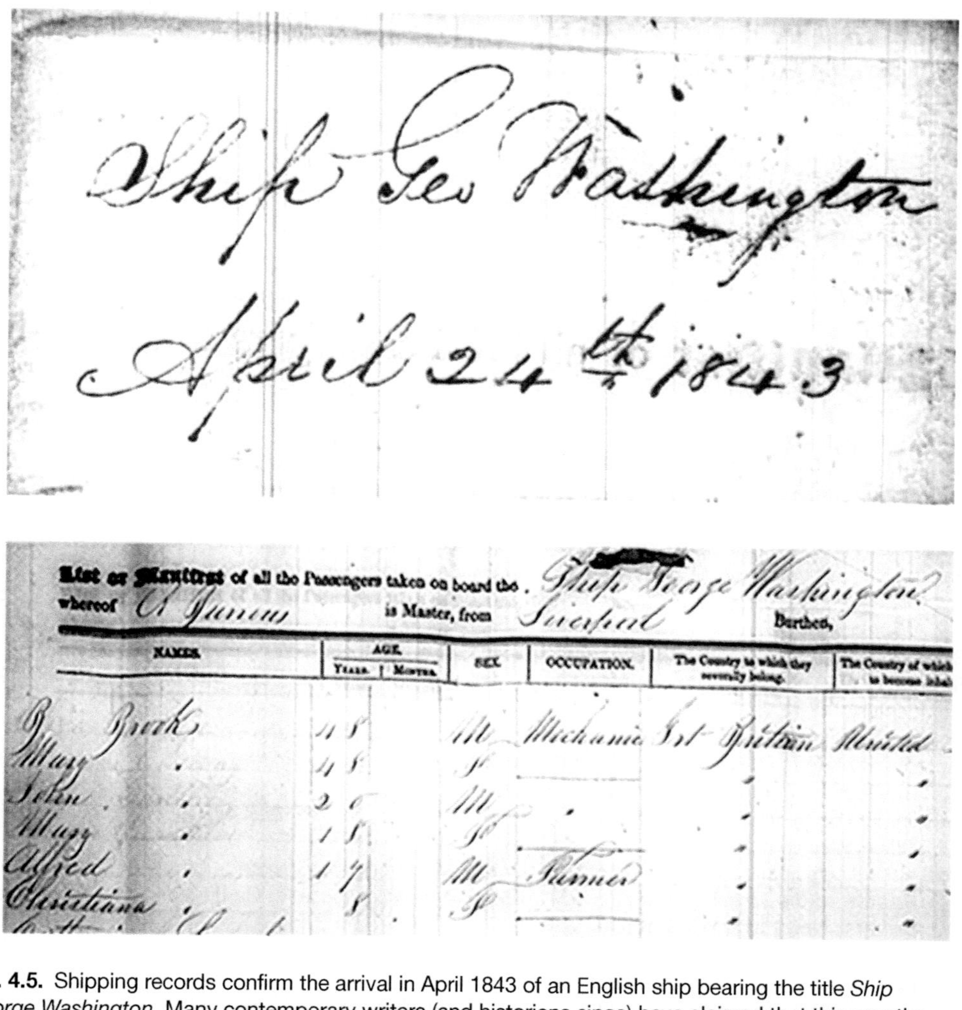

Fig. 4.5. Shipping records confirm the arrival in April 1843 of an English ship bearing the title *Ship George Washington*. Many contemporary writers (and historians since) have claimed that this was the vessel carrying the cow – perhaps originally of Dutch origin – that introduced CBPP into the USA. (From U.S. Bureau of Customs, 1957, National Archives and Records Service, Washington, DC, public domain via Internet Archive.)

came to infect other cattle on Long Island. In any case, within a few decades, the Brooklyn area and Long Island were home to many outbreaks of CBPP. In fact, at the height of a forthcoming trade dispute with Great Britain (see Chapter 5, this volume), these very environs would be investigated and indicted as the culprit for spreading CBPP and tarnishing the US cattle industry's reputation.

Conclusion

As explained in this chapter, the 1840s to 1860s witnessed multiple introductions of CBPP into the USA. These included, but were not limited to, two especially noteworthy importation events (1843 and 1859) that led to the harbouring of CBPP in American herds – especially dairy cattle – on Long Island in New York (specifically in and around Brooklyn), Massachusetts and other New England states. While veterinary leaders such as James Law sounded the alarm, national regulatory action by the US government was slow. However, international trade pressures would soon compel the US department of agriculture to take more serious action and, as Britain and continental Europe were modelling, take decisive action to stamp out the disease. This 'regulatory maturation' took place in the economic context of the US–British live cattle trade, explored in the next chapter.

References

39th Congress (1st Session) (1865) An act to prevent the spread of foreign diseases among the cattle of the United States. *United States Statutes at Large* 14, 1–2.

39th Congress (1st Session) (1866) An act to amend an act entitled "An act to prevent the spread of foreign diseases among the cattle of the united states. *United States Statutes at Large* 14, 3–4.

Abraham Lincoln Presidential Library (2018) *Chenery House*. [Online]. Springfield, Illinois: Abraham Lincoln Presidential Library. Available at: https://papersofabrahamlincoln.org/organizations/CH38598 (accessed 30 June 2024).

Anonymous (1860a) Pleuro-pneumonia epizootic. *Prairie Farmer* 21(22) (31 May), 340.

Anonymous (1860b) Pleuro-pneumonia in cattle. *Scientific American* 3(5) (28 July), 67–68.

Anonymous (1891) George B. Loring (obituary). *The New York Times* 15 September, 5.

Anonymous (2019) Dr. John Gamgee and his mechanically frozen ice rinks. *Veterinary Heritage* 42(2), 74.

Banks, N.P. and Warner, O. (eds) (1860) *House Misc. Doc. 93: Resolutions of the Legislature of Massachusetts, relative to the cattle disease or pleuro- pneumonia*. Government Printing Office, Washington, DC.

Bierer, B.W. (2019) The eradication of contagious pleuro-pneumonia. *Veterinary Heritage* 42(2), 67–72.

Bowers, D. (2025) Personal communication to Justin Kastner regarding Peter Dunn, milkman in the 19th century.

Bradley, O.C. (1923) *History of the Edinburgh Veterinary College*. Oliver and Boyd, Edinburgh.

Butterfield, M. (ed.) (1860) *House Report 651: House Agriculture Committee Report on Cattle Disease*. Government Printing Office, Washington, DC.

Capron, H. (1869) *Report of the Commissioner of Agriculture for the Year 1868*. Government Printing Office, Washington, DC.

Connecticut Legislature (1860) *Report of Testimony Heard by the Joint Standing Committee on Agriculture, Relative to the Disease of Cattle, Now Prevalent in Massachusetts*. Carrington & Hotchkiss (state printers), New Haven, Connecticut.

Converse, J.C. and Sabine, L. (eds) (1864) *Memorial of the Boston Board of Trade (1 March 1864)*. Massachusetts Legislature, Boston, Massachusetts.

Corbett, W.W. (1863) Beef and beef-cattle of the west. In: Newton, I. (ed.) *Report of the Commissioner of Agriculture for the Year 1862*. Government Printing Office, Washington, DC, pp. 326–335.

Dadd, G.H. (1869) *The American Cattle Doctor: A Complete Work of All the Disease of Cattle, Sheep, and Swine, Including Every Disease Particular to America, and Embracing all the Latest Information on the Cattle Plague and Trichina*. Orange Judd Company, New York, 1888 reprint.

Dodge, J.R. (1866) The cattle plague in Europe. In: Newton, I. (ed.) *Report of the Commissioner of Agriculture for the Year 1865*. Government Printing Office, Washington, DC, pp. 550–569.

Dodge, J.R. (1867) Report of the statistician. In: Newton, I. (ed.) *Report of the Commissioner of Agriculture for the Year 1866*. Government Printing Office, Washington, DC, pp. 51–96.

Dodge, J.R. (1868) Report of the statistician. In: Stokes, J. and Capron, H. (eds) *Report of the Commissioner of Agriculture for the Year 1867*. Government Printing Office, Washington, DC, pp. 77–128.

Eby, C.H. (1959) James Law 1838–1921. In: *Modern Veterinary Practice*. Royal Dick Veterinary College, Edinburgh.

Gamgee, J. (1857) *Diseased Meat Sold in Edinburgh, and Meat Inspection in Connection with The Public Health and with the Interests of Agriculture: A Letter to the Right Hon. The Lord Provost of Edinburgh*. Southerland & Knox, Edinburgh.

Gamgee, J. (1864) *Our Domestic Animals in Health and Disease: Organs of Circulation and Respiration*. MacLachlan & Stewart, Edinburgh.

Gamgee, J. (1869) The lung plague. In: Capron, H. (ed.) *Reports on the Diseases of Cattle in the United States, Made to the Commissioner of Agriculture, with Accompanying Documents*. Government Printing Office, Washington, DC, pp. 7–72.

Gamgee, J. (1871) Report of Professor Gamgee on the lung plague. In: Capron, H. (ed.) *Report of the Commissioner of Agriculture on Diseases of Cattle in the United States*. Government Printing Office, Washington, DC, pp. 3–63.

Goodwin, D.K. (2006) *Team of Rivals: The Political Genius of Abraham Lincoln*. Simon & Schuster, New York.

Gamgee, J. and Law, J. (1861) *General and Descriptive Anatomy of the Domestic Animals*. Thomas C. Jack, Edinburgh.

Hurt, D. (1994) *American Agriculture: A Brief History*. Iowa State University Press, Ames, Iowa.

Johnson, B.P. (1860) Cattle disease in Massachusetts. *Transactions of the New York State Agricultural Society* 777–785.

Kansas Legislature (1865) An act to prevent the bringing of stock into the State from the State of Texas, or territory south of the southern line of this State, and to seize and condemn the same when brought into the State (approved February 11). In: Barker, R.A. (ed.) *The Laws of the State of Kansas*. S.D. Macdonald & Co, Topeka, Kansas, pp. 159–160.

Kansas Legislature (1866) An act to repeal an act entitled ‘An act to prevent the bringing of stock into the State, from the State of Texas, or territory south of the southern line of this State, and to seize and condemn the same, when brought into the State’ (approved February 16). In: Barker, R.A. (ed.) *The Laws of the State of Kansas*. Speer & Ross, Lawrence, Kansas, p. 248.

Kennedy, J.C.G. (ed.) (1864) *Agriculture of the United States in 1860; Compiled from the Original Returns of the Eighth Census*. Government Printing Office, Washington, DC.

Law, J. (1876) *The Farmer's Veterinary Adviser: A Guide to the Prevention and Treatment of Disease in Domestic Animals*. Published by the author, New York.

Law, J. (1879) *The Lung Plague of Cattle, Contagious Pleuro-Pneumonia*. published by the author, Ithaca, New York.

Law, J. (1880) The lung plague – our danger and the remedy: Address of 21 January 1880. *Transactions of the New York State Agricultural Society* 33, 130–141.

Le Duc, W.G. (1878) *Report of the Commissioner of Agriculture*. Government Printing Office, Washington, DC, pp. 1–149.

Loomis, S. (1863) Distribution and movement of neat cattle in the United States. In: Newton, I. (ed.) *Report of the Commissioner of Agriculture for the Year 1863*. Government Printing Office, Washington, DC, pp. 248–264.

Lowe, J. (n.d.) *Posting about Chenery House* [online]. Ancestry.com, Lehi, Utah. Available at: https://sites.rootsweb.com/~ilmaga/newspapers/cheneryhouse.html (accessed 30 June 2024).

Macdonald, A.A. and Warwick, C.M. (2023) *The History of Veterinary Education in Edinburgh*. Edinburgh University Press, Edinburgh.

Meachen, G.N. (1936) *A Short History of Tuberculosis*. John Bale, Sons & Danielsson Ltd, London.

Morton, J., Banks, A. and Barker, R.A. (eds) (1867) *Senate Misc.15: Resolution of the Legislature of Kansas in Favor of an Appropriation to Enable the Department of Agriculture to Make a Scientific*

Investigation of the Disease among the Cattle of that and Adjoining States Commonly Known as 'Spanish Fever.' Government Printing Office, Washington, DC.

Nash, H. (ed.) (1860) *Extra Session: Commonwealth of Massachusetts*. Massachusetts Legislature, Boston, Massachusetts.

Newton, I. (1865) *Report of the Commissioner of Agriculture for the Year 1864*. Government Printing Office, Washington, DC.

Newton, I. (1866) *Report of the Commissioner of Agriculture for the Year 1865*. Government Printing Office, Washington, DC.

Newton, I. (1867) *Report of the Commissioner of Agriculture for the Year 1866*. Government Printing Office, Washington, DC.

North British Agriculturalist (1860) Pleuro-pneumonia. *Edinburgh Veterinary Review and Annals of Comparative Pathology* 2(6), 214–216.

Payson, H. (1850) *Williamsburgh Directory, Register, and Yearly Advertiser for 1849–1850*. L. Darbee & Son, Brooklyn, New York.

Sanford, H.J. (1866) Document 63: Mr. Sanford to Mr. Seward, February 5, 1866. In: U.S. Department of State Office of the Historian (ed.) *Papers Relating to Foreign Affairs, Accompanying the Annual Message of the President to the Second Session of the Thirty-Ninth Congress (1866, Part II)*, 2018 reprinted ed. U.S. Government Printing Office, Washington, DC, pp. 191–192.

Schwabe, C. (1984) *Veterinary Medicine and Human Health*, 3rd edition. Williams & Wilkins, Baltimore. Maryland.

Thayer, E.F., Preston, C.P. and Lincoln, F.D. (1867) *Report of the commissioners on contagious diseases among cattle*. Massachusetts Legislature, Boston, Massachusetts.

Thompson, R.D.A. (1974) *The Remarkable Gamgees: A Story of Achievement*. The Ramsay Head Press, Edinburgh.

U.S. Bureau of Customs. (1957) Reel 0051 – Passenger lists of vessels arriving at New York October 26, 1842–June 15, 1843. In: *Passenger Lists of Vessels Arriving at New York, 1820–1897 [Microform]*. National Archives and Records Service, Washington, DC.

Vincent, F. (ed.) (1860) *Vincent's Semi-Annual United States Register*. Published by the author, Philadelphia, Pennsylvania.

Warwick, C.M. and Macdonald, A.A. (2003) The New Veterinary College, Edinburgh, 1873 to 1904. *The Veterinary Record* 153(13), 380–386.

5 CBPP or Not CBPP? Trade Dispute between GB and USA

Abstract

During the second half of the 19th century, and with ever-increasing growth of US livestock and meat exports to Europe generally, and Great Britain specifically, veterinary regulators raised concerns about the transatlantic transmission of diseases including contagious bovine pleuropneumonia (CBPP). Indeed, by the 1850s and 1860s, CBPP was prevalent in along the US Eastern Seaboard. Particularly among dairy herds in such locales as Long Island, New York, the presence of CBPP posed a threat to commerce. While initially reluctant (and even argumentative, contesting British veterinarians' diagnoses of CBPP in American cattle landed at the port of Liverpool), the US government eventually accepted the need for better disease surveillance and control. After an intense trade row during 1878–1879, the 1880s and 1890s saw US and British veterinarians engaging in exemplary regulatory cooperation, information sharing and problem - solving. Trade continued, albeit with the restriction of American cattle being subject to immediate slaughter at British ports of entry.

Introduction

As explained in Chapters 3 and 4 (this volume), by the end of the 1850s, there were justifiable concerns about CBPP in both Great Britain and the US. In Britain, the half-decade of 1855–1860 witnessed the suffering or death of 1 million cattle, at a collective cost of £12 million (Fisher, 1980, p. 294). During this same time period, two key events – one in 1858 and one in 1859 – illustrate how the US itself was grappling with the consequences of CBPP. In 1858 in Brooklyn (where, as explained in Chapter 4, this volume, CBPP had been imported as early as 1843), a veterinary surgeon provided the following testimonial to a committee of the New York Board of Health:

> Q. Are you conversant with the disease which they say is among cows, such as has been among the various swill stables in New York and its vicinity? Will you state to the Committee what effect this disease has upon cattle – what occasions it – if you can...
>
> A. We have it at this present time near Fort Hamilton [southwestern area of Brooklyn, on Long Island], which is a pleasant, healthy place...
>
> ...
>
> Q. Is it general?
>
> A. Yes, sir.
>
> Q. In the city and country?
>
> A. Yes, sir.
>
> ...
>
> Q. Is it a local disease?
>
> A. It was brought here...Sometimes we find it in one lobe of the lung and sometimes in both lobes; the ordinary weight of a lung is six or seven pounds; I have seen them weigh twenty-five or thirty pounds—a solid mass. Sometimes there is a pus and a great deal of fluid to be seen.
>
> Q. Does this disease affect oxen, and steers, as well as cows?
>
> A. Yes, sir.
>
> Q. Is it prevalent in the country?
>
> A. That is according to the number of cattle that is kept together. The cows have the same chance to take it in the country as they have here; it is infectious. (New York Board of Health, 1858, pp. 164–165)

While the account above signalled some concerns about CBPP, the next year (1859) brought many more CBPP-related deaths to herds across several New England states. As explained in Chapter 4, this volume, a Dutch shipment of cattle, imported into Massachusetts by Winthrop Chenery, seeded several outbreaks of the disease across many farms in the region.

DOI: 10.1079/9781800627536.0005

In April 1860, one of America's first biosecurity laws was passed, with the Massachusetts state legislature appointing 'three commissioners, with authority to take such action as would, it was hoped, circumscribe and extirpate the disease' (Butterfield, 1860, p. 8).

Ad hoc state-by-state regulatory responses (detailed in Chapter 4, this volume) were not sufficient to control CBPP's spread in the USA. CBPP outbreaks persisted during the 1860s and 1870s, with dairy cattle in Brooklyn posing a stubborn 'hotbed' of disease. Both American and British veterinarians took note of this and nervously braced for a new and frightening phase of CBPP history in the transatlantic trading region. This phase had been anticipated by some, most notably British veterinarian John Gamgee (Fig. 5.1), who had been hired by the US government to investigate other diseases in the American Midwest (see Chapter 4, this volume). In the early 1870s, he authored a damning report on CBPP's prevalence in the USA (Gamgee, 1871), just as he had issued previous warnings in his home country (see Chapter 3, this volume).

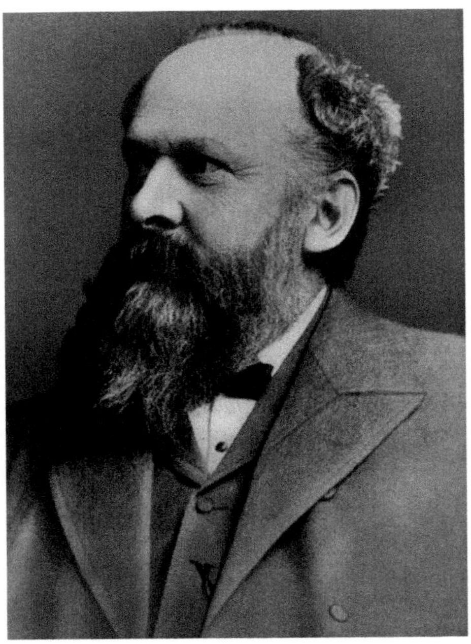

Fig. 5.1. Comments and writings by British veterinarian John Gamgee compelled regulators on both sides of the Atlantic to give attention to CBPP's presence in the USA. (From unknown, n.d., public domain.)

Gamgee's warnings, while reiterated by the likes of his protégé Dr James Law, were largely ignored in the USA, and CBPP continued to spread. In the growing urban area of New York, where perishable meat and milk were sourced from nearby farms, both beef cattle and dairy cattle were trafficked in ways that were in many ways objectionable. With respect to cattle destined for the beef supply, the Brooklyn Board of Health (BBH) remarked, 'The driving of cattle through the streets...is a greater nuisance than the slaughter-houses themselves' (Brooklyn Board of Health, 1877, p. 31). In addition to such nuisances, dynamics in the dairy sector posed a more serious disease-transmission threat, as suggested by the following account from the BBH:

> In April, 1876, the Board directed the Secretary to have an inspection and enumeration made of the stables in the city where cows were kept for the production of milk for sale, with a view to their more careful supervision and the enforcement of proper sanitary regulations with respect to both cattle and premises...In one of these stables, where 8 cows (several of them stumptails) were kept in a shanty 8 by 16 feet in size and 5 feet high without light or ventilation, with floor and surroundings in an inexpressly filthy condition, and with manure and pigs in heaps in sheds and yards adjoining, immediate orders were issued for the removal of the cattle and filthy and the destruction of the pens. (Brooklyn Board of Health, 1877, p. 33)

The term 'stumptails' in the previous excerpt refers to cattle that had been inoculated against CBPP; while this practice of inoculation was fiercely debated (see Chapters 2 and 3, this volume), the presence of such 'stumptails' confirms that CBPP had remained an omnipresent threat in New York dairy herds.

The account, documented by the BBH in the New York environs in the spring of 1876, took place a year prior to a major international trade shift involving cattle, CBPP, and Great Britain. In 1877, an outbreak of CBPP in continental Europe prompted the British government to significantly restrict – and rethink – its imports. While it had been accustomed to importing live cattle from the continent, it now turned to the US (Zimmerman, 1962, p. 46). However, and as explained below,

Britain would soon discover that this decision carried its own CBPP risks.

Trade Growth and Emerging Diseased Cattle Concerns

The relationship between Great Britain and the USA during the second half of the 19th century featured an ever-increasing growth in trade of agricultural food products. Both wheat and meat exports from the USA to Great Britain dominated this economic reality (Perren, 1978). Westward expansion of the USA brought with it increased agricultural output, which helped meet the economic and culinary needs of consumers in a growing British population. The decade of the 1870s – precisely when Britain turned to US livestock and meat imports – witnessed a robust trade in meat, including US livestock (cattle, sheep, and pigs) imported into Britain for further fattening and subsequent slaughter. Private investors in both countries seized on this profit making opportunity (Rippy, 1955).

In 1875, businessmen associated with the New York Central and Hudson River Railroad (see Fig. 5.2) paid for the construction of a stockyard to accommodate up to 4000 head of cattle. Located between New York City's 60th and 63rd Streets from 11th Avenue to the North River, this facility provided a place where steamships could retrieve American cattle destined for ports overseas in Liverpool and London (Zimmerman, 1962, p. 47). British economic stakeholders, such as the Liverpool Provision Trade Association (LPTA), enthusiastically welcomed US agricultural imports (Thompson, 1980). By the mid-1870s, the LPTA and others viewed

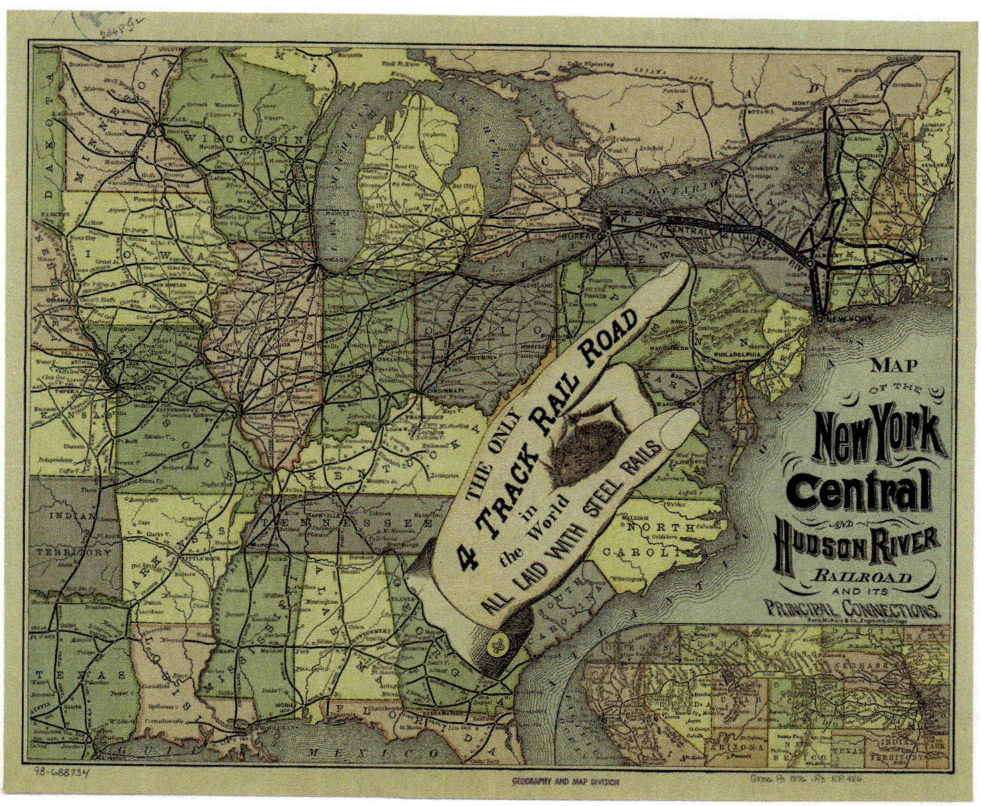

Fig. 5.2. A growing network of US railroads helped facilitate the growth of the cattle export trade to Great Britain. (From Rand McNally and Company, and New York Central and Hudson River Railroad Company, 1876, public domain via Library of Congress.)

with approval growing volumes of processed pork (including canned bacon and ham) as well as brine-preserved beef products. While the dead meat trade was inviting to capitalists, some in Britain were worried about the foreign competition. One Scotland based agricultural writer, James MacDonald, gave voice to this concern in his aptly titled publication of 1878: *Food From the Far West: American Agriculture with Special Reference to the Beef Production and Importation of Dead Meat From America to Great Britain* (MacDonald, 1878). MacDonald's investigation was commissioned by *The Scotsman* newspaper, and he concluded that cheap American meat imports posed a partial threat to the domestic British meat sector:

> [I]n reviewing for the *Scotsman* the perils facing the farmers of that period from the importation of meat, [MacDonald] told his fellow countrymen that the part of the domestic industry producing a high-class article would be free from any harmful effect from overseas supplies but that the inferior domestic product would be subjected to a destructive competition. (McFall, 1927, p. 162)

As it turned out, the rapid growth of the dead meat trade did eventually bring about depressed prices. Those involved in the meat trade saw a solution this new problem by switching to the importation of live animals (termed 'store cattle') from the US; these could be imported for further fattening. Store cattle also offered livestock raisers the ability to wait for optimal market prices (Perren, 1971, pp. 432–433). While it was arguably still less expensive to send dead meat products across the Atlantic in a steamship, they were often perishable and in need of rapid sale. In search of more marketing flexibility, investors perceived that more money could be made in the shipment of live store cattle. This fuelled the development of railroad networks (see Fig. 5.2), as well as portside infrastructure like that mentioned previously, in New York. Across the Atlantic, similar infrastructure improvements appeared in the 1870s – first at Deptford (Anonymous, 1872, p. 9) and later at Birkenhead, near Liverpool. Logistical support for this trade made good business sense, for the export of live animals offered a lucrative alternative to the trade in so-called 'dead meat'.

Due to these economic opportunities, the export of live animals became a new primary objective for many agriculturalists and businessmen on both sides of the Atlantic during the 1870s and 1880s. There was a risk lurking, however. The points of embarkation for these live cattle included such locales as New York (ominously next to CBPP-infected Brooklyn) and other port cities that had cases of CBPP: Boston, Massachusetts; Philadelphia, Pennsylvania; Baltimore, Maryland; and Portland, Maine). From these urban centres, cattle were loaded for their 3-week journey to British ports including, but not limited to, Birkenhead and Liverpool, Bristol, Glasgow, and London and Deptford (see Fig. 5.3) (Zimmerman, 1962, p. 47).

This trade-related risk of CBPP spreading was not entirely ignored by US government officials, who were beginning to conduct crude surveillance for animal diseases of various kinds. British diplomats based in the USA were also becoming concerned about animal diseases that might disrupt the profitable and growing trade (Fig. 5.4). In August 1877, one month after being appointed as the US Commissioner of Agriculture, William G. Le Duc wrote to prominent farmers and veterinary surgeons across the country, requesting information on the existence of animal diseases (Billings, 1879, p. 1). Several responded, and a later report refers to these individuals as 'regular correspondents' for the department of agriculture (Lyman, 1881, p. 582). In March 1878, Commissioner Le Duc was fully engaged with this issue, conferring with not only his veterinary colleagues but also some of the most prominent scientific and regulatory minds in Washington, DC, including the physician John Shaw Billings, founder of the National Library of Medicine (Le Duc, 1878). By the summer and autumn of 1878, Le Duc had good reason to panic about CBPP. One of his correspondents, writing from Virginia, indicated the extent to which CBPP was becoming a problem in both urban and rural areas: 'The principal disease among cattle in this locality is pleuro-pneumonia. The disease started from Georgetown, D.C., 2 years ago, and has gradually spread down the Potomac [River] for a distance of about 25 miles' (Billings, 1879, p. 2).

In late November 1878, New York's *Weekly Tribune* reinforced these types of concerns about CBPP's presence in herds in and around

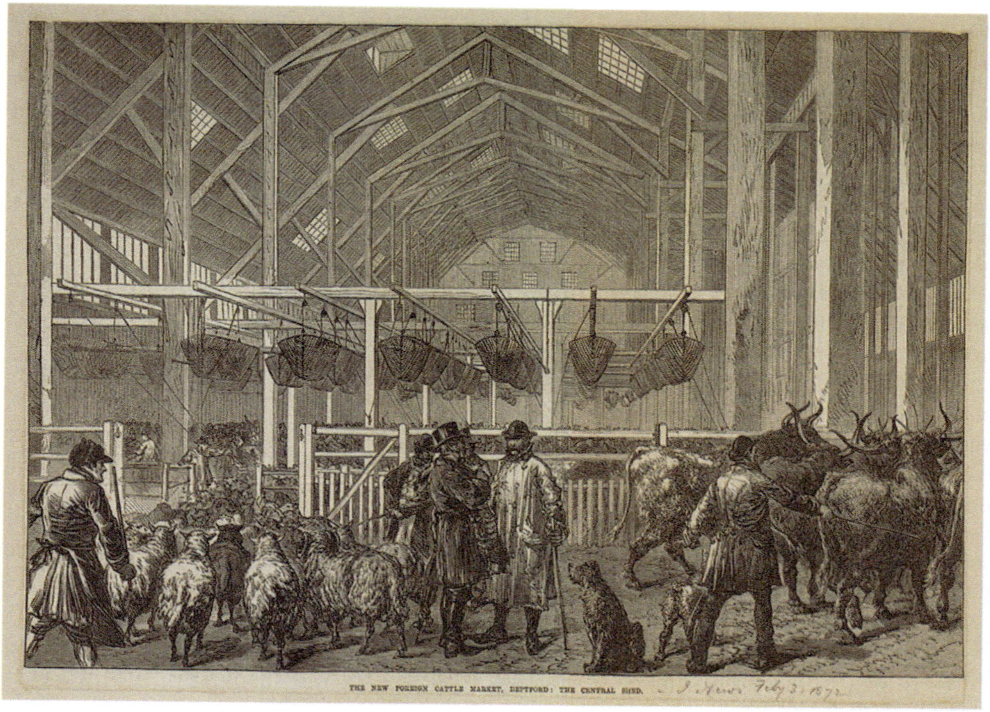

Fig. 5.3. Infrastructure improvements made in Britain in the 1870s would enable the growth of the live cattle trade. (From Anonymous, 1872, *Illustrated London News*, public domain.)

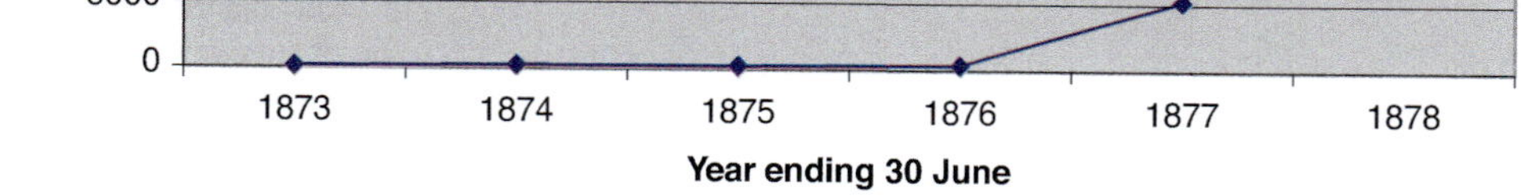

Fig. 5.4. Number of cattle exported from the USA to the UK, from 1 July 1872 to 30 June 1878. (Graph based on tabular data in House of Representatives Committee on Agriculture (ed.) 1880, *House Ex. Doc. 53: Pleuro-pneumonia in Neat Cattle*, Government Printing Office, Washington, DC, p. 7.)

Washington, DC. One British diplomat was keenly paying attention. Sir Edward Mortimer Archibald, the seasoned British consul in New York, asked if the disease might threaten cattle shipped from ports of embarkation in the city. Despite legitimate cause for concern, and in contrast to the prudent attitude of veterinarians like Dr Law, New York political and agricultural leaders (including the secretary of the state's agricultural society) downplayed the concerns, asserting that the *Weekly Tribune*'s reporting was faulty. 'I very much distrust the diagnosis given in that paper', the secretary for the New York Agricultural

Society wrote to Consul Archibald (Great Britain (Parliament), 1879).

While sometimes disputed, such reports of CBPP in the USA called for others across the Atlantic – especially veterinary inspectors working on behalf of the Privy Council – to be vigilant in their work at such ports as Birkenhead and Liverpool. In Britain, a newly adopted Contagious Diseases (Animals) Act of 1878 provided authority for the Veterinary Department of the Privy Council to issue, amongst other regulations, a new Foreign Animals Order (no. 452) that divided foreign livestock into three groups (Table 5.1). This was a newsworthy development that appeared in the press (Anonymous, 1878, p. 11). As indicated in Table 5.1, in late 1878, the USA was still exempt from *both* prohibition (applied to countries with rampant disease endemicity) *and* immediate slaughter (a regulatory tool reserved for countries where diseases like CBPP were common but not necessarily endemic). However, given the recent reports indicating (or at least suggesting) CBPP's presence in New York and Washington, the USA's exemption status was now in peril. In fact, in Liverpool, preparations were made for the likelihood that the USA would eventually become subject to at least the immediate-slaughter rule. It was agreed that port infrastructure improvements would be needed to accommodate large numbers of cattle held for slaughter. Therefore, in November 1878, the British government sanctioned the establishment of an officially designated Foreign Animals Wharf in Birkenhead (across the River Mersey from Liverpool). The wharf featured four sheds capable of holding 1000 head of cattle; a slaughterhouse was added soon thereafter (Perren, 1971, p. 434).

Table 5.1. The regulatory categorization of countries exporting livestock to Great Britain in late 1878 and early 1879, as outlined in Foreign Animals Order no. 452, made under the 1878 Contagious Diseases (Animals) Act. (From McCarron, 1991, pp. 19–21; Anonymous, 1878, p. 11.)

Prohibition of Imports: countries where one or more animal diseases were endemic and, therefore, not allowed to import animals into Britain	**Immediate-slaughter:** countries where disease was more or less common and, therefore, animal imports required to be landed at designated Foreign Animal Wharves where they were to be slaughtered 'immediately', that is, within 10 days	**Permitted, but Inspected:** countries where disease was uncommon or unknown and, therefore, animals were exempt from immediate slaughter but required to be held for 12 hours and inspected by a veterinary inspector of the privy council; if certified as disease-free, the animals permitted inland; if found to be or suspected to be diseased, subject to immediate slaughter and further inspection – in the case of CBPP, lung inspection
Austria-Hungary	Germany	Denmark
Greece	Holland	Norway
Italy	Belgium	Sweden
Montenegro	France	Spain
Romania	Argentina	Portugal
Russia	Uruguay	Canada
The Ottoman Empire		USA
Bosnia and Herzegovina		

Winter 1878–1879: US Cattle Become Subject to Immediate Slaughter

With its own diplomats paying attention to these developments, the US government was anxiously aware that US cattle might lose its privileged exemption. Indeed, on 18 December 1878, an ominous telegram was received by the US Treasury Department, the agency then responsible for the US export trade. The telegram, based on intelligence gathered by US state department officials based in Britain, was clear: 'Unless cattle shipped from United States have government health-certificate when embarked, slaughter probably compulsory on land, paralyzing trade' (Sherman, 1879, p. 4).

Although a number of shipments of American cattle would arrive in a healthy condition, a pivotal event took place on 26 January 1879 with the arrival into Liverpool of a cattle shipment aboard the steamship *Ontario*. The *Ontario*, which had departed Portland, Maine, on 11 January, was technically a Canadian vessel (the shippers being Messrs T. Crawford & Co., of Toronto); while the animals had been originally sourced from the USA, they had been transported through Canada, for they were reportedly 'examined by competent men at both Montreal and Portland' (Billings, 1879, p. 5). On 26 January, 199 cattle, two of which were dead, were landed at the port of Liverpool.

An inspector for the Privy Council examined the lungs of one of the carcasses, and declared it to contain pathological evidence of CBPP. In compliance with the procedure set forth by Foreign Animals Order no. 452 (see Table 5.1), a sample was taken from the supposedly diseased lungs and sent to the Privy Council Veterinary Department in London. In London, pathologists confirmed the diagnosis, and the remainder of the shipment was ordered to be slaughtered, with 12 more post-mortem examinations indicating CBPP. Within weeks, the British authorities changed the US cattle shipments' regulatory status. US cattle would soon be subject to immediate slaughter (that is, within 10 days of importation). For the next two decades, US cattle shipments would remain subject to this rule (Kastner, 2011).

Illustrating a high-stakes situation, both the diagnosis of CBPP and the decision to apply the immediate-slaughter rule were not without controversy. Four days after the *Ontario* arrived at Liverpool, the British Foreign Secretary, Lord Salisbury, announced that on account of detecting CBPP, the British government was now reconsidering its exemption of US cattle from compulsory slaughter (Great Britain (Parliament), 1879). In early February, *The New York Times* used the words 'alarm and anxiety' to describe the situation (Anonymous, 1879a, p. 5) (Fig. 5.5). US regulatory authorities haphazardly elaborated the semblance of an inspection and certification programme (initially administered by the Treasury Department), and Agriculture Commissioner Le Duc sent two of his correspondents to conduct inspection and certification activities at the New York ports and the Chicago stockyards (Sherman, 1879, pp. 6–8). Despite these efforts, the CBPP diagnosis had all but guaranteed that US cattle would become subject to immediate slaughter (Kastner *et al.*, 2005).

US business leaders, including the shipping mogul Timothy Eastman, adopted a new line of argument to try to persuade the British government to not apply the immediate-slaughter rule. While conceding that pleuropneumonia was present in certain eastern locations (e.g. dairies, like those on Long Island, where CBPP's presence was irrefutable), Eastman insisted that that disease did not actually threaten export cattle, which (based on his own business-operations knowledge) was sourced from the western states. Indeed, within a few years (by 1884), '95% of the cattle exported came from west of Chicago' (Zimmerman, 1962, p. 47). While Eastman had a point, Commissioner Le Duc and other veterinary leaders (especially Dr James Law) knew that epidemiological evidence would be needed for such an argument (Billings, 1879, pp. 5–6). However, this 'disease-free west' argument seemed somewhat legitimate – and, therefore, worth pursuing – in light of the rapidly emerging controversy about the CBPP diagnosis of the cattle landed at Liverpool on 26 January.

With Liverpool being home to a number of business interests (including those of importers), *The New York Times* (see Fig. 5.5) noted that these individuals had called in 'veterinary surgeons of high repute, to act as a check upon the Privy Council Inspectors' (Anonymous, 1879a, p. 5). These consultants included Drs James McCall of the Glasgow Veterinary College, Thomas Walley of Edinburgh's Royal (Dick) Veterinary College, and

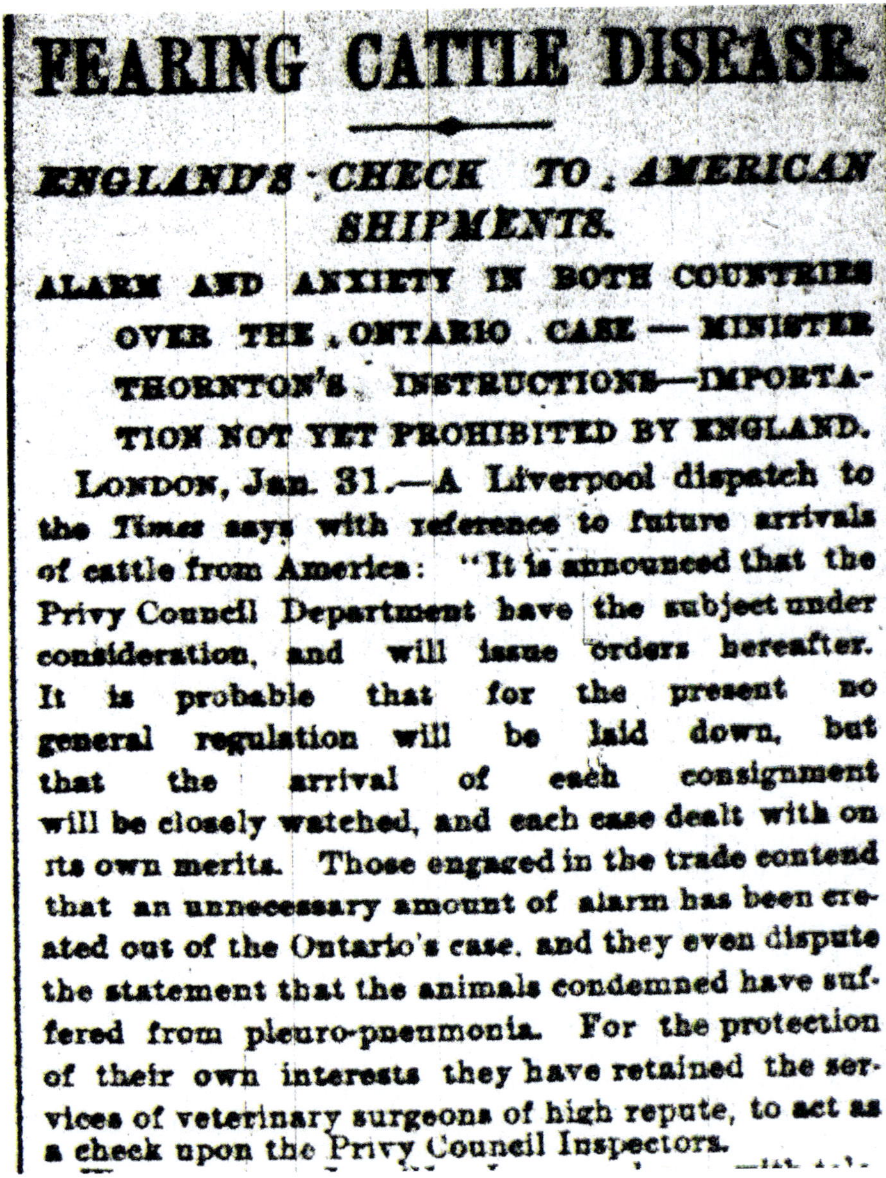

FEARING CATTLE DISEASE.

ENGLAND'S CHECK TO AMERICAN SHIPMENTS.

ALARM AND ANXIETY IN BOTH COUNTRIES OVER THE ONTARIO CASE—MINISTER THORNTON'S INSTRUCTIONS—IMPORTATION NOT YET PROHIBITED BY ENGLAND.

LONDON, Jan. 31.—A Liverpool dispatch to the *Times* says with reference to future arrivals of cattle from America: "It is announced that the Privy Council Department have the subject under consideration, and will issue orders hereafter. It is probable that for the present no general regulation will be laid down, but that the arrival of each consignment will be closely watched, and each case dealt with on its own merits. Those engaged in the trade contend that an unnecessary amount of alarm has been created out of the Ontario's case, and they even dispute the statement that the animals condemned have suffered from pleuro-pneumonia. For the protection of their own interests they have retained the services of veterinary surgeons of high repute, to act as a check upon the Privy Council Inspectors.

Fig. 5.5. This headline in the *New York Times* indicates the high-stakes consequences of the CBPP diagnosis in cattle landed aboard the *Ontario* at Liverpool. (From Anonymous, 1879a, *The New York Times*, 1 February, p. 5, public domain.)

William Williams of Edinburgh's New Veterinary College. Walley, who was accompanied by McCall, observed several of the detained *Ontario* cattle coughing and, after viewing two post-mortem lung samples, concluded the shipment definitely harboured CBPP. However, Professor Williams, who also observed the animals before and after slaughter, concluded that the animals had conventional bronchitis, not pleuropneumonia (House of Representatives Committee on Agriculture, 1880, pp. 3–4, Kastner *et al.*, 2005). Nor surprisingly, the US press continued to give voice to Williams's opinion, who insisted he had evidence for his claim: 'I have the specimens most carefully preserved, and am ready to show them to the whole world, and his wife, if necessary' (Anonymous, 1879b, p. 10).

While Williams's dispute about the CBPP diagnosis would endure for many years (and even be echoed in a similar controversy in 1892 over the so-called 'Deptford ox'; see Chapter 3, this volume), the inevitable occurred in February 1879. Writing from the Veterinary Department of the Privy Council Office at 44 Parliament Street, Westminster, the Clerk of the Council explained that they 'have no option' and would, effective 3 March, apply the immediate-slaughter rule to US cattle (Great Britain (Parliament), 1879, pp. 354–355).

Regulatory Maturation, Surveillance and Eradication

In January 1880, commissioner William Le Duc hired Dr Charles Lyman of Harvard University to provide more epidemiological detail on the prevalence of pleuropneumonia in the US. This was done, in part, to support the 'disease-free west' argument – the contention that American export cattle sourced west of the Allegheny Mountains were of no CBPP threat to Britain. Indeed, Lyman would even, later that summer, travel to Edinburgh and personally meet with Professor Williams and observe for himself the preserved lung samples, and then go to London to meet with Professor George T. Brown, head of the Veterinary Department of the Privy Council (Kastner *et al.*, 2005). More importantly, however, Lyman's epidemiological investigation was crucial for the longer-term objective of controlling the disease's spread in the USA. Together, Commissioner Le Duc and Dr Lyman would engage with the growing army of veterinary correspondents across the country. As illustrated in Fig. 5.6, the coming years would feature correspondents regularly reporting on CBPP-related matters as they sought to establish an epidemiological picture of the disease.

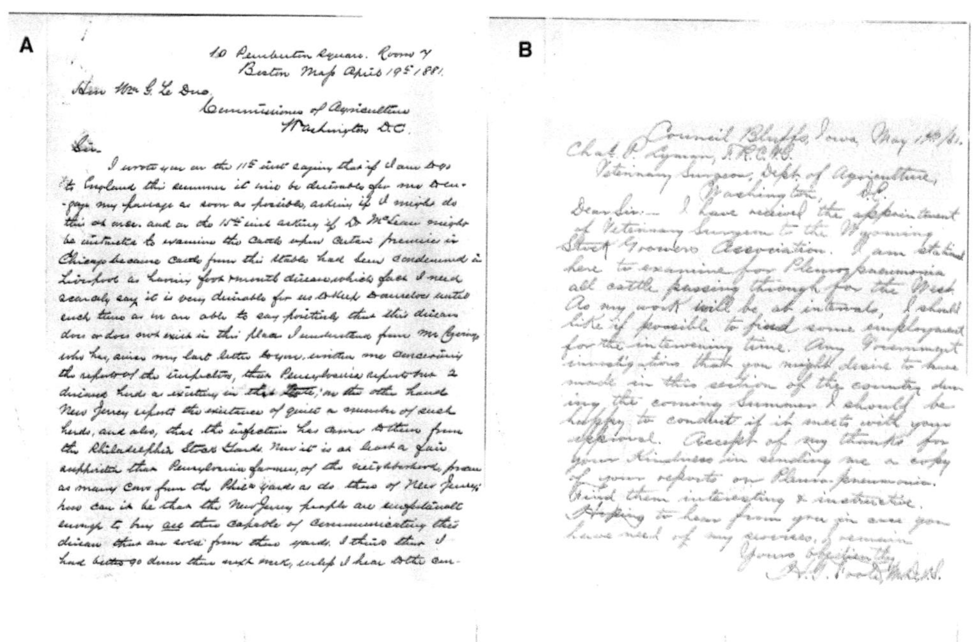

A

10 Pemberton Square. Room 7
Boston Mass April 19th 1881.

Hon Wm G. Le Duc,
Commissioner of Agriculture
Washington D.C.

Sir.

I wrote you on the 11th inst saying that if I am to go to England this summer it will be desirable for me to engage my passage as soon as possible, asking if I might do this at once. and on the 15th inst asking if Dr McLean might be instructed to examine the cattle upon certain premises in Chicago because cattle from this stable had been condemned in Liverpool as having foot and mouth disease, which fact I need scarcely say it is very desirable for us to keep ourselves until such time as we are able to say positively that this disease does or does not exist in this place. I understand from Mr [illegible] who has, since my last letter to you, written me concerning the reports of the inspectors, that Pennsylvania reports but 2 diseased herds as existing in that State; on the other hand New Jersey reports the existence of quite a number of such herds, and also, that the infection has come to them from the Philadelphia Stock Yards. Now it is at least a fair supposition that Pennsylvania farmers, of the neighborhood, draw as many cows from the Phila yards as do those of New Jersey; how can it be that the New Jersey people are unfortunate enough to buy all those capable of communicating this disease that are sold from these yards. I think that I had better go down there next week, unless I hear to the con-

B

Council Bluffs, Iowa, May 1st/81.

Chas. P. Lyman, F.R.C.V.S.
Veterinary Surgeon, Dept. of Agriculture,
Washington, D.C.

Dear Sir:— I have received the appointment of Veterinary Surgeon to the Wyoming Stock Growers Association. I am stationed here to examine for Pleuro-pneumonia all cattle passing through for the West. As my work will be at intervals, I should like if possible to find some employment for the intervening time. Any Government investigations that you might desire to have made in this section of the country during the coming Summer I should be happy to conduct if it meets with your approval. Accept of my thanks for your kindness in sending me a copy of your reports on Pleuro-pneumonia. I find them interesting & instructive. Hoping to hear from you in case you have need of my services, I remain

Yours obediently
[illegible] M.R.C.V.S.

Fig. 5.6. These letters, dated April and May 1881, are but two examples of the rich volume of CBPP-related correspondence between veterinarians in Western USA (in this case, Iowa) and agriculture commissioner William G. Le Duc and his colleague Dr Charles Lyman, originally from Harvard. (From Minnesota Historical Society, William G. Le Duc and family papers. Shelfmark location 149.B.19.8F (box 62), used with permission from the Minnesota Historical Society.)

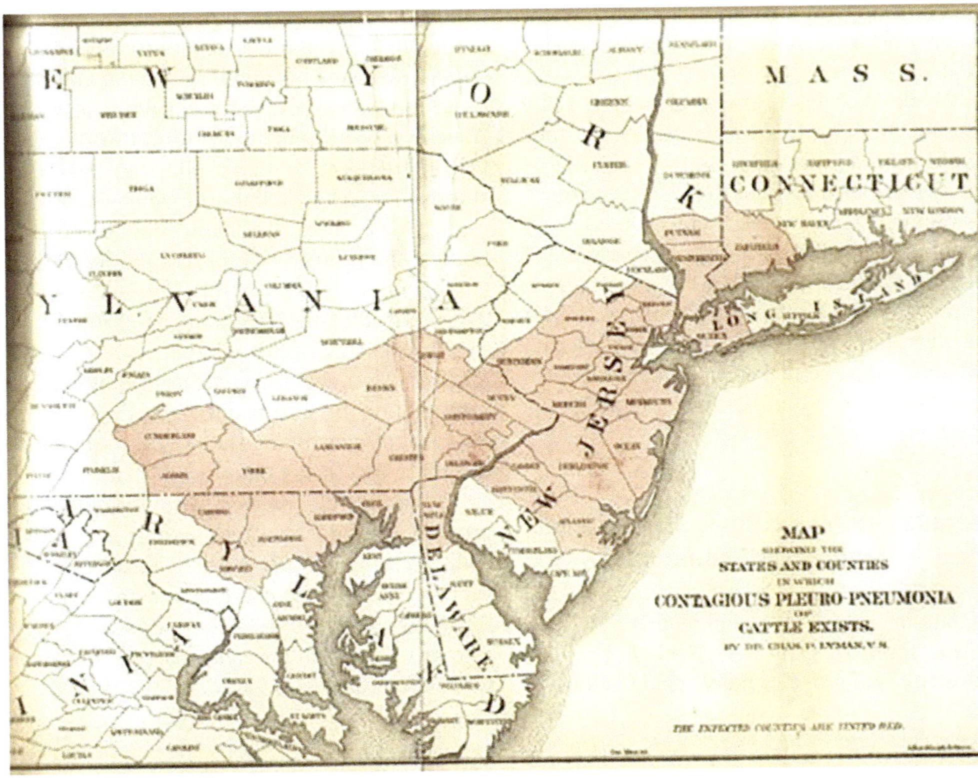

Fig. 5.7. Gathering data from Commissioner Le Duc's previously appointed veterinary correspondents, and performing his own investigative work, Dr Charles Lyman prepared the map shown here, the earliest known portrayal of CBPP's prevalence in the US. (From Lyman, C.P., 1880, Government Printing Office, Washington DC, map facing page 472, public domain.)

The institution of the immediate-slaughter order against US cattle had served to focus the minds of regulatory leaders in Washington, most notably Commissioner Le Duc. He must have been pleased when, in 1880, Dr Lyman provided a detailed map (Fig. 5.7) differentiating between counties where CBPP did exist and counties where it did not (Lyman, 1880, p. 472). This helped lay the groundwork for a decade-long effort to eradicate CBPP from US shores. Once again, the respected Dr James Law figured prominently in the effort. While Law was not the only key official (others included Dr Daniel Salmon), the following account illustrates how this important work was undertaken by the US Bureau of Animal Industry (BAI):

> James Law had been transferred to New York to direct eradication in that state in late 1887. Pursuing an approach he had used successfully in Illinois, he registered and tagged all cattle in the quarantine counties around New York City, the first attempt at animal identification for tracing purposes. Further, on farms where the disease had reappeared several times, Law began to tear down and burn the old barns that could not readily be disinfected properly. Strong opposition from livestock owners emerged against attempts of the BAI to prevent common pastorage of animals from infected and noninfected districts. This dangerous practice ceased only when Law seized and slaughtered over 100 head of cattle found grazing off their owner's premises without a veterinary permit. (Schwabe, 1984, p. 463)

Conclusion

In March 1892, the BAI completed the work begun by the likes of James Law and Daniel Salmon. Late that month, the last CBPP-infected cow was identified in New Jersey. Six months later, the US Secretary of Agriculture, J.M. Rusk, officially declared that, 'the United States is free from the disease known as contagious pleuropneumonia' (Schwabe, 1984, p. 463). Eradication of CBPP in the USA – to be mirrored 6 years later in Britain – was, to be sure, a victory for animal health. However, as elsewhere around the globe in the larger story of CBPP, the regulatory achievement had been motivated by trade-related (that is, economic) forces that demanded the attention of government officials.

References

Anonymous (1872) The new foreign cattle market, Deptford: The central shed. *Illustrated London News* 3 February.

Anonymous (1878) The foreign animals order. *The Times* 7 December, p. 11.

Anonymous (1879a) Fearing cattle disease. *The New York Times* 1 February, p. 5.

Anonymous (1879b) The pleuro-pneumonia scare: What prof. Williams, of Edinburgh, says of the American cattle. *The New York Times* 20 April, p. 10.

Billings, F.S. (ed.) (1879) *Senate Misc. Doc. 71: Information on the Subject of Pleuro-Pneumonia among Cattle*. Government Printing Office, Washington, DC.

Brooklyn Board of Health (1877) *Report of the Board of Health of the City of Brooklyn, 1875-1876*. Union-Argus Book and Job Printing Establishment, Brooklyn.

Butterfield, M. (ed.) (1860) *House Report 651: House Agriculture Committee Report on Cattle Disease*. Government Printing Office, Washington, DC.

Fisher, J.R. (1980) The economic effects of cattle disease in Britain and its containment, 1850–1900. *Agricultural History* 54(2), 278–294.

Gamgee, J. (1871) Report of professor Gamgee on the lung plague. In: Capron, H. (ed.) *Report of the Commissioner of Agriculture on Diseases of Cattle in the United States*. Government Printing Office, Washington, DC, pp. 3–63.

Great Britain (Parliament) (1879) Correspondence connected with the detection of pleuro-pneumonia among cattle landed in Great Britain from the United States of America. *Sessional Papers* LVIII(1878–1879), 349–364.

House of Representatives Committee on Agriculture (ed.) (1880) In: *House Ex. Doc. 53: Pleuro-Pneumonia in Neat Cattle*. Government Printing Office, Washington, DC.

Kastner, J. (2011) Chapter 2: Food and agriculture security: An historical illustration of contemporary challenges. In: Kastner, J. (ed.) *Food and Agriculture Security: An Historical, Multidisciplinary Approach*. Praeger, Santa Barbara, California, pp. 5–32.

Kastner, J., Powell, D., Crowley, T. and Huff, K. (2005) Scientific conviction amidst scientific controversy in the transatlantic livestock and meat trade. *Endeavour* 29(2), 78–83.

Le Duc, W.G. (1878) Letter of 15 March 1878 from agriculture commissioner William Le Duc to Dr J.S. Billings. Washington.

Lyman, C.P. (1880) Contagious pleuro-pneumonia – extent of its prevalence. In: Le Duc, W.G. (ed.) *Report of the Commissioner of Agriculture for the Year 1879*. Government Printing Office, Washington, DC, pp. 456–472.

Lyman, C.P. (1881) Report on contagious pleuro-pneumonia. In: Le Duc, W.G. (ed.) *Annual Report of the Commissioner of Agriculture for 1880*. Government Printing Office, Washington, DC, pp. 571–584.

MacDonald, J. (1878) *Food from the Far West: American Agriculture with Special Reference to the Beef Production and Importation of Dead Meat from America to Great Britain*. William P. Nimmo, London.

McCarron, K. (1991) *Meat at Woodside: The Birkenhead Livestock Trade 1878–1981*. Merseyside Port Folios and the National Museums and Galleries on Merseyside, Birkenhead.

McFall, R.J. (1927) *The World's Meat*. D. Appleton and Company, New York.

New York Board of Health (1858) *Majority and minority reports of the Select Committee of the Board of health, appointed to investigate the character and condition of the sources from which cows' milk is derived, for sale in the city of New York. Together with the testimony and the chemical and microbiological analyses of milks. Also, letters from distinguished physicians, &C., &C., &C.* C.W. Baker, New York.

Perren, R. (1971) The North American beef and cattle trade with Great Britain, 1870–1914. *The Economic History Review* 24(3), 430.
Perren, R. (1978) *The Meat Trade in Britain 1840–1914*. Routledge & Kegan Paul Ltd, London.
Rippy, J.F. (1955) British investments in Texas lands and livestock. *Southwestern Historical Quarterly* 331–341.
Schwabe, C. (1984) *Veterinary Medicine and Human Health*, 3rd edition. Williams & Wilkins, Baltimore, Maryland.
Sherman, J. (ed.) (1879) *Senate Ex. Doc. 71: Letter from the Secretary of the Treasury, in relation to the exportation of live animals to foreign countries, and recommending legislation providing for an inspection of the same before shipment*. Government Printing Office, Washington, DC.
Thompson, R. (1980) The Liverpool Provision Trade Association Ltd.: Commercial history. In: *Provision Trade Association Archives*. Mersey Docks and Harbour Board, Merseyside Maritime Museum Archives, Liverpool.
Zimmerman, W.D. (1962) Live cattle export trade between United States and Great Britain, 1868–1885. *Agricultural History* 36, 46–52.

6 CBPP: Never Out of Africa?

Abstract

Despite eradication from Europe and probably the rest of the world, contagious bovine pleuropneumonia (CBPP) continues to plague sub-Saharan Africa, affecting at least 20 countries, including those where it is most prevalent: Ethiopia, Ghana, Tanzania, Cameroon, Angola, Nigeria and Zambia. It is widely believed that CBPP first appeared in South Africa from Europe in the mid-19th century and spread rapidly reaching Central and East Africa in the next two decades, causing huge losses of local cattle. However, anecdotal and recent genetic evidence strongly suggests that CBPP may have already been present in West and North-East Africa before European colonization. By the end of the 19th century, the disease was present in most sub-Saharan countries. In the 1970s and 1980s, there was some optimism that CBPP could be eradicated, as international projects provided funds for vaccination, test and slaughter; movement controls and improved surveillance, leading to a marked reduction in cases. Unfortunately, many factors such as economic crises, civil wars and droughts impeded control efforts and outbreaks broke out again across sub-Saharan Africa. Numerous new CBPP vaccines have been trialled over the last 20 years to improve on the protection afforded by the T1/44, a live vaccine in continuous use in Africa for over 70 years, but none have so far succeeded; indeed, many exacerbate the disease.

Origin and Breakout

The upcoming storm that was to be CBPP made landfall in September 1854 at Mossel Bay (Fig. 6.1) 400 km west of Cape Town in the independent Cape Colony of southern Africa (Salmon, 1896). It was carried by a Friesen bull imported from the Netherlands at the request of the Dutch Ambassador. It seems that no control measures were imposed or were successful for the affected animal, as 3 years later CBPP had spread rapidly into Transkei in Eastern Cape (Fig. 6.2); it was then trekked into the Transvaal and Natal by oxen driven by Boer farmers where it was estimated to have killed over 100,000 local cattle (Davies, 1991). The indigenous African tribes, known collectively as the Xhosa, were said to be 'suffering dreadfully' from this 'new and unknown disease' which they were treating with 'bleeding, purging and separation of the diseased herd' (Anonymous, 1856).

The high mortality rate seen was because it occurred in local cattle that had never experienced the disease before. The loss of cattle was compounded between 1856 to 1857 by an extraordinary and unprecedented voluntary event known as the 'Xhosa cattle killing' during which a local girl, named Nonggawuse, had been told by her ancestors in a dream to slaughter all their remaining cattle (Mares, 2011). In doing so, they would rid themselves of the colonists who would be replaced by new people (thought to be Russians) bringing fresh healthy cattle. While not all her people were convinced by her prophecy, the cattle were killed leading, unsurprisingly, to much suffering and deprivation. Whether this far-sighted though catastrophic action was an inadvertent attempt to stamp out CBPP will never be known, but slaughter, where practical, became an important tool for control, particularly in Europe. Sadly, for the Xhosa, the colonists remained, and the Russians never arrived. In 1874, CBPP was still killing thousands of cattle annually in Natal, according to its first official veterinary surgeon Samuel Wiltshire, who said: 'Lung sickness spread like an evil fire as infected oxen transported it along the wagon trails of the Cape Colony' (Pieres, 1989, p. 166).

CBPP spread north by other cattle movements as European settlers grew in number and infected animals were transported into Southern and Northern Rhodesia (now Zimbabwe and Zambia, respectively). Others blame British troops for its dissemination during the Anglo-Zulu Wars (Tambi *et al.*, 2006). An outbreak

DOI: 10.1079/9781800627536.0006

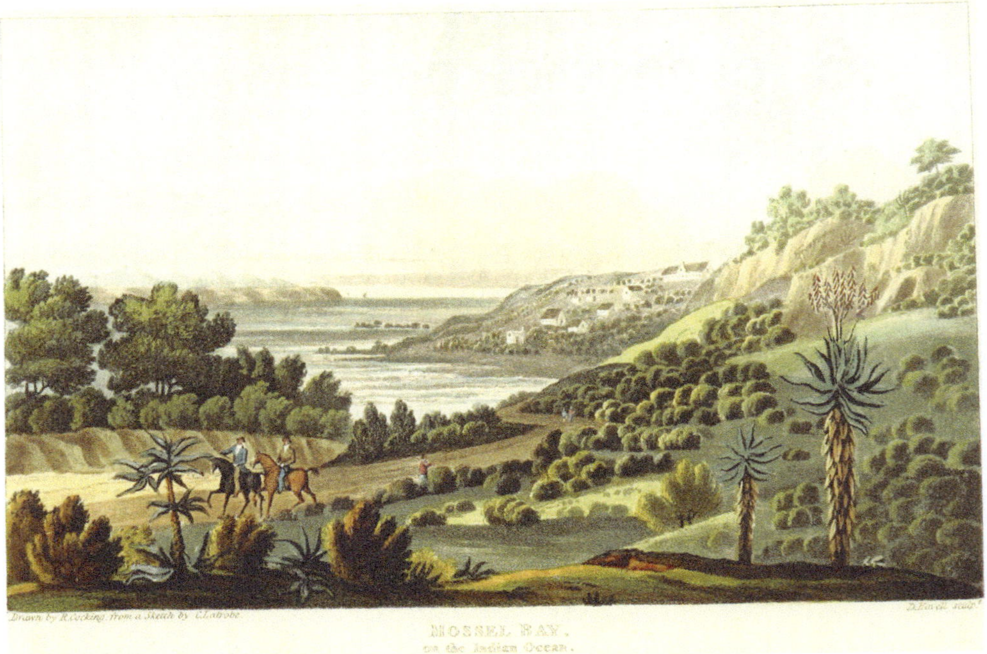

Fig. 6.1. Mossel Bay, South Africa where CBPP first came ashore after the journey from the Netherlands in 1853. (From Cocking, R. (from a sketch by Latrobe, C.I.), 1818, The British Library, public domain via Wikimedia Commons.)

of African horse sickness in 1856, killing 60,000 horses, exacerbated the already dire circumstances by restricting the movement of goods and supplies by horse and adding more burden for oxen. The disease eventually entered the Kenyan highlands by the end of the 19th century (Egwu *et al.*, 1996) and was officially reported there in 1905 (Bygrave *et al.*, 1968). The disease was said to be common in both Uganda and Tanzania by the 1920s when there were extensive outbreaks involving thousands of cattle with one-quarter of the Masai cattle population undergoing quarantine (Kusiluka and Sudi, 2003).

A large outbreak of CBPP during the First World War, when British troops were engaged in hostilities with Germans in East Africa, threatened food supplies and required a call to the War Office in Britain for five veterinarians to help control it (Anonymous, 1917).

CBPP also escaped west via infected oxen from Cape Colony to South-West Africa (now Namibia) in 1856, but strict control measures limited its impact to the south until it was re-introduced a few years later and spread to the whole country. It caused great losses to the cattle of the indigenous Herero people who referred to 1860 as the year of the 'Otjipunga' or 'lung'. It spread north into Angola with Boer migrants from the Transvaal, in 1882, – an extraordinary journey of some 3000 km – who settled in Humpata, the chief town of the province of Huīla in the south of the country (Duarte, 1969). At the time, Angola was nominally controlled by the Portuguese who diagnosed the disease some 5 years after the Boers settled. By then, CBPP was present in a huge area extending south to Namibia and east to Zambia. In the following years, it moved north as a result of the constant displacement of the indigenous peoples and their cattle, as well as the continued movement of the oxen trains of the Boers (Sousa *et al.*, 1975). It would be another 50 years before eradication was achieved in Namibia, though sporadic outbreaks still occur on the borders with Angola and Zambia.

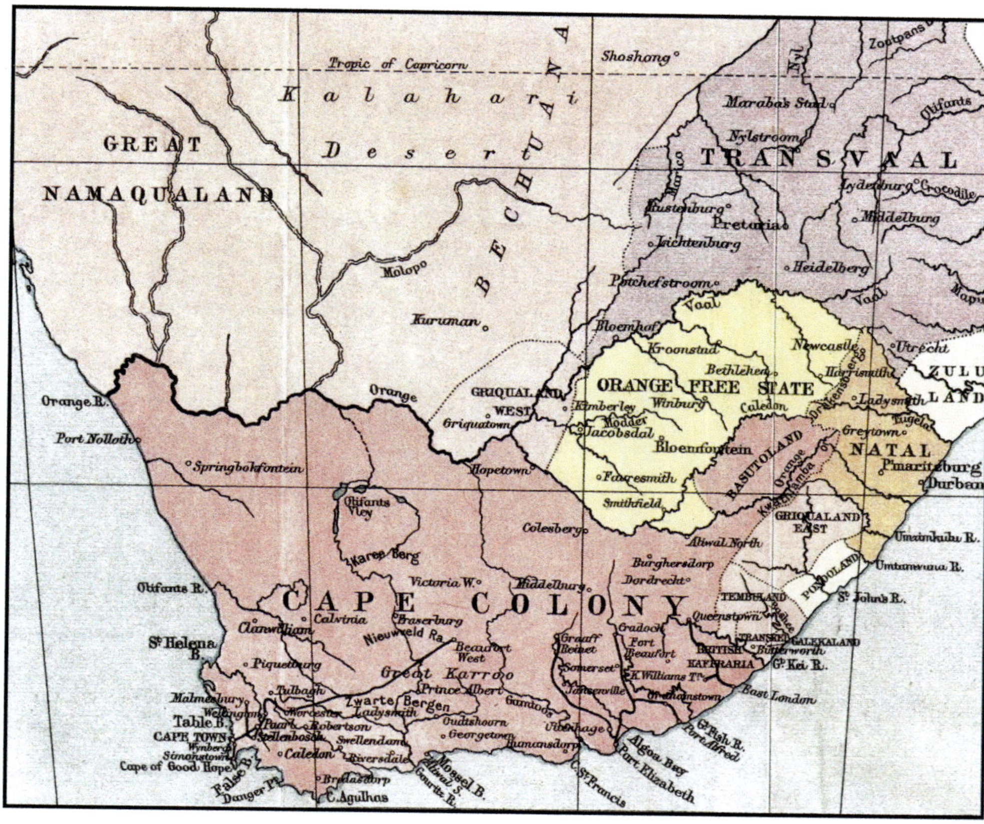

Fig. 6.2. Map of Cape Colony which existed between 1806 and 1910. (From Anonymous, 1900, public domain via Wikimedia Commons.)

The importance of CBPP was emphasised by its prominent inclusion in one of the first conferences on animal diseases held in Cape Town in 1904, attended by veterinary officials from affected regions including German South-West Africa. All reported large losses and the difficulty in 'getting natives to kill their animals by compulsion, or voluntarily for the purpose of preparing material to prepare vaccine'.

Where slaughter was not possible, the conference recommended branding infected animals and keeping them in isolation until the disease died out (or presumably when the animals died).

Emergence in the Rest of Africa

How CBPP originated or spread into the rest of Africa is less well known. There is good evidence that it was already present in Nigeria in the 1920s. G.E Owen, acting chief deputy veterinary officer in the northern provinces, recorded its presence in the markets of Kano, northern Nigeria in his first departmental report of 1924 (Owen, 1926). He stated unequivocally that the source of the disease was:

> [T]he French Territory more especially among [trade cattle] entering from the north and northeast. That the disease had existed in those herds for some time was proved by the detection of chronic lesions on postmortem and from the presence of facial disfiguration which is the usual sequelae of the native method of vaccination. (Owen, 1926)

However, it is clear from this British report that the disease was well known among the local people who, as can be gathered from his remarks, were already practising a crude but effective vaccination against it (Fig. 6.3). But, whether Niger

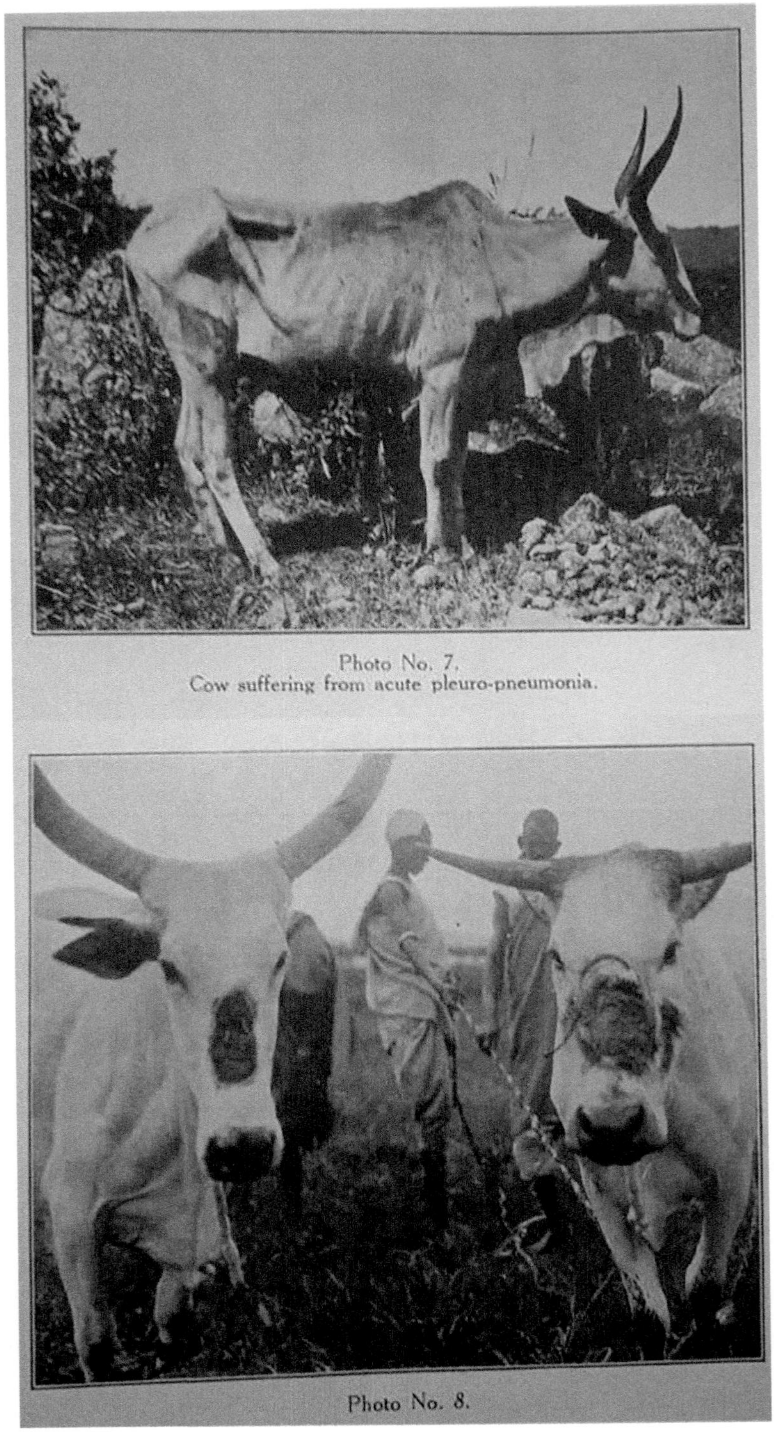
Photo No. 7.
Cow suffering from acute pleuro-pneumonia.
Photo No. 8.

Fig. 6.3. A cow with clinical signs (top); cattle showing vaccination lesions on faces of cattle (bottom) in Nigeria in the 1920s. (From Owen, 1926, public domain.)

and Chad, the neighbouring French colonies at the time, were the source of infection for Nigeria or whether it was present in West Africa before European annexations is not clear, though it seems highly likely it was already there. While, according to Owen's report, 1925 appeared to be a relatively quiet time for CBPP, it soon made its impact on the Nigerian herds, killing more cattle than rinderpest between 1925 and 1929; Owen blamed this on the uncontrolled movements of trade livestock and, probably unfairly, on the cattle owners themselves: 'The natives recognise [CBPP] as a serious disease...they dispose of the affected and suspected animal to anyone who will buy it; this is how the disease spreads' (Owen, 1926).

Considering this reliable evidence, it would strongly suggest that CBPP was present in West and Central Africa long before its introduction to South Africa, thus pointing to a multi-origin scenario for CBPP for which there is some genetic and anecdotal evidence. Molecular epidemiological studies were initially hampered by the very close homogeneity of strains of the causative mycoplasma but are now beginning to shed light on the spread of CBPP worldwide.

Using a molecular typing method called multilocus sequence typing (MLST), analysis of 20 *M.m.mycoides* strains, the CBPP Reference Laboratory in Montpellier, France divided African strains into three distinct groups (Yaya *et al.*, 2008): (i) Central and East African; (ii) West African; and (iii) southern African. Variable number tandem repeat (VNTR) analysis at the Animal Health and Veterinary Laboratories Agency, Weybridge, UK, appeared more discriminatory and showed clear differences between strains from southern and East Africa (McAuliffe *et al.*, 2007). These and other molecular typing studies, showing differences between strains from different regions of sub-Saharan Africa, have been limited by a lack of recent and historical strains which prevents drawing too many firm conclusions about the origin and dissemination of CBPP. Moreover, without the very strict eradication programmes seen in Europe during the 20th century, CBPP in Africa has been largely allowed to go unchecked and strains isolated today show a much greater heterogeneity than recent European strains. However, what is known using next-generation sequencing and Bayesian analysis is that all strains circulating in sub-Saharan Africa today so far have evolved from a common ancestor present in Europe in the early 19th century (Dupuy *et al.*, 2012) providing some supporting evidence for the Dutch origin of CBPP in southern, central and East Africa.

Other Possible Routes of Infection

Interestingly, these molecular studies could provide further support for a multi-origin theory for CBPP in Africa which may become clearer when more strains are isolated and sequenced, ideally from West and Central Africa (Fig. 6.4). So, other than the direct European origin, what other routes could CBPP have taken to invade Africa?

There is some early published evidence that supports the hypothesis that CBPP was already present in Africa before colonial times from the German explorer Gustav Nachtigal, who, in 1869, described 'lungenseuche' (the great cattle death), which was decimating cattle populations around Lake Chad. Nachtigal reported that these outbreaks were regular occurrences and appeared to have spread from the west (Weiss, 1998). This may be linked to the imaginative suggestion by Dupuy *et al.* (2012) that CBPP may have been introduced into Africa via cattle from the Portuguese bases along the West African coast, possibly as early as the 17th century, assuming Portugal itself was infected at that time. The disease may then have migrated eastwards along Arab trade routes through Mali, Niger and Chad. Of course, without diagnostic tests, unavailable then, or clear descriptions of clinical or pathological signs, it is not possible with any certainty to say whether this was CBPP. However, further evidence of a pre-colonial origin of CBPP was given by the British explorer Joseph Thompson, who in the 1880s reported Masai cattle dying of a disease with signs similar to CBPP; these outbreaks would certainly have been too early for the disease to have reached Kenya from South Africa (Davies, 1991). Mares (2011), too, was convinced that CBPP was already prevalent in sub-Saharan Africa as he said it was known among the Samburu pastoralists of north-east Kenya in 1870, present in

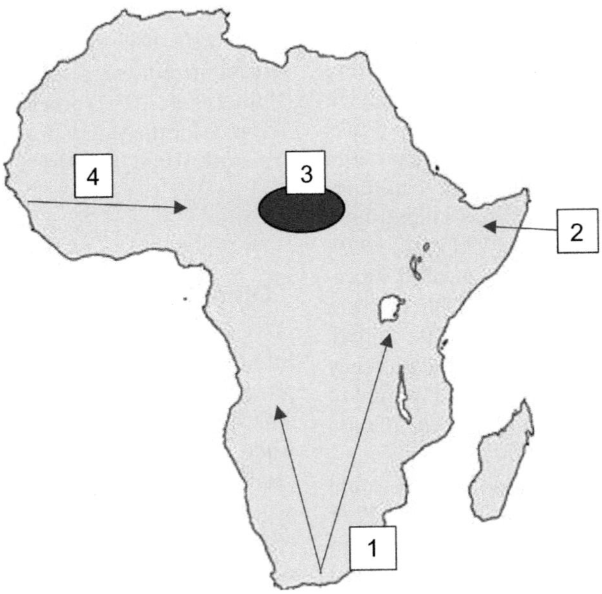

Fig. 6.4. Possible routes of CBPP spread through Africa. 1) Via infected cattle from the Netherlands in 1858. 2) Via infected cattle with General Napier's expedition into Abyssinia 1868 from India. 3) Infection predates European colonization. 4) Via infected cattle from Portuguese bases on the West African coast 17–18th century.

the Rift Valley in 1882 and 'was well established among the Masai by 1883'.

According to Harold Baskerville Williams, a British veterinary officer writing during the early part of the Second World War, CBPP was recorded in Sudan between 1875 and 1889, first appearing in Darfur in the west of the country and later spreading east to Khartoum causing massive cattle losses. It then re-emerged in 1912 in the central region of Kordofan (Williams, 1940). Again, this would suggest that the disease had spread from the west from an unknown source.

More convincingly, writing in Nocard and Leclainche, 1898, Nocard and Leclainche, provided 'published evidence' of what seemed to show that preventative inoculation against CBPP (i.e. vaccination) had been practised 'since time immemorial in Senegambia' [a historical name for a geographical region in West Africa, between Senegal River in the north and Gambia River in the south] and southern Africa (Blancou, 1996). This immunisation involved inserting virulent material from an animal that died of CBPP beneath the skin either on the bridge of the nose, the tail tip or the thigh. In fact, the practice had also been reported in 13 other sub-Saharan countries where traditional vaccination was carried out long before the first European publication of vaccination by Willems in 1852, thus predating the arrival of CBPP in South Africa. Early 19th-century travellers in eastern and western Africa could only say that the procedure they witnessed 'was very ancient'. Furthermore, it was thought that this knowledge had been acquired from the Persians who used similar methods for centuries to fight the goat equivalent of CBPP, contagious caprine pleuropneumonia also caused by a mycoplasma.

A fascinating account of early vaccination attempts against CBPP, or 'lung sick' as it was known then, appeared in the novel *King Solomon's Mines* by H. Rider Haggard (1885) (Fig. 6.5). The following extract shows both the severe post-vaccinal response that could occur and the fear that CBPP provoked.

> As for 'lung sick' which is a dreadful form of pneumonia, very prevalent in this country, they [oxen] had all been inoculated against it. This

is done by cutting a slit in the tail of an ox, and binding piece of the diseased lung of an animal which has died of the sickness. The result is that the ox sickens, takes the disease in a mild form, which causes its tail to drop off, as a rule about a foot from the root, and becomes proof against future attacks. It seems cruel to rob the animal of his tail, especially in a country where there

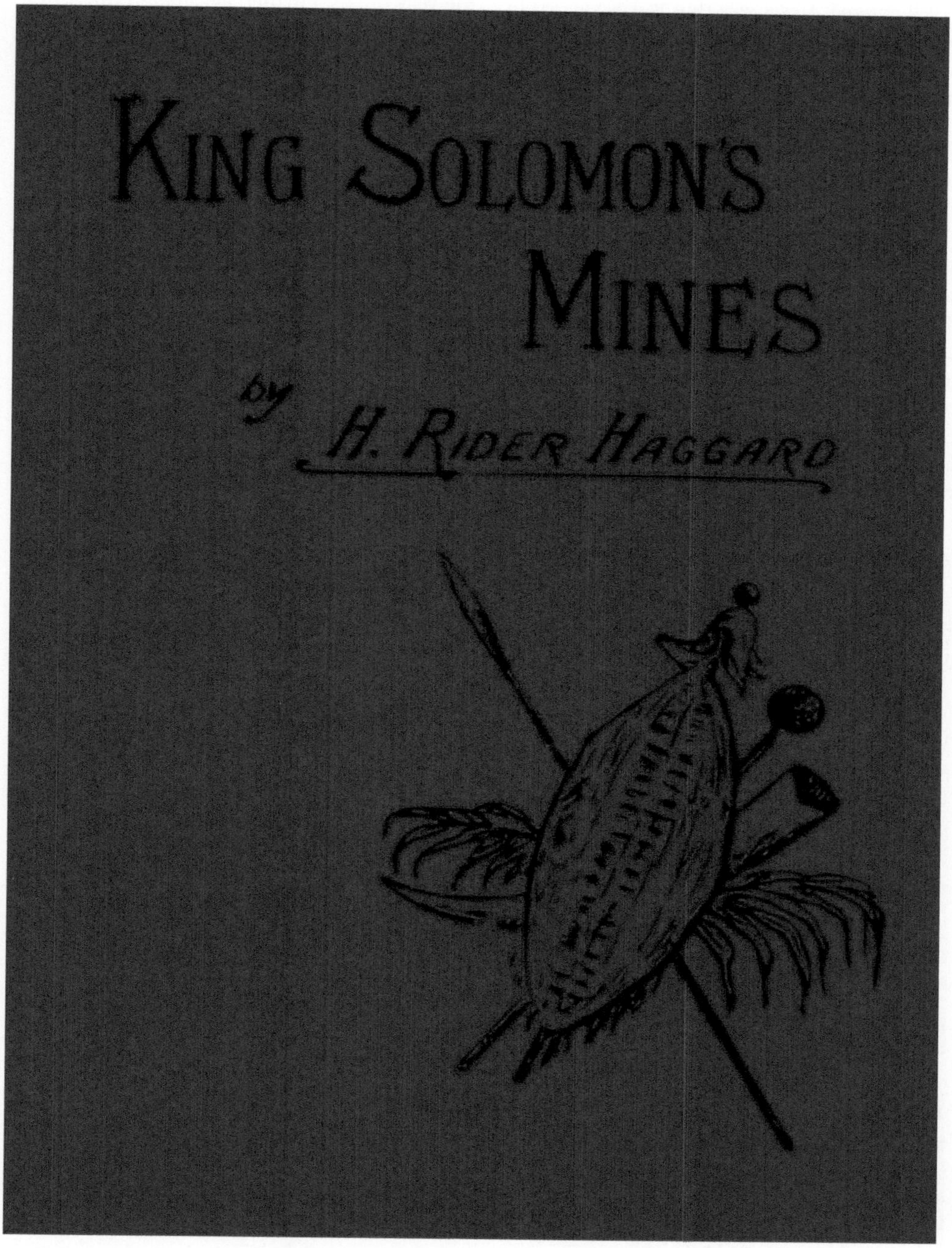

Fig. 6.5. *King Solomon's Mines* with its detailed account of CBPP vaccination. (From Haggard, 1885, public domain.)

are so many flies, but it is better to sacrifice the tail and keep the ox than to lose both tail and ox, for a tail without an ox is not much good, except to dust with. (Haggard, 1885, p. 42)

Probably the least likely theory of how CBPP entered Africa was that it was carried in oxen with a huge invading force by the British army between 1866 and 1867, led by the buccaneering and colourful character, Field Marshall Charles James Napier, to rescue (successfully as it turned out) a handful of European hostages held by the Abyssinian Emperor Theodore (Masiga *et al.*, 1996). Sadly, for this hypothesis, Henry Morton Stanley, a reporter for *The New York Times* and later an explorer of Africa, makes no reference in his detailed account of the expedition to any outbreaks of respiratory disease, let alone CBPP, in the oxen accompanying the army, besides the fact that mules were the main beasts of burden for supplies (Stanley, 1896). Crucially, there was no evidence at all that India, from where the expedition began, was infected with CBPP at the time; indeed, CBPP was not reported there until the 1930s (Nicholas, 2023). Incidentally, Stanley did describe a severe outbreak of 'glanders', caused by the bacterium *Burkholderia mallei*, which was highly fatal in the mules and nearly sabotaged the mission at the very outset. Further speculation that CBPP came with cattle traded from India in the 19th century (Alhaji *et al.*, 2020 is also very unlikely for the same reason that it was not present in the subcontinent at the time.

There is, clearly, still a lot of uncertainty about the exact arrival of CBPP into Africa, but it seems inconceivable that the disease seen in the Central African Republic and Nigeria, where cases were first reported in 1920 and 1924, respectively, could have had the same origin as countries in the south and east of Africa – Lagos is 7000 km from Cape Town! Rivers, jungles and deserts all present formidable obstacles to cattle movements. The British had annexed an area later to become Nigeria in 1861 so would have been aware of any new respiratory diseases of cattle in the late 19th century. So, at this time,

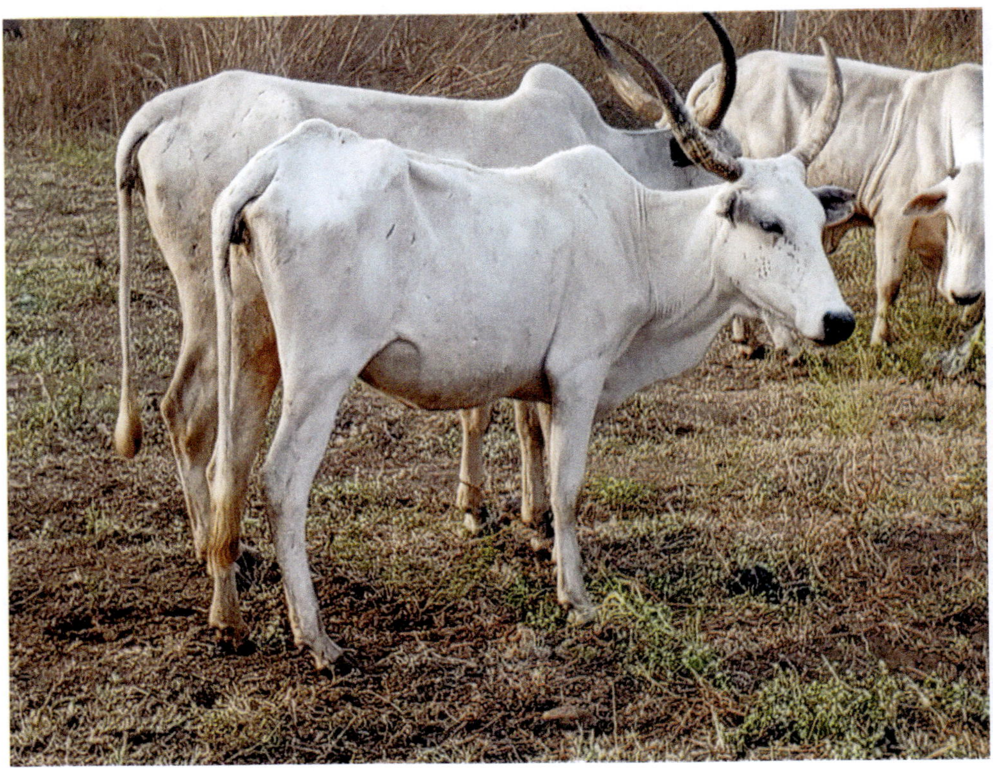

Fig. 6.6. White Fulani Zebu cattle main cattle breed in West Africa. (From Robin Nicholas.)

several entry points must be the best hypothesis until more information is available.

Current Status

CBPP is a transboundary disease of sub-Saharan Africa that extends from Senegal and Gambia in the west through Somalia in the east and as far south as Namibia, Zambia and Tanzania. The disease is well known today by local peoples in sub-Saharan Africa where it is called *samba* or *fofi* in different regions of Ethiopia, *chiwu huhu* in Nigeria by the Fulani nomads; in Zambia depending on the stage of the disease it is *butuku bwamasafu*, or *mahunyungu*, and in Uganda it is known as *adeka na iwukooi*. In Angola during Portuguese-rule it was known as *caonha*. It is mostly characterized by a chronic endemicity with occasional severe outbreaks when naïve herds are exposed to infected animals moved, often illegally, across borders. Moreover, due to the weak economies of many affected countries, stamping out, movement control, slaughter and compensation as practised in Europe are not options (Nicholas, 2009). Additionally, systematic detection of infected clinically silent cattle is impossible in regions where extensive husbandry is the main type of cattle rearing. More importantly, cattle raised in pastoral systems are an important source of livelihood for families and contribute to national food security (Fig. 6.6). Consequently, cattle owners are reluctant to slaughter even where it is clear the sick animals are potent sources of infection to the rest of the herd (Fig. 6.7).

Despite great advances in diagnostic technology and improved epidemiological tools over the last 30 years, it is fair to say that eradication of CBPP in Africa is as far off as when the OIE put forward a plan to eradicate it in 1994. The disease is endemic in over 20 countries, although more are probably affected as many do not carry out regular or comprehensive surveillance (Fig. 6.8). Consequently, it is probably more accurate to list the sub-Saharan countries free of CBPP, at least at the time of writing in 2025. These are: South Africa and its enclaves, Lesotho and Eswatini, Botswana, Zimbabwe, Malawi and Mozambique; Namibia is essentially free but is prone to isolated outbreaks on the borders with Angola and Zambia. The countries with the highest prevalence include Ethiopia, Ghana, Tanzania and Angola. Indeed, this has hardly changed over the last 20 years, showing that most attempts at control have been unsuccessful. Occasional outbreaks are seen in Saudi Arabia following the importation of cattle for festivals from neighbouring African countries like Ethiopia and Sudan, but these rarely spread to local cattle as they are slaughtered shortly after arrival.

The following regional reports must be taken as selective and descriptive as few recent updates have emerged from many African countries partly due to the COVID-19 pandemic.

West Africa

CBPP was first reported in Nigeria ('the giant of Africa') in 1924 and is believed to have originated in the neighbouring French colonies of Niger or Chad, or possibly both (Owen, 1926). Eradication was nearly achieved in the early 1980s thanks to the large international projects Joint Project 28 and Pan African Control of Epizootics (PACE). This was carried out through a policy of compulsory mass vaccination in the endemic foci followed by quarantine and test and slaughter, crucially, with compensation for owners of slaughtered cattle; reporting of outbreaks was also greatly strengthened leading to significant advances in eradication. Despite this, success was limited because pastoralists were reluctant to have their cattle vaccinated for fear of adverse reactions. Furthermore, any progress was quickly undone when the disease re-emerged probably from one or all of the bordering countries of Niger, Chad and/or Cameroon. Then to make matters worse an economic crisis hit; Nigeria introduced a Structural Adjustment Programme with World Bank loans, which resulted in a 1000% devaluation of local currency. As a consequence, costs of vaccine production, vaccination programmes and all services became prohibitively expensive, and budgetary provisions fell well short of requirements. Diagnostic services, essential for the serological detection of chronic carriers, ground to a halt and compulsory slaughter and compensation could not be carried out

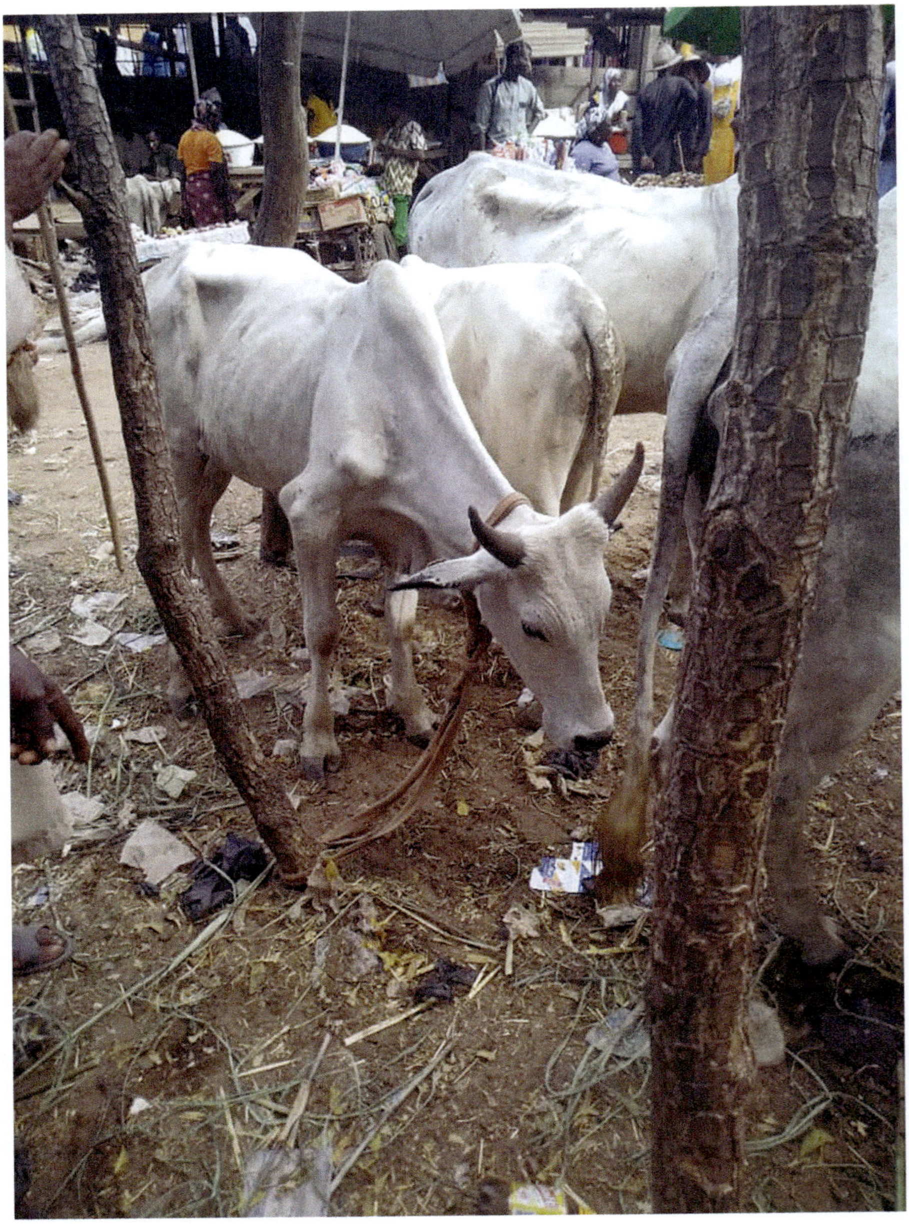

Fig. 6.7. Cattle showing anorexia and breathing difficulties. (From Robin Nicholas.)

for lack of funds. As a result, outbreaks rose rapidly from 1986 onwards to a peak in 1989 when over 10,000 cattle died. Presently, the disease is widespread in Nigeria and the recent wave of civil and religious unrest has enabled the spread of the disease in the northern part of the country where 75% of the country's 16 million cattle are kept. The recent CBPP prevention programme that involved vaccination, test, slaughter and abattoir surveillance has suffered major setbacks as a result of inconsistent policies from the government, as well as insecurity in some regions in Nigeria (Olorunshola *et al.*, 2021). The nomadic nature of local pastoralists

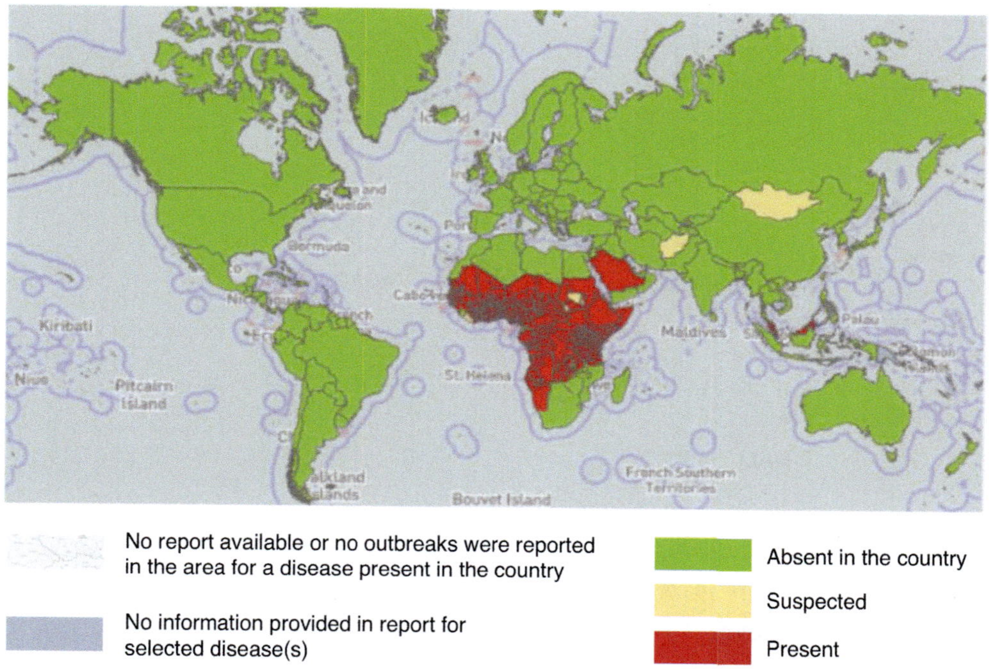

Fig. 6.8. Countries affected or suspected of being affected by CBPP between 2005 and 2023. (Image courtesy of Dr Patrick Bastiaensen, WOAH.)

which involves migrating cattle great distances for grazing purposes has further exacerbated the spread of CBPP.

Coordinated research aimed at improving the quality of vaccines for controlling CBPP has virtually stopped because the National Veterinary Research Institute leading such studies is located in a region badly affected by the geopolitical disturbances that have resulted in serious tribal and religious conflicts leading to loss of life (Olorunshola *et al.*, 2021).

On Nigeria's northern border lies Niger, 80% of it occupying the Sahara Desert. Despite the challenging environment, 87% of the population relies on raising livestock. Unfortunately, CBPP, which has been enzootic for years, takes a heavy toll on cattle though these are hard to estimate because of its insidious nature. Like other African countries, some degree of control was exerted by the combined rinderpest/CBPP vaccine but since rinderpest's eradication, there has been an upsurge of CBPP cases. The main CBPP risk areas close to Nigeria, Mali and Benin, as measured by a serological survey, are shown in Fig. 6.9 (Yansambou *et al.*, 2018).

The other countries just south of the Sahara appear in an even worse state. The World Bank-funded *Regional Sahel Pastoralism Support Project* report1 (PRAPS and World Bank, 2019) calculated herd prevalence levels of CBPP as ranging from 37% in Mali, 46% in Niger, 63% in Mauritania, 73% in Chad, to 75% in Senegal. The Gambia has also reported recent outbreaks while Somalia, which neighbours both Kenya and Ethiopia, must be suspect for CBPP. The situation in the region has almost certainly not improved now following the COVID-19 pandemic with the reduction in vaccination and surveillance.

North-East Africa

Livestock is an integral part of agriculture in Ethiopia, contributing about 45% of the total value of agricultural production and providing livelihoods for a large part of the population. In addition, the country's livestock population is large with an estimated 70 million cattle, 52

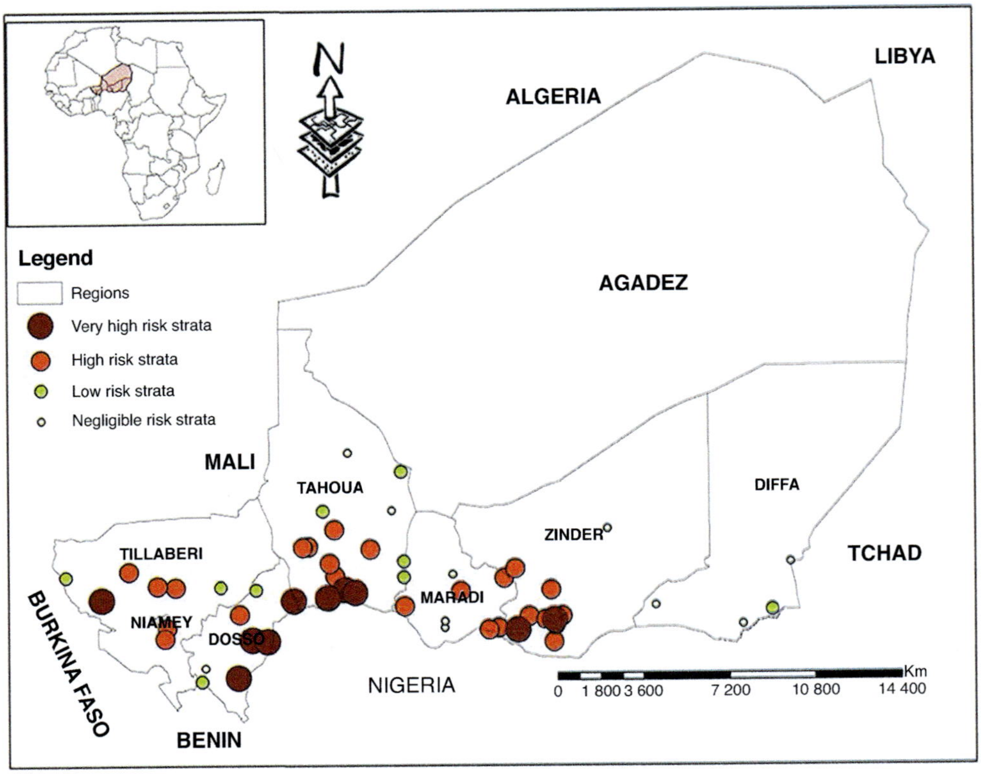

Fig. 6.9. Map of Niger showing CBPP risk areas. (From Yansambou *et al.*, 2018.)

million goats, and 43 million sheep. After rinderpest was eradicated, CBPP became Ethiopia's most important cattle disease greatly impeding livestock development (Molla *et al.*, 2021). Prevalence surveys revealed the presence of the disease in many parts of the country with prevalence varying from nearly 2% in southern and eastern lowlands to 96% in Western Gojjam. The disease is causing high economic losses in the agricultural sector, which impacts on the national economy, costing over US$4 million per year. Available data on the distribution of the disease in Ethiopia show the north-western part of the country, especially the western part of the North Gondar zone (where livestock production is very important), as free or of unknown status. This area is adjacent to the endemic zone of West Gojjam and Awi. The situation in other regions is unknown too. As there are no animal movement restrictions in place, the disease will likely continue to spread.

In 1940, over 100 outbreaks were reported in six states of Sudan affecting over 16,000 cattle leading to about 250 deaths (Williams, 1940). Although several outbreaks occurred between 2007 and 2008, none were reported in the northern region of Sudan, which could be attributed to the limited movement and small animal numbers living in the harsh environment. A small serological survey carried out in 2017 found 13% of 200 sera from cattle in Khartoum state to be positive; interestingly, the OIE-approved competitive ELISA gave the same results as the rapid penside latex agglutination test which takes just a few minutes to complete and can be carried out directly on blood (Hassan and Ismail, 2017). A recent, as yet unpublished study (due to the ongoing civil war), calculated seroprevalence at 7% around Khartoum where the largest concentration of cattle is held (Eslah Abdelhabib, personal communication). While CBPP prevalence remains low, Sudan is threatened by the endemic countries of Ethiopia, Chad and the Central African Republic because of the large cross-border movements of peoples and livestock due to droughts and civil disturbances including the present one affecting Khartoum.

Southern Africa

CBPP was re-introduced into Botswana, probably from Angola, after 55 years of freedom, and led to the slaughter of 320,000 cattle at a cost of US$100 million. Further indirect losses were estimated at over US$400 million before CBPP was eradicated in 1997, and remains free today. Botswana is a model for the successful eradication of CBPP in Africa but was greatly incentivised by its lucrative trade with the EU, which requires disease-free carcasses.

CBPP has been endemic in Angola for many years but was controlled where possible by the Portuguese veterinary services, which carried out periodic surveys and vaccination programmes. After independence in 1975, years of civil wars fragmented the veterinary services ensuring disease control was ineffective and information on its prevalence largely unknown. Ironically, the outbreak of peace in the early 1990s saw security fences being damaged, often by elephants, enabling illegal cattle movements to spread CBPP and other diseases to Namibia, Zambia and the Democratic Republic of Congo. One of the first post-independence insights into CBPP in Angola was reported by Daniel *et al.* (2017) who carried out a study in three areas of the Namibe province, which is located next to the Namibian border and is home to the majority of the national herd belonging mostly to the Herero people. Thirty-five herds made up of over 1000 cattle were tested by ELISA; these comprised one epidemiological unit as cattle intermingle uncontrollably at pasture and watering holes. Herd seroprevalence was over 94% and almost certainly due to field infection rather than vaccine antibody as vaccination had not been practiced for several years in the region and when carried out was often random and poorly administered. Despite Angola having one of the fastest-growing economies in the world because of its vast mineral and oil reserves, problems are numerous and arise primarily due to wealth being concentrated in a disproportionally small sector of the population. Agriculture has been starved of financial resources and central and regional laboratories lack many basic services such as water and energy with frequent power cuts so are incapable are carrying out even the simplest of diagnostic and control activities.

The main farming areas of Namibia are free of CBPP but sporadic outbreaks, which are quickly stamped out, are reported in the northern communal regions bordering Angola, where half the Namibian population lives. This area is separated by the Trans Veterinary Cordon Fence, which prevents movement of infected cattle south. However, a large outbreak killing several hundred cattle occurred in the Caprivi (now the Zambezi region) in the early 2000s following the illegal movement of cattle from Zambia across the Zambezi River. The outbreak was controlled by a combination of slaughter, vaccination and, for the first time, chemotherapy (Nicholas *et al.*, 2007).

CBPP is the major contributor to cattle death in Zambia, particularly in the Western and North-Western provinces (Muuka *et al.*, 2019); these outbreaks adversely affect the livelihood of livestock owners who depend on cattle for survival, which is compounded by movement restrictions leading to a shortage of beef on the Zambian market and ultimately to higher meat prices. The disease was first recorded in 1915 and is blamed on the British Army bringing in infected oxen from Angola during the boundary settlement with the other colonist, Portugal. These outbreaks persisted for 30 years during which a quarter of a million cattle were reported to have died. The British authorities eventually eradicated it through a mixture of movement restrictions, vaccination and slaughter (crucially with compensation). The disease then reappeared in 1965 again from Angola because of refugees escaping with their cattle at the beginning of the civil war which was to tear the country apart for the next 30 years. The number of outbreaks was initially suppressed by a 10 km buffer zone imposed on the Angolan border, but this was often porous and eventually broke down as the number of refugees increased when the Angolan war intensified. To make matters worse, the northern provinces have become threatened from Tanzania by illegal cattle movements leading to sporadic outbreaks. As recently as May 2024, Zambia was reporting outbreaks affecting a herd of 5000 cattle just 70 km north of Lusaka, in which 2% had died or were sick but the slaughter of the whole herd was required (Muuka, personal communication).

East Africa

The Karamoja, a semi-arid cattle-rearing area in north-east Uganda and north-west Kenya, bordering South Sudan, Ethiopia and Somalia, has been the traditional home of CBPP since it re-entered the region from southern Sudan in 1956. Uganda had also been infected from the south sometime early in the 1920s and may have eradicated it shortly afterwards. Recent surveys show a quarter of all cattle tested in the region were seropositive, indicating the need for serious control interventions, in particular vaccination which has not been applied here for nearly 5 years (Tweyongyere *et al.*, 2024). Outbreaks here are thought to be instigated by animal movements during dry seasons, when animals are stressed due to poor nutrition and exhaustion from trekking in search of pastures and water.

In Kenya, CBPP is present in the Karamoja region bordering Uganda, Southern Sudan and Somalia. Over a recent ten-year period, the incidence of CBPP in Kenya was 2.8% and 12.7% in endemic and epidemic situations, respectively, and up to 47% in the event of sporadic outbreaks (Kairu-Wanyoike *et al.*, 2014). Test and slaughter were used extensively to control CBPP in the Masai lands in the south, backed by strict movement control. However, it can be lengthy and difficult to achieve in the absence of adequate quarantine and compensation. But some success has been seen by detecting infected animals at meat inspection, tracing back the disease, testing suspected herds and slaughtering infected animals. This approach was used very effectively in Italy during the re-emergence of CBPP in Europe at the end of the 20th century.

CBPP reappeared in Arusha, Northern Tanzania in 1990 after a 25-year absence, having been introduced from Kenya (Kusiluka and Sudi, 2003); it then spread unnoticed to southern Tanzania in 1994, where it had not been recorded for 50 years. The disease spread rapidly to the Mara region through the rustling of sick or infected animals. An unrelated outbreak occurred in Kagera, having spread from Southern Uganda but appeared to be confined to Kagera and Arusha until it was seen in Morogoro region, south of the central railway line. Thereafter, the disease spread throughout western Tanzania. Later, further disease occurred in the Southern Highlands and Central regions. The direct losses incurred as a result of animal mortality, vaccination campaigns and disease surveillance have been assessed at over US$11 million. Abattoir and market surveillance carried out in 2014 showed at least 13% of randomly slaughtered cattle had lesions suggestive of CBPP; many of which were acute cases showing the disease to be widespread.

The Rwandan genocide of 1994 was a catastrophe not just for 800,000 Rwandans who were killed but also for its impact on the country's agriculture with thousands of farmers fleeing to the northern part of Uganda with their livestock (Masiga *et al.*, 1996). These exiles returned later, bringing back their cattle and, with them, CBPP. Large numbers of outbreaks resulted in morbidity rates as high as 70% and mortality rates between 20 and 50%. The movement of herds south and west led to the infection of the whole country and into Northern Burundi. Cases were still being reported in Eastern Rwanda a decade later where 20% of cattle examined were positive following laboratory examination of an outbreak in 2011 (Enyaru *et al.*, 2012).

Central Africa

The Central African Republic (CAR) became infected in 1920 '*from the west*' (Ngounda *et al.*, 2021, italics added). Today it is enzootic despite control campaigns using live T1 vaccines, which have shown little efficacy due to poor implementation in the field (Ngounda *et al.*, 2021). New strategies combining controlled use of antibiotics and inactivated vaccines, with increased thermostability, have been welcomed by livestock keepers and have allowed better control of CBPP in the region. Three strains isolated from different regions shared the same genomic sequence showing that they were closely related to a strain isolated in CAR in 1991, also sequenced in this study; they clustered with *M.m.mycoides* strains originating from East and Central Africa. The recent isolates showed increased microbial inhibitory values though they were still sensitive to tetracyclines. The national prevalence in the CAR was estimated at 12.5% with no significant differences observed between cattle breeding regions, nor between males and females. However, zebu had a significantly higher prevalence than taurine cattle, most likely because of their herding system based on cattle transhumance and nomadic pastoralism.

An abattoir study between 2009 and 2010 (Wade *et al.*, 2015) in the northern region of Cameroon, an important crossroads for cattle movements, showed nearly 30% of cattle being slaughtered there had lesions suggestive of CBPP. However, confirmation of results by culture and PCR was not always successful in part due to poor mycoplasma isolation and excessive therapeutic use of antibiotics in the cattle according to the authors. The report also found no significant differences in cattle breed between Red Mbororo and White Fulani though many more Reds passed through the slaughterhouse.

Little reliable data emerges from the Congo and the Democratic Republic of Congo, but significant numbers of outbreaks were reported in 2012 (Alhaji *et al.*, 2020) and both countries are still believed to be affected.

Control

The COVID-19 pandemic of 2020 has had a dramatic impact on CBPP control with national surveillance and vaccination rates decreasing significantly, leaving exposed many vulnerable and susceptible herds. Before the pandemic, several studies had attempted to estimate the losses incurred by CBPP. In 2006, Tambi *et al.* (2006) calculated losses of US$47 million over 14 countries while in Nigeria alone, one of the largest cattle-raising countries in Africa, Musisi *et al.* (2006) estimated over $2 billion. More recently and at much more of a local level, Kairu-Wanyoike *et al.* (2017) showed that cattle owners in Kenya could lose more than twice their annual income, due to vaccination, post-vaccine reactions, treatment costs, morbidity and mortality. With the reduction in vaccination and surveillance seen since the pandemic, it can be expected that losses will rise significantly.

In 2003, the Nigeria Animal Diseases Information System (NADIS) classified Nigeria as an endangered zone based on its CBPP status. The value of these losses was assessed nationally and across the four agro-ecological zones of Nigeria to be US$8.7 million (Olorunshola *et al.*, 2021). Economically, Nigeria suffers direct losses through infection and deaths of cattle, while indirect losses include exclusion from participation in international livestock and livestock product trade.

The impact of CBPP in Africa has not always been so bleak. South Africa, Zimbabwe (then known as Rhodesia), Tanzania and Botswana were all able to eradicate CBPP by mixed policies of movement controls, vaccination and slaughter. Indeed, in the 1960s and 1970s, a huge international effort known as Joint Project 16 (JP16) mainly aimed at rinderpest, also resulted in a dramatic reduction in clinical CBPP. Unfortunately, the eradication of rinderpest negatively impacted CBPP control particularly in the Horn of Africa as the bivalent rinderpest/CBPP vaccine was no longer being administered. In East Africa, after an absence of 25 years, CBPP returned to Tanzania in 1994 spreading throughout the country where it remains endemic, costing the country at least US$3 million per year though these estimates are over 30 years old. Furthermore, an incursion of CBPP in 1996 into Botswana led to the slaughter of over 300,000 cattle at the cost of between US$100–400 million enabling the re-establishment of its disease-free status and protecting the lucrative EU export market.

Unlike Europe, where a single strategy of movement control, test and slaughter was imposed following the re-emergence of the disease in southern Europe in the 1980s enabling the eradication of CBPP by the end of the 20th century, the lack of sustained cooperation between countries in sub-Saharan Africa seriously constrains control of this transboundary disease. In addition, a panoply of other factors compounds control efforts including a need for an improved safer and more robust vaccines and greater national vaccine coverage, lack of versatile diagnostic field tests, a greater awareness of the socio-economic impact of CBPP, poor private and public funding, climate change, particularly drought and even terrorist activities.

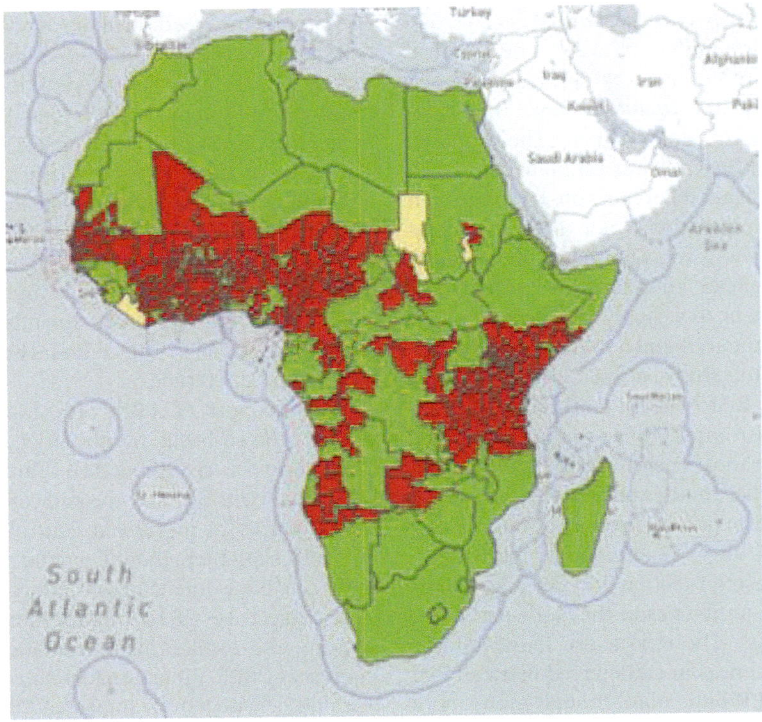

Fig. 6.10. WOAH-WAHIS composite map (2005–2019) of the distribution of CBPP in Africa (red = present; yellow = suspected); map generated on 5 April 2022. (Image courtesy of the kind permission of WOAH.)

Prevalence and distribution studies are urgently required to locate the disease both nationally and within countries to protect clean zones and limit losses in high-prevalence areas (Fig. 6.10). Despite the difficulties in controlling CBPP in Africa, the disease does have some advantages compared to others: it is not very contagious – the reproductive number (R0) (which measures the contagiousness of an infectious agent) is low at 2, though estimates vary and further studies should be carried out; lesions are pathognomonic at post-mortem by experienced personnel; identification of the causative organism *M. m. mycoides* is relatively easy by PCR; there is only a single serotype so vaccines are cheap and largely effective if given regularly and on a large scale; antibiotics are effective presently with no signs of the development of antimicrobial resistance; and, generally, the environment and wildlife appear to play little role in the epidemiology of the disease. Consequently, mixed control strategies can be implemented.

On the other hand, the T1/44 vaccine has well-known flaws, including serious though infrequent adverse reactions at the inoculation site (so-called Willem's reaction), short-term protection and lack of thermostability. Incidentally, it is worth noting that during a large vaccination campaign in the Caprivi following the unexpected outbreaks in the early 2000s, no adverse reactions were seen among 1200 vaccinated cattle (Dr Ortwin Aschenborn, personal communication). This was put down to hygienic and careful inoculation technique suggesting that many of these effects may be the result of hurried and sloppy injection. Antibiotics rarely eliminate the pathogen completely and more recently there is concern over the role of buffalo as a reservoir of infection in Kenya. Encouragingly, with such a low R value any attempts to reduce transmission such as vaccination, culling, isolation or antibiotic treatment should lead to R0 >1 which will help lead to eradication.

Vaccines

An OIE scientific conference in Gaborone in 1994 concluded that vaccination of cattle remained the best way of controlling CBPP, but a vaccine that would confer better immunity than the T1 strain vaccine was urgently needed (OIE, 1994). Over a quarter of a century later, Jores *et al.* (2020) came to the same conclusions. Studies into the immunology of the disease have failed to provide sufficient insight to improve vaccines. No inactivated, sub-unit or attenuated vaccines have been developed which improve upon the live T/144 vaccine developed in the 1950s.

The T1/44 vaccine has been in constant use in Africa for over 70 years and was mainly responsible for the large reduction in CBPP cases in the 1970s and 1980s when the disease was probably restricted to only a few East African countries. It is worth reviewing the qualities of the T1/144 vaccine that made it effective, as these can often be forgotten in the haste to develop more speculative and expensive vaccines. Despite various attempts to, inadvertently, compromise the potency of the vaccine over the years – developing a bivalent product with rinderpest, producing a streptomycin-resistant vaccine and a deleterious reconstitution procedure (Nicholas *et al.*, 2008) – the OIE concluded that the vaccine can effectively protect herds when vaccination is performed annually (WOAH, 2018); evidence has also been presented to show that regular vaccination can significantly reduce adverse effects in cattle (Schieck *et al.*, 2014). Moreover, March (2004) showed that simple and inexpensive changes to the current vaccine, such as the use of HEPES buffer systems and the inclusion of pH indicators together with restrictions in the use of 1M MgSO4 as a vaccine diluent, can increase vaccine yields 10-fold and stability several 100-fold, producing a vaccine which should improve its effectiveness in the field. Little work has continued this promising approach.

A new vaccine with none of the disadvantages of T1/44 would help but there would still be the problem of achieving the required 80% coverage needed to have an impact on CBPP control. Work has been reported on the development of new vaccines that include sub-unit, attenuated and killed vaccines with variable reports of success. Using reverse vaccinology, the team at VIDO, Canada identified immunogenic recombinant proteins that appeared to provide similar protection to T1/44 in cattle using an improved aerosol challenge model. The vaccine is going through further trials in Kenya but progress has been slow.

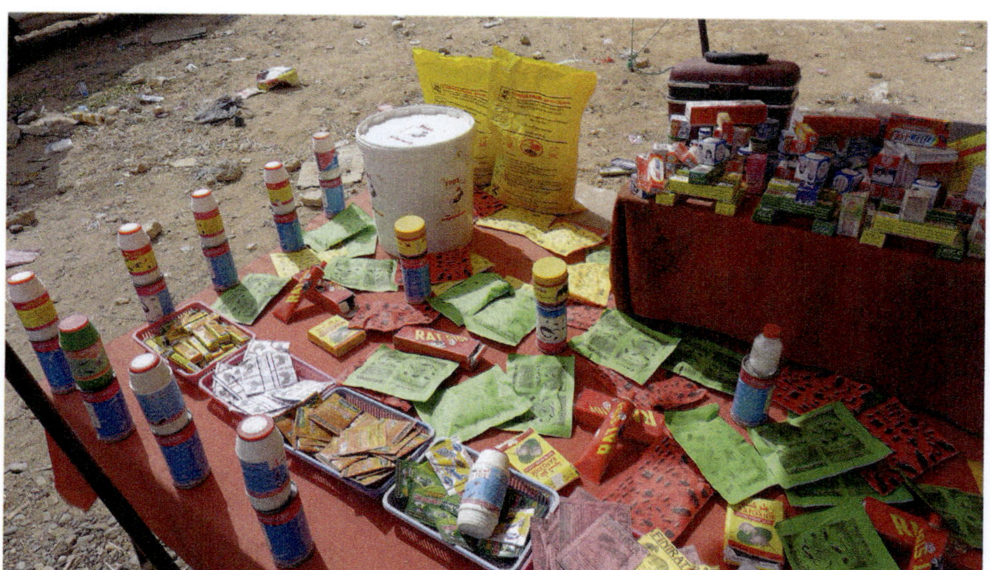

Fig. 6.11. Antibiotics and other commercial chemicals are freely available in markets across Africa. (From Wikimedia Commons, CC BY 4.0.)

Therapeutics

Recognition that vaccination alone will not bring about eradication led to a reconsideration of the use of antibiotics (begun at the FAO CBPP meeting in Rome in 2005, titled 'CBPP: antibiotics to the rescue') ideally in a targeted setting. Previously, it was believed that mycoplasma infections did not respond well to antimicrobial treatment and indeed their use was discouraged or prohibited because of the fear of creating carrier animals that could spread infection (Provost *et al.*, 1987). However, it is common knowledge that in the absence of an effective vaccine, its availability or sufficient coverage, farmers and field veterinarians will use antibiotics as the only control option which, of course, are available in markets across Africa (Fig. 6.11).

In vitro susceptibility testing of mycoplasmas to conventional and novel antibiotics in the early 2000s showed a marked difference between the sensitivity of *Mycoplasma bovis*, a cause of calf pneumonia in intensive cattle rearing, and *M. m. mycoides*, a problem in more extensive cattle farming (Ayling *et al.*, 2000). Strains of *M. bovis* from most countries were largely resistant to nearly all antibiotics currently used for the treatment of respiratory disease as a result of their widespread and indiscriminate use in intensive farming. In contrast, *M. m. mycoides* was sensitive to all despite their universal availability.

Later work confirmed these findings. *In vitro* antibiotic susceptibility testing of a wide range of isolates of *M. m. mycoides* has shown that at least ten antimicrobials were still effective against CBPP (Ayling *et al.*, 2005) and antimicrobial resistance was not yet evident. Further proof of the effectiveness of oxytetracycline, danofloxacin and tulathromycin was provided by Mitchell *et al.* (2012) who showed that these antibiotics could inhibit *M. m. mycoides* even in biological matrices.

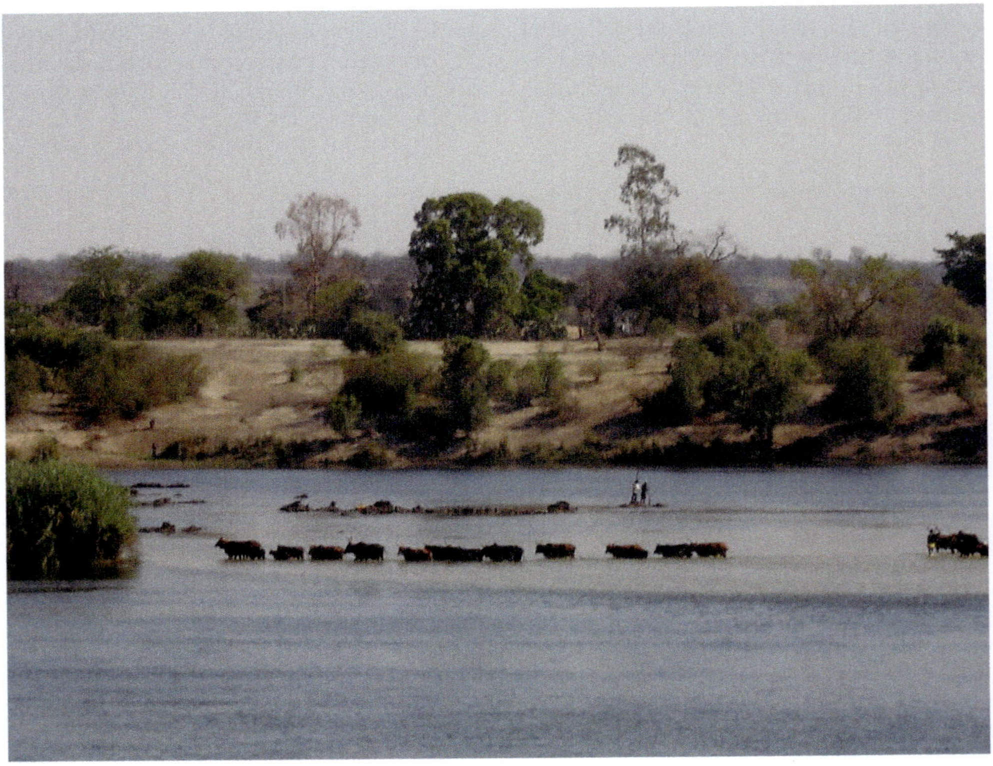

Fig. 6.12. During the dry season cattle can easily move across the Zambezi, which forms the border between Zambia to Namibia. (From Robin Nicholas.)

In 2006, the first official use of antimicrobial treatment to control an outbreak of CBPP was reported in the Caprivi region of Namibia (Nicholas *et al.*, 2007). The disease had been introduced across the Zambezi river from Zambia (Fig. 6.12) in 2003 and outbreaks were very severe, with mortality as high as 50% in the small herds of the region. In total, there were 37 outbreaks, which killed many cattle. Vaccination was immediately implemented but animals continued to die and there were serious concerns that the disease would become endemic and spread to other cattle-rearing areas of Namibia (Hübschle *et al.*, 2004a). It had previously been shown experimentally that treatment of all CBPP-affected cattle with the antimicrobial danofloxacin (Advocin; Pfizer Animal Health) could significantly reduce transmission of the mycoplasma to other cattle (Hübschle *et al.*, 2004b). Consequently, all clinically affected or seropositive herds were treated with the antimicrobial according to the manufacturer's instructions. The number of new cases fell immediately with only three animals dying within the first 3 months after treatment and no more overt cases appearing after that (Fig. 6.13). Clinical monitoring continued for 2 years during which no more cases were reported. Annual vaccination was instigated following the last outbreak.

In the years following antimicrobial treatment there were only sporadic and minor outbreaks in the east of Caprivi, where it was not possible at the time of the outbreaks to treat all cattle because of the seasonal flooding of the Zambezi; importantly there were no cases in the main cattle-rearing region in the south-west of Caprivi. The eradication of CBPP from this region, where some 100,000 cattle are kept, represents a significant achievement as it is known that CBPP can persist indefinitely in small populations (Mariner, 2009). Evidence has also been advanced that the effect of antimicrobial treatment is to accelerate the healing process by promoting fibrosis in the lung, further

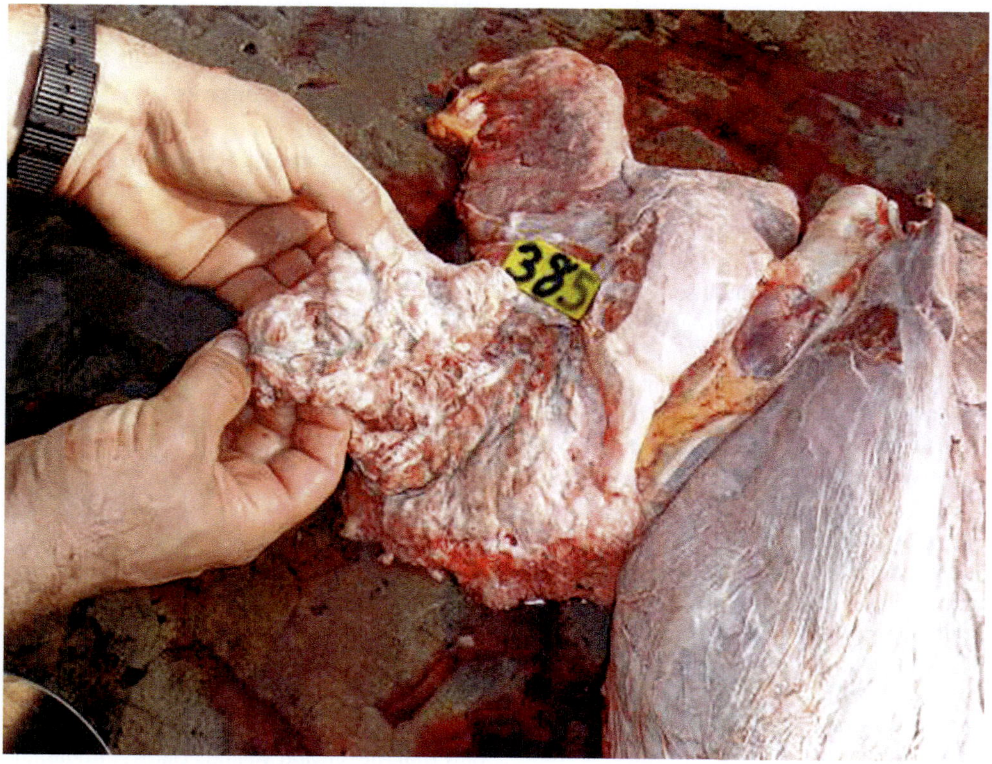

Fig. 6.13. CBPP-affected fibrotic lung following antibiotic treatment; no mycoplasmas could be isolated. (From Robin Nicholas.)

inhibiting mycoplasma transmission (Nicholas *et al.*, 2008).

The results of the Caprivi study supported the concept that strategic and targeted antimicrobial treatment can play a critical part in the control of CBPP alongside regular and comprehensive vaccination. Mariner (2009) has been an advocate of this approach and concluded: 'this is an example of innovation in civil society leading to the development of an evidence base for an institutional shift in policy' (Mariner, 2009).

The metaphylactic approach of antibiotic treatment is also the most effective way of preventing the development of antibiotic resistance (Peter Lees, personal communication).

More recently, controlled *in vivo* experiments in Zambia and Kenya showed that the macrolide, tulathromycin, could achieve metaphylactic protection of up to 80% and prevent the spread of CBPP to untreated controls (Muuka *et al.*, 2019). Further studies are required to evaluate antibiotic strategies with and without vaccination.

AMR surveillance of animal mycoplasmas has been hampered for many years because of lack of harmonized methods for antimicrobial sensitivity testing and interpretative criteria, resulting in a severe shortage of data. Recently, attempts have been made in Europe to address this deficiency by participating in an existing clinical surveillance network system to monitor antibiotic sensitivity in the field. Results show that *Mycoplasma bovis*, the cattle respiratory pathogen, had high MICs for all classes of antibiotics except the fluoroquinolones probably because of their use in intensive production of European livestock; members of the *M. mycoides* cluster including *M. m. mycoides* on the other hand, show predominantly low MICs reflecting their use on smaller more extensive livestock operations. Further work is required to establish breakpoints for animal mycoplasmas to provide clinical guidance for treatment. This work should be extended to Africa to monitor *M. m. mycoides* strains to provide an early warning of the emergence of AMR. The establishment of strain banks and surveillance networks would complement this approach.

Other means of control

A WOAH group of surveillance experts concluded that the most efficient method of detecting CBPP is through effective meat inspection at abattoirs followed by laboratory testing of suspect samples. These were the major tools in the eradication of the disease in Italy in the 1990s which was accomplished in 3 years involving the trace-back and slaughter of over 24,000 cattle and buffalo. Lesions of this largely unilateral pulmonary disease, in the most part, are pathognomonic. In Africa, PMs can be carried out in bush abattoirs and even at festivals where cattle are slaughtered enabling trace-back to affected farms. Rigorous training is, of course, essential for staff unfamiliar with all stages of the pathology. Nonetheless, mobile technology can also be used to send images from remote locations to diagnostic laboratories, so-called telediagnosis, greatly saving time. This training can be given not just to veterinary officials but also to private vets, traditional leaders and cattle breeders.

Final remarks

Despite frequent meetings of FAO on CBPP over the last 20 years, including one titled 'CBPP: Antibiotics to the rescue' in 2006, aimed at discussing new approaches to control based on targeted use of chemotherapy, very little real activity is evident in the field, partly due to the lack of funds but more often as the result of the inability of countries to cooperate. Despite the approval of FAO for UK to perform antibiotic susceptibility testing, The World Reference Laboratory for CBPP in the early 2000s refused to release its reference strains. There are reports that *in vivo* antibiotic trials are beginning but progress has been painfully slow. Furthermore, a trial of a live CBPP that had been effective in controlling the disease in China in the 1970s showed no improvement over the T1/44 vaccine though its production and use had to be modified for the more ethical conditions met in Africa. There are hopes that progress will accelerate now that the Bill and Melinda Gates Foundation, Canada and the USA have identified CBPP disease as a priority for funding. Indeed, a gap analysis meeting was held in Cambridge in 2023 to identify priorities for future USDA funding, in particular the development of sensitive, rapid farm-side diagnostic tests.

If international and national bodies are serious about eradicating, or even controlling, CBPP then extra funds must be set aside to improve vaccine coverage using the T1/44 with targeted use of antibiotics in outbreaks overseen by international experts. The development and use of increasingly sensitive diagnostic and epidemiological tests will only confuse what is a relatively easy disease to identify and will divert funds to where it is really needed. Although slow in identifying the disease, the Italian veterinary control authorities eradicated the disease in less than 3 years by movement control, a policy of test and slaughter mainly based on abattoir surveillance and enabled by an effective animal identification system. This is presently not feasible among the numerous affected countries of sub-Saharan Africa. However, rinderpest was a much more difficult disease to eradicate but was eventually successfully cleared from the world. As outlined nearly 30 years ago in Paris, an eradication plan for CBPP is eminently achievable if the will and cooperation are there. For now, it seems that the elimination of CBPP in Africa is as far away now as it was then.

References

Alhaji, N.B., Ankeli, P.I., Ikpa, L.T. and Babalobi, O.O. (2020) Contagious bovine pleuropneumonia: Challenges and prospects regarding diagnosis and control strategies in Africa. *Veterinary Medicine: Research and Reports* 11, 71–85.

Anonymous (1856) On the prevalence of pleuro-pneumonia at the cape of good hope. *The Veterinarian* 29, 729–731.

Anonymous (1917) Memo from GOC, Africa to war office 11/10/1917. German east Africa. September to December volume 8, p. 223.

Ayling, R.D., Baker, S.E., Nicholas, R.A.J., Peek, M.L. and Simon, A.J. (2000) Comparison of in vitro activity of danofloxacin, florlenicol, oxytetracycline, spectinomycin and tilmicosin against *Mycoplasma mycoides* subp. *mycoides* small colony type. *Veterinary Record* 146(9), 243–246.

Ayling, R.D., Bisgaard-Frantzen, S., March, J.B., Godinho, K. and Nicholas, R.A.J. (2005) Assessing the in vitro effectiveness of antimicrobials against *Mycoplasma mycoides* subsp. *mycoides* small colony type to reduce infections of contagious bovine pleuropneumonia. *Antimicrobial Agents and Chemotherapy* 49(12), 5162–5165.

Blancou, J. (1996) Early methods of surveillance and control for contagious bovine pleuropneumonia. *Revue Scientifique et Technique. International Office of Epizootics* 15, 1263–1282.

Bygrave, A.C., Moulton, J.E. and Shifrine, M. (1968) Clinical, serological and pathological findings in an outbreak of contagious bovine pleuropneumonia. *Bulletin of Epizootic Diseases of Africa* 16(1), 21–46.

Daniel, S., Abeledo-Abreu, M.-A. and Lobo-Rivero, E. (2017) Seroprevalencia de pleuroneumonía contagiosa bovina en tres municipios de la provincia Namibe, Angola. *Revista de Salud Animal* 39(1), 62–67.

Davies, G. (1991) Contagious bovine pleuropneumonia: What every veterinarian ought to know. *State Veterinary Journal* 1, 9–11.

Duarte, V.M.S. (1969) La Péripneumonie contagieuse des bovins en angola. [XXXVII Session Genérale, Rapport n.° 120], *Bulletin de l'Office International Des Épizooties* 72, 89–94.

Dupuy, V., Manso-Silván, L., Barbe, V., Thebault, P., Dordet-Frisoni, E. *et al.* (2012) Evolutionary history of contagious bovine pleuropneumonia using next generation sequencing of *Mycoplasma mycoides* subsp. mycoides 'small colony'. *PloS ONE* 7(10), e46821.

Egwu, G., Nicholas, R.A.J., Ameh, J.A. and Bashiruddin, J.B. (1996) Contagious bovine pleuropneumonia: An update. *Veterinary Bulletin* 66, 195–208.

Enyaru, J.C.K., Biryomumaisho, S., Balyeidhusa, A.S.P., Ebong, C., Musoni, A. *et al.* (2012) Comparison of competitive ELISA, PCR and loop mediated isothermal amplification of mycoplasmal DNA in confirmatory diagnosis of an outbreak of contagious bovine pleuropneumonia in eastern Rwanda. *International Journal of Animal and Veterinary Advances* 4(1), 22–28.

Haggard, H.R. (1885) *King Solomon's Mines*. Penguin Classics, p. 137. Available at: https://archive.org/details/king-solomons-mines-henry-rider-haggard (accessed 4 June 2025).

Hassan, O.S. and Ismail, H.M. (2017) Sero-prevalence of contagious bovine pleuropneumonia (CBPP) in Khartoum state, Sudan. *Journal of Applied Science and Research* 5(6), 42–46.

Hübschle, O., Godinho, K. and Nicholas, R.A.J. (2004a) Danofloxacin treatment of cattle affected by CBPP. *The Veterinary Record* 155(13), 404.

Hübschle, O.J.B., Ayling, R.D., Godinho, K., Lukhele, O., Tjipura-Zaire, G. *et al.* (2004b) Danofloxacin (AdvocinTM) reduces the spread of contagious bovine pleuropneumonia to healthy in-contact cattle. *Research in Veterinary Science* 81(3), 304–309.

Jores, J., Baldwin, C., Blanchard, A., Browning, G.F., Colston, A. *et al.* (2020) Contagious bovine and caprine pleuropneumonia: A research community's recommendations for the development of better vaccines. *NPJ Vaccines* 5(1), 66.

Kairu-Wanyoike, S.W., Kiara, H., Heffernan, C., Kaitibie, S., Gitau, G.K. *et al.* (2014) Control of contagious bovine pleuropneumonia: Knowledge, attitudes, perceptions and practices in Narok district of Kenya. *Preventive Veterinary Medicine* 115(3–4), 143–156.

Kairu-Wanyoike, S.W., Taylor, N.M., Heffernan, C. and Kiara, H. (2017) Micro-economic analysis of the potential impact of contagious bovine pleuropneumonia and its control by vaccination in Narok district of Kenya. *Livestock Science* 197, 61–72.

Kusiluka, L.J.M. and Sudi, F.F. (2003) Review of successes and failures of contagious bovine pleuropneumonia control strategies in Tanzania. *Preventive Veterinary Medicine* 59(3), 113–123.

March, J. (2004) Improved formulations for existing CBPP vaccines – recommendations for change. *Vaccine* 22, 4358–4364.

Mares, R.G. (2011) First appearance of bovine pleuropneumonia in southern Africa and some of its consequences. *Veterinary History* 11, 33–40.

Mariner, J.C. (2009) More appropriate disease control policies for the developing world. *The Onderstepoort Journal of Veterinary Research* 76(1), 135–140.

Masiga, W.N., Domenech, J. and Windsor, R.S. (1996) Manifestation and epidemiology of contagious bovine pleuropneumonia in Africa. *Revue Scientifique et Technique de l'OIE* 15(4), 1283–1308.

McAuliffe, L., Ayling, R.D. and Nicholas, R.A.J. (2007) Identification and characterization of variable-number tandem-repeat markers for the molecular epidemiological analysis of *Mycoplasma mycoides* subspecies *mycoides* SC. *FEMS Microbiology Letters* 276(2), 181–188.

Mitchell, J.D., McKellar, Q.A. and McKeever, D.J. (2012) Pharmacodynamics of antimicrobials against *Mycoplasma mycoides* small colony, the causative agent of contagious bovine pleuropneumonia. *PLOS ONE* 7(8), e44158.

Molla, W., Jemberu, W.T., Mekonnen, S.A., Tuli, G. and Almaw, G. (2021) Seroprevalence and risk factors of contagious bovine pleuropneumonia in selected districts of north Gondar zone, Ethiopia. *Frontiers in Veterinary Science* 8, 626253.

Musisi, F.L., Dungu, B., Twala, R., Mogajane, M.E. and Mtei, B.J. (2006) The threat of contagious bovine pleuropneumonia and challenges for its control in SADC region. Rome FAO. *Towards Sustainable CBPP Control Programmes for Africa*. Available at: www.fao.org//docrep/007/y5510e/y5510e0d.htm?sfgdata=4 (accessed 5 February 2025).

Muuka, G., Otina, B., Wesonga, H., Bowa, B., Gicheru, N. *et al.* (2019) Evaluation of new generation macrolides for the treatment and metaphylaxis of contagious bovine pleuropneumonia (CBPP) in cattle experimentally infected with *Mycoplasma mycoides* subspecies *mycoides*. *BMC Veterinary Research* 15(1), 451.

Ngounda, P., Manso-Silván, L. and Thiaucourt, F. (2021) Situation actuelle de la péripneumonie contagieuse bovine en République Centrafricaine. DOI: 10.48327/mtsibulletin.2021.100.

Nicholas, R.A.J. (2009) Contagious bovine pleuropneumonia: In search of the origins and virulence of lung sickness. *Microbiologist* 10, 41–43.

Nicholas, R.A.J. (2023) Contagious bovine pleuropneumonia: A passage to india. *Animals* 13, 2151.

Nocard, E. and Leclainche, E. (1898) *Les maladies microbiennes des animaux*, 2nd edition. Masson, Paris.

OIE (1994) *Meeting of the Ad Hoc Group on CBPP: Recommended Standards for Epidemiological Surveillance for CBPP*. OIE, Paris.

Nicholas, R.A.J., Aschenborn, H.K.O., Ayling, R.D., Loria, G.R., Lukhele, O. *et al.* (2007) Effect of Advocin on the elimination of CBPP from the Caprivi Region of Namibia. In: *CBPP Control: Antibiotics to the rescue. Proceedings of FAO-OIE-AU/IBAR-IAEA. Consultative Group Meeting on CBPP in Africa, 2006*, FAO, Rome, Italy, pp. 33–40.

Nicholas, R.A.J., Ayling, R.D. and McAuliffe, L. (2008) Contagious bovine pleuropneumonia. In: *Mycoplasma Diseases of Ruminants*. CABI, Wallingford, UK, pp. 69–97.
Olorunshola, I.D., Daodu, O., Lawal, A.N., Oloweni, F.R., Adegboye, D.S. *et al.* (2021) Prevalence and risk factors of contagious bovine pleuropneumonia in Kwara state. *Tropical Veterinarian* 39, 2–18.
Owen, G.E. (1926) First annual report of the veterinary department for the year 1925. London.
Pieres, J.B. (1989) *The Dead Will Arise*. James Currey, London, pp. 166–167.
PRAPS and World Bank (2019) Disclosable Version of the ISR Regional Sahel Pastrolism Support Project-P147674. Available at: https://documents1.worldbank.org/curated/en/519791555625275805/pdf/Disclosable-Version-of-the-ISR-Regional-Sahel-Pastoralism-Support-Project-P147674-Sequence-No-09.pdf (accessed 14 March 2025).
Provost, A., Perreau, P., Bréard, A., Le Goff, C., Martel, J.L. *et al.* (1987) Contagious bovine pleuropneumonia. *Revue Scientifique et Technique. International Office of Epizootics* 6, 625–679.
Salmon, D.E. (1896) Contagious pleuro-pneumonia. Special report on diseases of cattle and on cattle feeding. Government Printing Office, Washington, DC.
Schieck, E., Liljander, A., Hamsten, C., Gicheru, N., Scacchia, M. *et al.* (2014) High antibody titres against predicted mycoplasma surface proteins do not prevent sequestration in infected lung tissue in the course of experimental contagious bovine pleuropneumonia. *Veterinary Microbiology* 172(1–2), 285–293.
Sousa, M.F., Duarte, V.M.S. and Soares, A.E. (1975) Le problème de la Péripneumonie Contagieuse des bovins en Angola. *Bulletin de l'Office International Des Épizooties* 84, 451–462.
Stanley, H.M. (1896) *Magdala: The Story of the Abyssinian Campaign of 1866–7*. Sampson Low, Marston and Company, London.
Tambi, N.E., Maina, W.O. and Ndl, C. (2006) An estimation of the economic impact of contagious bovine pleuropneumonia in Africa. *Revue Scientifique et Technique. International Office of Epizootics* 25, 999–1011.
Tweyongyere, R., Nkamwesiga, J., Etiang, P., Mugezi, I., Wamala, H. *et al.* (2024) Seroprevalence of contagious bovine pleuropneumonia (CBPP) in cattle from Karamoja Region, north-eastern Uganda. *BMC Veterinary Research* 20(1), 97.
Wade, A., Yaya, A., El-Yuguda, A.D., Unger, H., Nafarnda, D.W. *et al.* (2015) The prevalence of contagious bovine pleuropneumonia in Cameroon: A case study Garoua Central Abattoir, Cameroun. *Journal of Veterinary Medical Research* 2(4), 1029.
Weiss, H. (1998) Dying cattle: Some remarks on the impact of cattle epizootics in the Central Sudan during the nineteenth century. *African Economic History* 26(26), 173.
Williams, H. (1940) *Annual Report of the Sudan Veterinary Service, 1939*. Sudan Veterinary Service.
World Organisation for Animal Health (WOAH) (2018) *Annual Report*. Paris, OIE. Available at: https://www.oie.int/scientific-expertise/reference-laboratories/annual-reports/ (accessed 25 June 2024).
Yansambou, M.S., Diallo, A.A., Idi, M., Gagara, H., Haido, A.M. *et al.* (2018) Serological prevalence of contagious bovine pleuropneumonia in Niger in 2017. *Frontiers in Veterinary Science* 5, 238. DOI: 10.3389/fvets.2018.00238.
Yaya, A., Manso-Silván, L., Blanchard, A. and Thiaucourt, F. (2008) Genotyping of *Mycoplasma mycoides* subsp. *mycoides* small colony by multilocus sequence analysis allows molecular epidemiology of contagious bovine pleuropneumonia. *Veterinary Research* 39(2), 14–18.

7 Pleuro Goes Down Under

Abstract

The introduction of CBPP into Australia in 1858 became a slowly unfolding tragedy that would persist for over a century, infecting all states, killing hundreds of thousands of cattle and ruining the livelihoods of countless livestock owners, while the authorities often appeared indifferent, and actions taken, if any, were mostly ineffective. To make matters worse globally, the Australian livestock industry soon began to export cattle and was the source of infection for many Pacific Ocean countries including New Zealand, perhaps as early as 1861, and the Far East where it had a major impact on herds in China. While the history of the disease in Australia is relatively well known, its invasion of New Zealand has attracted less attention. But, unlike Australia, New Zealand eradicated the disease within a decade of infection using a mixture of movement control, stamping out and crude vaccination.

Australia

The Arrival of CBPP

Much is known about the circumstances surrounding the introduction in a single animal of CBPP or 'pleuro', as it became known to Australian farmers. The infected heifer, bred by Mr Jefferson of Preston Hall, was named 'St Bees' after the village in Cumbria, in the north of England, where she had originated. She was shipped in the *Copenhagen*, arriving in the newly established independent state of Victoria in October 1858, after 99 days at sea with a group of other Shorthorn cattle destined for Mr Boadle's farm at Darebin Creek, just outside the fast-growing town of Melbourne (Fig. 7.1). Some uncertainty exists over the condition of the animal during the passage, some saying she was silently incubating CBPP but, according to Bruce and Loir (1891), two French veterinarians visiting a few years later, she was infected before purchase, 'treated and cured', then relapsed shortly after arriving in Australia and died within a few weeks. Before dying, she infected Mr Boadle's resident cattle but, presumably, her Shorthorn shipmates on that long journey must also have been infected, though there is no record of their condition. So, perhaps the 'single infected animal infecting Australia' hypothesis must be questioned. Nonetheless, reports of sickness and death began to emerge from Boadle's farm and a meeting was held in September 1859 (nearly a year after St Bees had arrived) by local farmers concerned it was CBPP. Under their instruction, a local veterinarian, John Miscamble, confirmed their worst suspicions after post-mortem examination of the infected cattle (Newton, 1992). A decision was subsequently taken to slaughter the herd and pay compensation but this did not happen for another 11 months. Remarkably, the disease had remained confined to Boadle's farm for several months despite 23 of his cattle dying and 5 showing clinical signs; inevitably, the disease broke out in a neighbouring farm owned by a Mr Hooper. Hooper's herd was slaughtered, revealing nearly half of his 123 animals to have CBPP lesions. It was later discovered that the breakout was due to the trespassing on Boadle's land of working bullocks owned by another neighbour. Two of the bullocks died, the remainder were sold and dispersed and the rest, as they say, is history. The CSIRO website excellently describes it as: 'like a flame running after a trail of spilled paraffin, pleuropneumonia roared up the overland route to New South Wales.'

At the time, there was no legislation to control animal disease in Victoria and it was difficult to interest the government, despite urgent petitioning by livestock associations seeking 'prompt measures to arrest the ravages of the disease' even with further evidence of spread.

DOI: 10.1079/9781800627536.0007

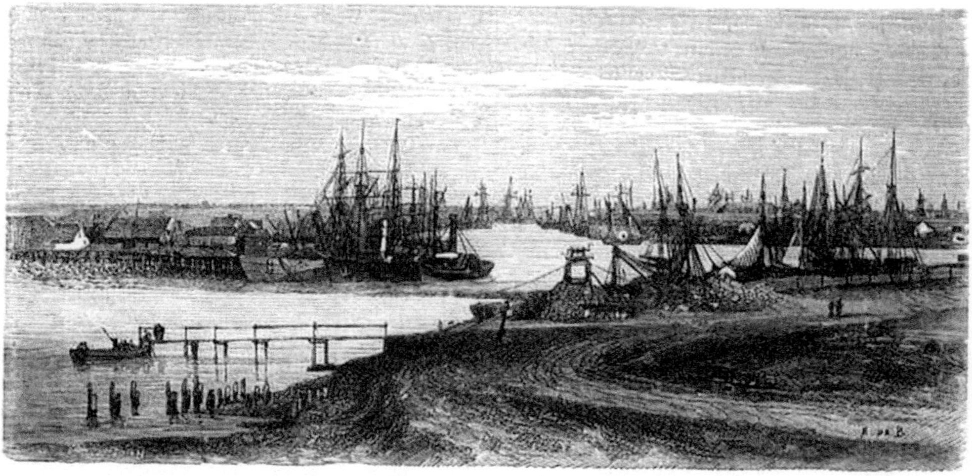

Fig. 7.1. Melbourne Harbour in the 19th century where CBPP was first introduced. (From Évremond de Bérard, 1861, *Le Tour du Monde*, public domain via Wikimedia Commons.)

Finally, an Act was passed in April 1861 but, by then, the barn door had been closed and the infected cattle had long since bolted.

The requirement for cattle to feed an ever-increasing population in Victoria, some of whom had been attracted by the discovery of gold in 1851, meant the acquisition of animals from all over Australia, including the northernmost territories and southern Queensland. Breeding cattle was also sourced from Britain, some of which, like 'St Bees', were not always in the best health upon landing. These conditions provided a perfect environment for disease spread, accelerated by the reliance on bullock teams to transport goods around the country (Fig. 7.2). And, within months of its escape from Boadle's farm, CBPP spread rapidly along the entire track from Melbourne to Beechworth, a distance of 200 miles (Pullar, 1965).

The state government's inaction at the spread of CBPP throughout the country is not too difficult to understand. These were early days in the understanding of 'contagion', and disease at that time was generally thought to be caused by 'miasmic influences or cold foggy weather' or spontaneous generation (Anonymous, 2024). The term 'virus' was used initially as a synonym for poison but gained a more scientific meaning when French researchers later discovered that the CBPP 'virus' could pass through filters that usually held back micro-organisms.

A royal commission, exclusively of medical men, had been set up as early as 1862 to investigate whether CBPP was contagious, whether inoculation was beneficial and whether the consumption of meat from infected cattle was safe. The omission of veterinarians from the committee was criticized but may have reflected the divergent opinions of the veterinary profession at the time. Extraordinarily (well at least from a 20th-century perspective), the commission could find: 'no evidence of contagion and considered the slaughter of diseased animals and restrictions on movements were unnecessary and undesirable, ...saw no value in inoculation, and [correctly] believed the meat from affected animals was wholesome' (Newton, 1992, p. 306).

The commission seemed intent on agreeing with an earlier British inquiry that had reached similar conclusions. Based on this evidence, the state government allowed its 1861 legislation to lapse, setting back control of CBPP for several decades.

The great escape

Very soon, diseased herds (or mobs, as they are called in Australia) crossed the border into the

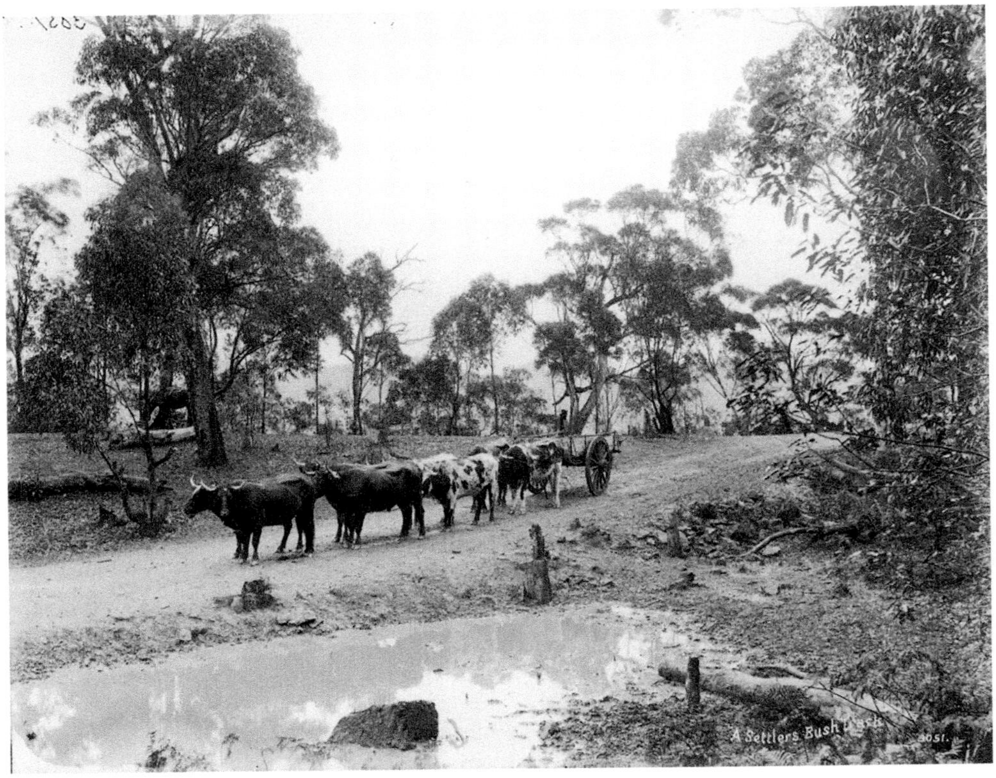

Fig. 7.2. Bullock teams were the primary means of moving goods and CBPP around Australia in the mid 19th century. (From Anonymous, c.1900, Powerhouse Museum, public domain via Wikimedia Commons.)

neighbouring colony of New South Wales and from there into South Australia in 1863. CBPP was then trekked north to Queensland and the Northern Territory before reaching Darwin in 1881, 23 years after its arrival on Australian soil, amounting to an extraordinary distance of 4200 km by road. Having no railways at the time, cattle were subjected to huge journeys across Australia on specially marked trails varying in length from 500 to 1500 miles, with one epic journey covering 3000 miles from New South Wales to Kimberley taking an extraordinary 2 years to complete (Fig. 7.3). On average, herds would cover 8–10 miles a day often over unforgiving ground, taking some 2–6 months to reach their destination. If they became infected on the way or had contained CBPP-incubating animals at the start, a herd of 1500–2000 may have expected to lose a quarter to a third of its stock (Bruce and Loir, 1891). Later shiploads of cattle would be transported from Melbourne and Darwin to Perth in Western Australia, and from Darwin to Brisbane, taking CBPP with them.

By the end of the 19th century, pleuro was enzootic throughout northern Australia, home to nearly 5 million cattle. From here, it would frequently find its way south again and, even more alarmingly, to Pacific countries far and wide, including New Zealand, China, Japan and Korea; Hong Kong then a British colony may have been infected as early as 1885 (Newton, 1992). As a result, overseas markets were either closed for varying periods of time to Australian cattle, or animals were admitted only after being tested, causing considerable damage to the export trade (Paterson, 1998).

In the early years when CBPP began to spread rapidly, it behaved as a virulent epidemic with losses of up to 75% in newly infected herds, but soon mortality began to decrease and its virulence abated – a common feature of this disease in Africa – largely as a result of herds

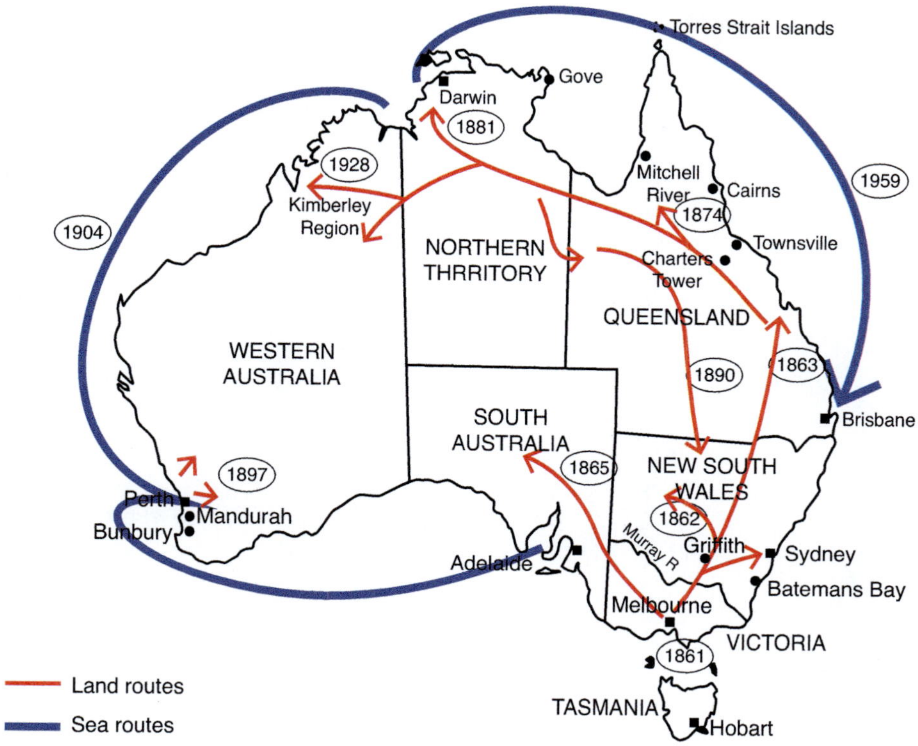

Fig. 7.3. Main routes of CBPP that spread within Australia between 1861 and 1959. (From Robin Nicholas.)

gaining immunity through exposure. Only in naïve herds did it continue to cause severe losses. It has been estimated that in the first 15 years, CBPP was responsible for the deaths of 1.4 million cattle valued, at the time, at £8.5 million; and in Queensland alone, 4% of the cattle population died within 2 years (Newton, 1992). The only other livestock disease having a similar impact at the time was tick-borne fever.

The huge size of the country meant that the authorities had to battle the disease in two different climatic zones: (i) the south and east, largely similar to British conditions with small intensively managed stock where well-tried control measures could be applied successfully; and (ii) a much larger tropical region in the north where holdings were huge, often unfenced with thinly populated stock able to move freely from one farm to another especially during the rainy seasons. In some respects, these latter conditions were similar to sub-Saharan Africa but vastly different in that Australian cattle could only be rounded up once or twice a year; in contrast, herdsman, particularly in East Africa, constantly tend their animals, collecting them together in kraals at night. Such conditions in the Northern Territory and Queensland made CBPP control an almost impossible task and explains why it continued for so long.

The Queensland government was becoming alarmed at the rapid spread of CBPP through New South Wales and quickly passed legislation to prevent its introduction. Inspectors, appointed specifically for this task, examined 27,000 cattle in the 5 months beginning January 1862 but failed to detect a single case. One must ask today what training these officials had because this is a very difficult disease to detect clinically, even for veterinarians. Despite this, it was not until the following year, after the suspension of the legislation due to pressure from pastoralists, that the first outbreak occurred on the border with New South Wales; then, more worryingly, it appeared at Rockhampton 500 miles deep into

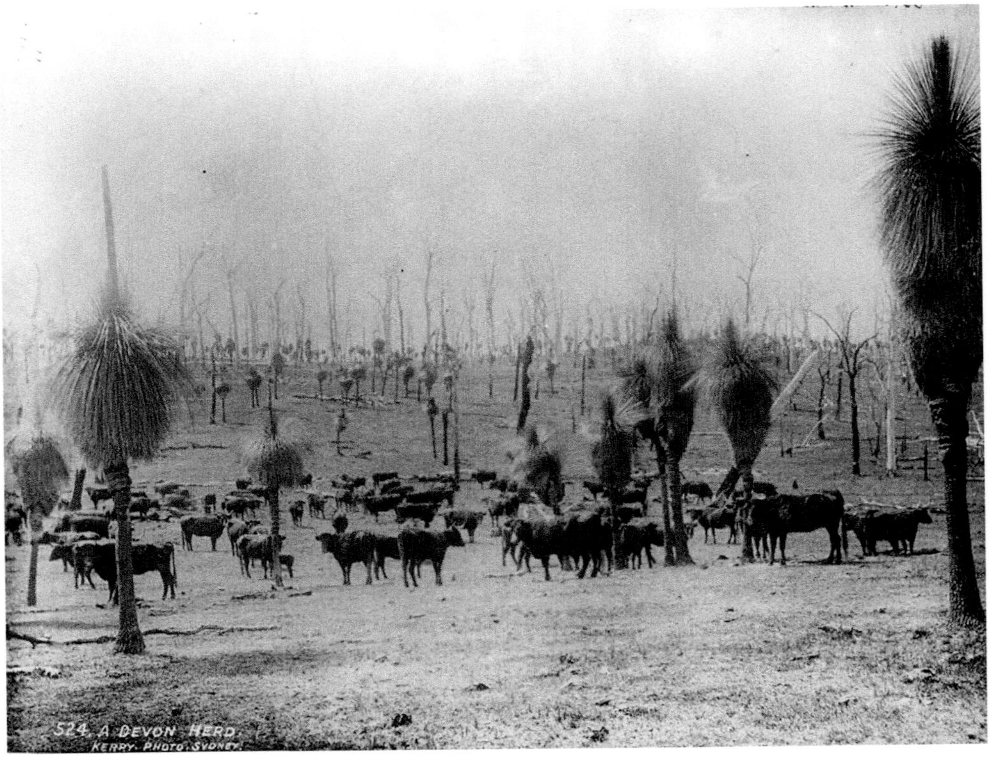

Fig. 7.4. Australian cattle assembling in Victoria for the long trek northwards. (From Anonymous, c.1900, Powerhouse Museum, public domain via Wikimedia Commons.)

Queensland. Re-establishment of the widely ignored legislation, appointments of select committees and even enabling compensation had no effect and, as Newton described:

'The disease spread out from the great north road like branches of a tree and most of Queensland was involved by 1870' (Newton, 1992, p. 307).

The spread of the disease into the Northern Territory was accelerated by the Australian government's granting of land leases in the late 1870s (Fig. 7.4). Very quickly, stock moved from Queensland into the new lands and with them, inevitably, CBPP, with first outbreaks seen near Darwin in 1881. Two years later, it had crossed the border into the Kimberley region of Western Australia and CBPP's conquest of Australia was complete. Its impact would ebb and flow for the next few decades while the authorities were slowly forced to intervene. Indeed, until 1889 there was no coordinated action between the fiercely independent states.

First attempts to control 'Pleuro'

In the absence of any meaningful state involvement, stockowners quickly took the means to control the disease into their own hands. In August 1860, Graham Mitchell, a Scottish veterinarian practising near Melbourne, became the first to use 'inoculation' following a method pioneered by Louis Willems a decade earlier in Belgium. Willems had shown that injecting small drops of inflammatory exudate or 'virus' from diseased lungs into the tip of the tail of healthy cattle protected the majority from acquiring CBPP. While this crude vaccination had been met with suspicion and disbelief by the veterinary profession in Great Britain, it was eagerly and widely taken up in Australia.

Another early proponent of 'inoculation' was John Miscamble, who treated his first severely affected herd 2 years later with a mixture of lung and trachea extract from a

CBPP case using the tail tip method (Miscamble, 1863). Losses were reported to have been reduced immediately, which is rather surprising given that many of the cattle must have been incubating the disease. Regardless, Miscamble saw the commercial potential of this approach and marketed a product curiously called 'absorbent' – 'No other remedy, less expensive, so easy of application, or giving better results has ever been recommended' (Miscamble, 1863).

It was mainly due to the adoption of vaccination by the Victoria State Veterinary Services that the disease came under reasonable control by the end of the century. Miscamble was not modest about his achievement and, although reporting some adverse reactions in about 1% of vaccinated cattle, declared: 'My mode has proved harmless....and a sure preventative of pleuro-pneumonia- the worst scourge that has ever attacked the cattle on a thousand hills' (Miscamble, 1863, p. 111).

Independently minded New South Wales (as all Australian states would become in their control of CBPP) took a more circuitous, though perhaps more rational, route to control when the disease broke out there in 1861. It appointed an inspector of cattle, Alexander Bruce, a poundkeeper from Holbrook, who quickly recognized the futility of culling only overtly sick cattle and instigated whole herd slaughter with compensation. He also took a much more scientific approach to 'inoculation' comparing many methods before recommending one that involved inserting a thread soaked in 'virus' into the tail using a spaying needle (Fig. 7.5). He advocated the compulsory use of vaccination and was one of the first Australians to believe the disease was contagious.

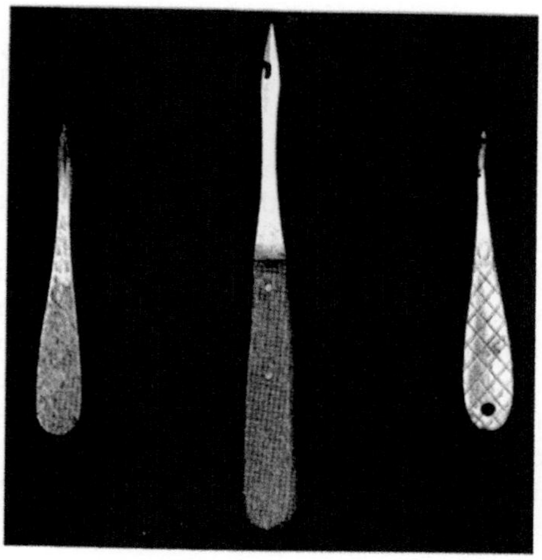

Fig. 7.5. Knives used for inoculation of cattle. (With permission from CSIRO Australia.)

In the southern states where farms with high stocking density and restricted cattle movement, vaccination was highly successful together with other measures such as quarantine, movement controls and slaughter. This approach was impractical in the big herds of the north as 'virus' could not be stored for any length of time. The solution conducted by the visiting French veterinarians from the Pasteur Institute, Bruce and Loir (1891), was to inoculate the virus into the so-called *'partie défendue* [forbidden parts]' of the animal, that is in a place other than the tail and usually behind the shoulder resulting in an oedema which contained large quantities of the pathogen. Thus, a supply of inoculum was always at the disposal of 'inoculators' by maintaining a calf in an infected state. Bruce and Loir reported that the material could be harvested from the oedema before the calf died which usually occurred within 2 weeks of inoculation. Owners wishing to send their cattle to market would obtain the virus from a vaccine-producing station and inoculate their herd via the tail route. It was recorded that, in one instance, after a journey of 1500 miles, all vaccinated cattle in a large herd arrived in good condition while just about half of unvaccinated cattle had died, proving the value of inoculation.

However, these attempts to control the disease were no more than pinpricks as the disease spread into the huge trackless pastures of the north. The following gives an accurate and tragic insight into the havoc CBPP was causing:

> Farmers felt panic and despair that is hard to comprehend these days. For many of them, living in hand-hewn huts on properties that were little better than virgin bushland, their cattle were their only asset and livelihood. Pleuropneumonia struck their stock with a swiftness and contagion that seemed uncanny. (Only quite recently it has been found that a coughing cow can spray infection for nearly 100 metres.) Diseased cattle would cough, slobber and stand with necks outstretched, gasping for air. They went off their milk as soon as they

became sick. Those that did not die were often disease-carriers and would have been safer dead, but before 1925 there was no compensation and slaughtered cattle were a total loss. (CSIRO, n.d.)

Some consensus among the states began to emerge following the Australian Stock Conference in 1889, chief of which was compulsory vaccination when the disease appeared and that vaccinated cattle, distinguished by an inoculation earmark, should be allowed freedom of movement. This was a neat compromise between disease control and commercial interests though this was slow to get off the ground. Finally, a decade later, the following measures were put in place by all states.

1. Compulsory notification of CBPP.
2. Destruction of affected animals.
3. Quarantine of infected herds.
4. Vaccination of all in-contact animals.

As seen with vaccination earlier, these measures were much easier to apply in the south. Here, the *coup de grâce* for CBPP was the passing of the Cattle Compensation Act in 1925, whereby owners of both diseased and in-contact cattle were compensated, leading to cases plummeting particularly in Victoria at the end of the 1920s (Table 7.1).

Sporadic outbreaks would continue in the south for the next 30 or so years but these, mostly originating in the north, were manageable. During the first half of the 20th century, the endemic areas of CBPP covered the north-east part of Western Australia, north-west Northern Territory and a large part of Queensland. It was here that a major effort to control and eradicate CBPP would be directed but this would need more than policy and homemade vaccine: it would require the appliance of science.

Table 7.1. Number of cases of CBPP recorded in Victoria between 1924 and 1929. (From Robin Nicholas.)

Year	Outbreaks
1924	48
1925	86
1926	84
1927	60
1928	14
1929	4

The age of technology

Although the teaching of veterinary science began at Melbourne University in 1888, Australia was highly dependent on British and other European assistance to deal with disease outbreaks during the late 19th and early 20th centuries. And so it was with CBPP, with experts from the Pasteur Institute and Edinburgh University, in particular, advising on control strategies often with mixed and confusing messages. The first significant step to developing its own expertise was the establishment of the Commonwealth Scientific and Industrial Research Organisation (CSIRO) in 1916. To combat the increasing risk and realities of tick-borne diseases and CBPP, a research station was built in 1932 at Oonoonba, Townsville, in Queensland, to study these animal diseases in a tropical environment.

Until well into the early 1930s, the only way to diagnose CBPP was to observe variable and often non-specific clinical signs and the detection of pathological lesions in the lungs at post-mortem which were not always pathognomonic. Other respiratory diseases like tuberculosis and pasteurellosis could resemble CBPP, particularly in the early stages of infection. Furthermore, cattle carrying the disease would often show no clinical signs at all.

A great deal of work had been going on from the late 19th century, especially in France, to culture the causative pathogen, and cell-free bacteriological media had been developed to grow and study the 'virus' morphologically (Nocard and Roux, 1990). Microscopic examination revealed long-branching mycelium-like filaments, from which tiny particles that could pass through filters were produced.

While these studies were fundamental in understanding the pathogen and would later enable the growth of vaccine antigens, an urgent requirement at this stage of the epidemic in Australia was an accurate and specific test that could detect infected animals.

A breakthrough came in the early 1930s from a group working at the newly established

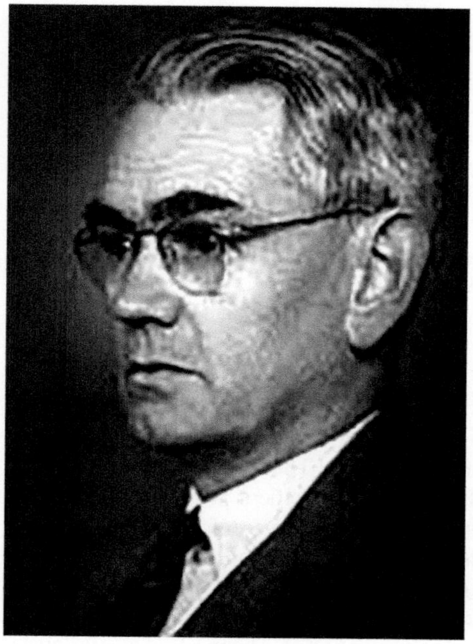

Fig. 7.6. Arthur William Turner studied the CBPP pathogen and developed many diagnostic tests. (Photo courtesy of Australian Academy of Science.)

research station at Oonoonba, led by Drs Campbell and Turner (Fig. 7.6) who adapted a partly developed serological test, the complement fixation test (CFT), for CBPP using an *M. m. mycoides* antigen extracted from the pleural fluid of an infected animal. The test was modified later when a culture-grown antigen was produced enabling a much more reliable and consistent test for detecting specific antibodies in the sera of infected cattle. The Campbell – Turner CFT, as it became known, was used worldwide and, indeed, is still used across Africa though modified later to a much more convenient microtitre system (Campbell and Turner, 1953).

Once standardized and interpretation established using an experimentally infected herd kept near the station, the CFT was rolled out to test sera from the field. Large numbers of sera were tested from Western Australia from 1934 onwards, enabling the movement of herds free of CBPP antibodies to markets. This proved very successful and soon up to 4000 animals were being tested yearly. It was so successful, in fact, that the states of Victoria and New South Wales, unhappy with the adverse reactions and incomplete protection of the current vaccine, began to use the CFT to eliminate outbreaks using test and slaughter. Results were only partially successful so vaccination was re-established in tandem with test and slaughter. Strict movement controls and quarantine lines were also set up to provide greater protection from infected cattle from Queensland.

To supplement the CFT, Turner developed an antigen-detection test, called the tube precipitin test, that could be carried out on acute and chronic lung lesions to enable more accurate diagnosis. Though less sensitive than the CFT, the precipitin could be used on animals that gave false-negative reactions in the CFT due to excessive production of CBPP antigen by an infected animal, not an infrequent occurrence.

A major logistical problem remained the transport of samples over hundreds, if not thousands, of miles to laboratories capable of CBPP testing. Samples could deteriorate due to the climate or poor storage conditions and provide material not fit for testing. Additionally, the time from sampling to testing could mean that the herd may have moved great distances by the time the results were available – this being especially true in sub-Saharan Africa. A test that could be carried out and interpreted in the field would be desirable. In 1963, Turner described a simple slide agglutination test in which serum or blood could be mixed with stained *M. m. mycoides*; clumping or agglutination on a slide reaction would indicate the presence of specific CBPP antibodies (Turner and Etheridge, 1963). Despite a lack of sensitivity, the test could detect most positive herds and could be perfomed in mobile laboratories that were being increasingly used across the states. This test was shown later to be highly effective in Portugal and Nigeria when improved by Ayling *et al.* (1999) using antigen-coated coloured latex beads. It should be remembered that CBPP control is primarily aimed at the herd level so developing expensive tests of ever-increasing sensitivity for mass screening is not necessary or helpful (Olorunshola *et al.*, 2017).

Turner's work on the growth of the CBPP agent logically turned to vaccine development in 1932. Vaccines up to this time were crude lung extracts or pleural fluid from diseased animals which had highly variable outcomes sometimes leading to adverse reactions and, it was believed, CBPP itself, though hard evidence for this was lacking. An acid digest liquid medium with added bovine serum, formulated by Turner and colleagues, allowed the fast growth of various local isolates of *M. m. mycoides* which could be used to produce 'cleaner' vaccines. Finding one that had the right balance of virulence and immunogenicity was not easy but trials led eventually to the stable V5 strain isolated in Victoria in 1936. The vaccine was made from 4-day-old cultures and continued to be used until CBPP was eradicated. Early batches of the vaccine had a shelf life of only a couple of months so frequent quantities were required until lyophilization greatly improved stability.

The road to eradication

It would be a mistake to get the impression that the various control measures introduced in the 1930s led to immediate improvements. Outbreaks continued to occur and, in 1952, one of the worst occurred in New South Wales and spilled over to Victoria via a carrier animal from Queensland (Newton, 1992). Smaller epidemics again occurred in 1956–1957 which led to a tightening of regulations. So, by a range of measures including compulsory vaccination of travelling stock, the establishment of quarantine, protected and CBPP-free areas where cattle could be carefully monitored, abattoir surveillance and extra funding from both state and federal government, CBPP was slowly coming under control. But what really accelerated the process was the development of road and rail transport systems for moving cattle to abattoirs and other properties. It began in the 1930s when a small road train was introduced in the Northern Territory to move cattle to markets quickly and by 1965 three-quarters of the Territory's animals were transported in this way. Similar improvements in transport took place in Queensland in the early 1960s. It was believed, correctly, that by reducing stress, transport time and fatigue, animals were less likely to become infected by contact (Newton, 1992).

In 1965, Henry Edward Albiston, one of the longest-serving members of the Veterinary Faculty of Melbourne University and long-time editor of the *Australian Veterinary Journal*, wrote: 'It is now at least 7 years since pleuropneumonia was active in southern Australia and during this period New South Wales, Victoria, South Australia and Western Australia with the exception of the Kimberleys have been free from disease' (Newton, 1992).

After 1967, no further cases were seen and Australia was declared free of CBPP in 1972, some 110 years after its arrival.

New Zealand

On the 5th April 1864, a well-attended meeting of New Zealand settlers at the Criterion Hotel, Otahuhu, a few kilometres from Auckland on the North Island discussed the as yet unsubstantiated rumours that CBPP (referred to as 'this dreadful scourge') was infecting cattle in the country (Anonymous, 1864). The meeting was organized by the Agricultural Society and chaired by the president of the association, John Grigg. In a letter of apology read out by Grigg at the meeting, the veterinary superintendent, Thomas Spencer, said he was on his way to the 'Front' (as he described it) to see for himself and was dreading what he would find; he was most concerned about a report that: 'working bullocks belonging to the Transport Corps taking the disease which of all cattle are most predisposed to take and propagate it' (Anonymous, 1864, p. 488).

Unambiguous evidence was then presented by Grigg shocking many of the farmers and graziers. He then pointed out the startling truth: 'that the meeting would therefore have no effect on preventing the introduction of the disease, but might nevertheless be useful in arresting its progress' (Anonymous, 1864, p. 488).

Grigg had drawn up a series of clear and farsighted resolutions that he hoped would find agreement amongst the interested parties.

Given the very close trading links, shared ownership and similar farming conditions between Australia and New Zealand, it was inevitable that CBPP would be exported to New Zealand during its pastoral expansion of agriculture. And, in 1863, CBPP was introduced via affected cattle to the provinces of Otago and Southland on the South Island (Fig. 7.7). Cattle numbers had increased rapidly particularly in

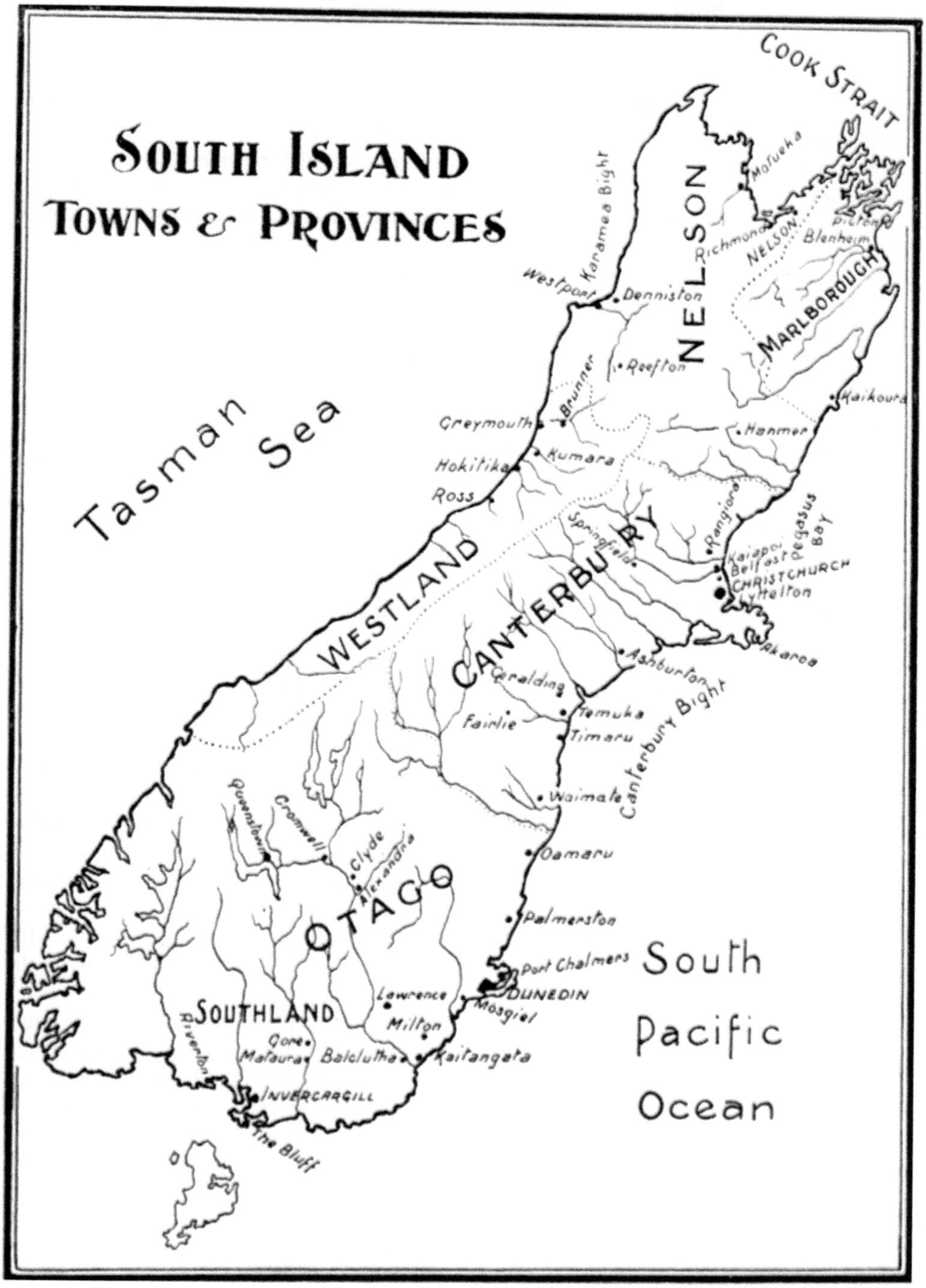

Fig. 7.7. New Zealand in the mid-19th century showing the CBPP-infected provinces of Otago and Southland following its arrival from Australia through the port of Dunedin. (From MacDonald Gill, 1931, The Empire Marketing Board, public domain via Wikimedia Commons.)

Otago in the 1860s, in part to satisfy the high demand caused by the huge influx of miners during the gold rushes of the time and to feed the army embroiled in the war with the Maoris.

While, in theory, live cattle imports from Australia had been banned by the central government, pressure, both commercial and political, on the Otago provincial administration ensured an easing of the restrictions, leading inevitably to the introduction of infected cattle among the nearly 8000 animals imported in 1863 alone (Fisher, 2006). Probably the first of many infected batches were shipped from New South Wales in the *Tessie May* during the year along with dubious animal health certificates. Two weeks later the disease had spread widely and over the porous border to Southland, and its local newspaper, *The Southland News*, complained sarcastically 'that Southland is indebted to Otago for the introduction of pleuro-pneumonia' (Fisher, 2006).

This statement was to prove somewhat unfair as a separate outbreak occurred in Southland itself shortly afterwards. There were no barriers to the dissemination of the disease: grazing between the two provinces was contiguous, no accepted method of branding had been established and rustling or *duffing*, as it was known locally, was common (Fisher, 2006). The official response, as seen also in Australia, was ineffectual with widely different interpretations of the legislation made by the provinces, some of whom, like Canterbury, imposed complete bans on live importation from Australia; others like Southlands were more selective as to which part of Australia they bought their cattle from. Marborough, on the other hand, banned all meat imports even from the other New Zealand provinces though this had more to do with commercial advantage than disease threat.

Control of the disease throughout the South Island was beyond the experience of local inspectors, unsure of their arbitrary powers, as they watched helplessly as bullock teams, one of the main means of disease spread, passed through their districts with impunity. There were also economic considerations in both provinces anxious to do things on the cheap which hampered inspection. But many interests had to be catered for including the livestock agencies who found the restrictions on movement to be too disruptive to business and consumers who complained about the rising costs of meat and all associated provisions. In opposition to easing controls were the graziers who fattened cattle in disease-free areas and paid inspectors to check all cattle entering their districts. In the end, William Logie, Chief Inspector of Livestock for Otago, strongly recommended opening up the whole province as well as lifting the ban on live imports from Australia. To some, it seemed the completely wrong strategy to attempt eradication or even contain the disease, though to be fair the province maintained a system of inspection and enforced quarantine on live imports.

Paradoxically, and inexplicably to some, as restrictions were lifted the disease began to abate from both Otago and Southland where control had only ever been superficial, and by 1865 only a handful of cases were reported. Its rapid disappearance was ascribed at the time to the disease 'exhausting its virulence' and CBPP faded quickly from the farming memory.

The province of Canterbury which maintained an import ban, a strict exclusion policy, and was geographically protected by the Waitara River which could be easily policed, remained CBPP-free throughout the epidemic and helped prevent the spread of the disease northwards. Of course, no testing was available to chart the decline of the disease and cases continued sporadically into the mid-1870s probably from fresh Australian imports or, indeed, from pedigree cattle from Britain where CBPP was still ravaging the country.

So what was the explanation for the unprecedented decline in CBPP cases in the absence of any major control measures being applied even after many of these measures had been lifted? The answer appeared to be 'inoculation', as described by the Belgian veterinarian Louis Willems in 1852 and adapted widely in Australia very shortly after the epidemic took hold there. The injection of lung exudate on absorbent cotton, from a recently killed diseased animal, into the tail was widely practised as early as 1865 in Australia and the close links with New Zealand ensured that vaccination of cattle began apace, encouraged by the livestock agencies. They advised all cattle owners to adopt this preventative measure without delay as it is useless after pleuro-pneumonia has shown itself.

The procedure, often crudely applied, did not always 'take', particularly if the animal was already infected and was never more than

Table 7.2. Differences in factors concerning the CBPP epidemic between Australia and New Zealand. (From Robin Nicholas.)

Risk Factors	Australia	New Zealand
Disease duration	100 years	10 years
Herd size	30,000–50,000	100
Geography	Few barriers	Southern Alps/ Waitara River
Infected area	Extensive	Restricted
Transport/draft	Bullocks	Horse
Vaccination	Sporadic	Comprehensive
Climate	More variable	Milder

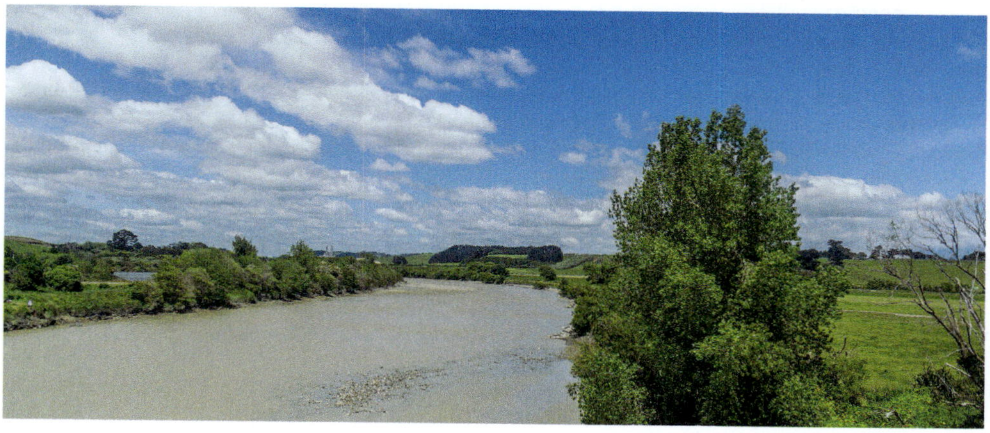

Fig. 7.8. River Waitara prevented the spread of CBPP northwards. (From Golik, 2017, Wikimedia Commons, CC BY 4.0.)

60–70% protective even when healthy cattle were vaccinated. Despite this, 'inoculation' was a 'game-changer' in the New Zealand pastoral environment, possibly as a result of the smaller herd sizes of an average of 100 animals; in comparison, Australian herds were massive, sometimes exceeding 40,000–50,000, making control much more difficult (Table 7.2).

There were even reports of Australian 'inoculators' providing this service to New Zealand farmers, for which they were reported to be satisfied as it greatly reduced losses to CBPP (Fisher, 2006). According to an Australian livestock owner, Mr Weston, who attended the Auckland meeting and had settled in New Zealand in the previous few months, inoculation could save at least 95% of vaccinated cattle (Anonymous, 1864), if done properly – a far higher protection rate than the T1/44 vaccine used today in Africa. Weather appeared to be an issue and he felt the milder winters in New Zealand could mitigate losses. Not everyone, however, was convinced that the method was safe and many veterinarians were openly hostile but as case numbers reduced, interest in CBPP and 'inoculation' waned.

Other unique features facilitated the control and eventual eradication of CBPP from the South Island. Geography was a major factor with the Southern Alps and the Waitara River providing an obstacle to disease spread (Fig. 7.8). Naturally, small numbers of outbreaks continued after 1865 but containment by vaccination and close monitoring backed up by slaughter of infected cattle ensured the end game was close.

The disappearance of CBPP, Fisher (2006) believed came without any concerted public action. New Zealand was probably the only country in the world, where once CBPP had become established, it was essentially private action that disposed of the threat.

References

Anonymous (2024). Available at: www.science.org.au/academy/memoirs/turner.htm (accessed 20 June 2024).

Anonymus (1864) Pleuropneumonia in New Zealand. *Edinburgh Veterinary Review* 6, 488–492.

Ayling, R.D., Regalla, J. and Nicholas, R.A.J. (1999) A field test for detecting antibodies to *Mycoplasma mycoides* subsp. *mycoides* SC using the latex slide agglutination test. In: Stipkovitis, L., Rosengarten, R. and Frey, J. (eds) *Mycoplasmas of Ruminants: Pathogenicity, Diagnosis, Epidemiology and Molecular Genetics*, Vol. 3. EU, Brussels, Belgium, pp. 155–158.

Bruce, A. and Loir, A. (1891) Les maladies du betail en Australie. *Annales de Institut Pasteur* 12, 177–183.

Campbell, A.D. and Turner, A.W. (1953) Studies of contagious bovine pleuropneumonia of cattle: IV. An improved complement fixation test. *Australian Veterinary Journal* 29, 154–163.

CSIRO (n.d.) Available at: https//csiropedia/csiro.au/contagious-bovine-pleuropneumonia-eradication (accessed 1 July 2024).

Fisher, J. (2006) The origins, spread and disappearance of contagious bovine pleuro-pneumonia in New Zealand. *Australian Veterinary Journal* 84(12), 439–444.

Miscamble, J. (1863) Pleuro-pneumonia in Australia. *Edinburgh Veterinary Review* 5, 109–112.

Newton, L.G. (1992) Contagious bovine pleuropneumonia in Australia: Some historic highlights from entry to eradication. *Australian Veterinary Journal* 69(12), 306–317.

Nocard, E. and Roux, E. (1990) The microbe of pleuropneumonia. *Reviews of Infectious Diseases* 12(2), 354–358.

Olorunshola, I.D., Peters, A.R., Scacchia, M. and Nicholas, R.A.J. (2017) Contagious bovine pleuropneumonia: Never out of Africa? *CABI Reviews* 12, 1–7.

Paterson, A.B. (1998) Contagious bovine pleuropneumonia (*Mycoplasma mycoides*). In: Parsonson, I. (ed.) *The Australian Ark: A History of Domesticated Animals in Australia*. CSIRO Publishing, Collingwood, Australia, pp. 187–207.

Pullar, E.M. (1965) Contagious bovine pleuropneumonia in Victoria 1858–61: Fate or folly? *Victorian Veterinary Proceedings* 66, 12–17.

Turner, A.W. and Etheridge, J.R. (1963) Slide agglutination tests in the diagnosis of contagious bovine pleuropneumonia. *Australian Veterinary Journal* 39(12), 445–451.

8 China: The Impact of CBPP on the Great Leap Forward

Abstract

Contagious bovine pleuropneumonia (CBPP) caused by *Mycoplasma mycoides* subsp. *mycoides*, was once the most damaging infectious animal disease in China. Between 1949 and 1989, the Chinese authorities estimated that nearly 180,000 cattle and yaks died of CBPP, causing estimated losses of 356 million Yuan (approximately US$52 million) that seriously impacted Mao Zedong's Great Leap Forward. In 1956, in an effort to control the disease, a virulent strain (Ben-1) isolated from a cow that had died of CBPP was attenuated by multiple passages of infected pleural fluid in rabbits. This vaccine was reported to have achieved a remarkable, if unlikely, protection rate of 100% in cattle with a duration of immunity of 28 months. To increase antigen yield, a vaccine was also prepared in domestic sheep (*Ovis aries*) but produced some adverse reactions in yaks. A modified vaccine prepared in Tibetan sheep (*Ovis ammon*) was adopted because it resulted in fewer complications in yaks and related species. However, despite making a significant impact on control, these vaccines would be ethically unacceptable these days. The last CBPP-infected animal was identified in 1989; since then no more cases have occurred and, in 1992, vaccination of cattle was stopped. In 2014, China was declared CBPP-free by the OIE. Unlike Africa, China had the advantage of a centrally controlled surveillance and eradication campaign which enabled a high level of vaccine coverage.

Introduction

From the beginning of the Chinese communist revolution in 1949 until relatively recently, China was a black hole of reliable information. What light did emerge showed a country in chaos, as disastrous agricultural reforms created one of the largest famines in human history, killing anywhere from 15 to 55 million people. CBPP exacerbated the disaster producing meat shortages and greatly reducing the numbers of draft cattle available for ploughing and as beasts of burden. This catastrophe was barely known outside China, and CBPP experts as late as 1987 felt confident in saying say that, while CBPP had been exported to China from Australia at around the 1920s, it had not become established (Provost *et al.*, 1987).

Slowly, however, papers emerged in English in the early 2000s providing insights into the damage that CBPP had done in China, often with surprising precision. First came discussions on the possible routes of infection, then appeared very detailed accounts of how many cattle died or were vaccinated, and finally how the Chinese authorities eradicated the disease.

According to Chen (1993), there were two possible routes by which CBPP was introduced into China. First, it could have been introduced to north-east China from the Lake Baikal region of Siberia in 1918, but this seems unlikely as CBPP was prevalent only in a few provinces of Northern China when surveillance was performed in 1949. Furthermore, the movement of cattle from the north to the rest of China would have been inhibited by the near-continuous wars in the regions between 1920 and the late 1940s. Secondly, and more likely, is that CBPP was introduced into China with the well-documented importation in 1919 of high-quality dairy cattle to Shanghai from Australia, which was widely infected at that time (Hudson, 1971). Some genetic evidence to support the Australian route of infection was described by Li *et al.* (2009) who compared Chinese mycoplasma strains isolated between 1953 and 1960 with two African and two recent European strains. Sequence analysis of the *lppB* gene, which codes for a lipoprotein unique to African/Australian strains, showed the Chinese and African strains to be identical. Their similarity was confirmed using multilocus sequence analysis and by immunoblotting using anti-*lppB* antiserum. The European strains tested

DOI: 10.1079/9781800627536.0008

here were isolated following the re-emergence of CBPP in Europe between 1980 and 1999 and were distinguished by an, as yet, unexplained 8.84 kb genomic deletion which was lacking from the Chinese strains.

Was Australia the Source of CBPP in the Far East?

There is compelling evidence to suggest that *M. m. mycoides* was carried to parts of Asia in Australian cattle. Its livestock producers were among the first of the nation's exporters, with live shipments beginning as early as 1829. Indeed, the opening of large cattle stations in the Northern Territory and Kimberley, the northernmost region of the state of Western Australia in the 1880s, was driven by the potential of exports to the newly emerging Asian markets. In 1889, large cattle shipments were sent to Hong Kong, Singapore, Indonesia and later the Philippines, but were suspended shortly afterwards because of a disease outbreak in the Northern Territory. Newton (1992) describes an outbreak of CBPP in a consignment of cattle destined for Hong Kong as early as 1885 but whether it became established in the British colony is unknown. It is not difficult to identify this disease as CBPP, which was ravaging Australia at the time, and there is little doubt that infected cattle were carried in those early consignments to contaminate those importing countries. The exporters must have convinced the Asian countries, somehow, that Australian cattle were CBPP-free because live trade appears to have resumed though on a smaller scale through the first half of the 20th century. And, as Hudson (1971) confirmed, high-quality dairy cattle entered Shanghai in 1912, initially with unreported consequences. While little is known about the fate of CBPP in those other early importing countries, it can be assumed that it died out shortly after its introduction. In China, however, the disease spread silently until the intensification of the cattle industry took place in the early 1950s with explosive results.

The impact of CBPP on the cattle population in China following its introduction has not been well researched in the West. However, in 1949, when the Chinese government began to intensify agricultural production during the Great Leap Forward, subsequently increasing the number and movements of cattle, the number of CBPP cases rose significantly. According to reports, over the next 40 years, the Chinese authorities, with remarkably detailed figures, recorded the loss of 178,570 cattle that had died from CBPP, reaching a peak of mortality in 1959 (Xin *et al.*, 2012) (Fig. 8.1). Like other countries, China began vaccinating against CBPP using locally isolated strains which were attenuated initially in rabbits then, to boost production, in two different sheep breeds: domestic sheep (*Ovis aires*) and the Tibetan sheep (*Ovis ammon*), also known as the argali or mountain sheep. These vaccines were extensively applied throughout affected regions of China to over 74.5 million cattle and yaks and helped to prevent the spread, and eventually led to the eradication, of CBPP.

1949–1962: CBPP Prevalence Before Vaccination

Between 1949 and 1962, the Chinese veterinary authorities calculated that a total of 153,771 cattle had died of CBPP, causing very severe economic losses. In 1949, CBPP outbreaks were reported in ten counties of the Chinese-controlled regions of Inner Mongolia, Heilongjiang, Xinjiang, Sichuan and Hebei, which affected just over 3000 cattle and killed about one-third (Fig. 8.2). The spread of CBPP continued in the 1950s with increased cattle movements. In 1958, CBPP was prevalent in 377 counties of Inner Mongolia, Liaoning, Jilin, Heilongjiang, Xinjiang, Qinghai, Shandong, Shanxi, Henan, Hebei, Beijing and Jiangsu, affecting 274,750 cattle of which 93,371 died. In 1958, following the introduction of CBPP-affected cattle from Inner Mongolia to the Anyang District of Henan Province, nearly 1000 cattle in 70 villages of 11 counties in Anyang were infected, of which 610 died, representing a mortality rate of over 60% (Hou *et al.*, 1994). The direct economic losses for Anyang were 1.1 million RMB and resulted in a severe shortage of animal labour and great damage to agricultural production. In 1959, the CBPP epidemic reached a peak in China with outbreaks reported in 325 counties of Hebei, Inner Mongolia, Liaoning, Jilin, Shandong, Henan,

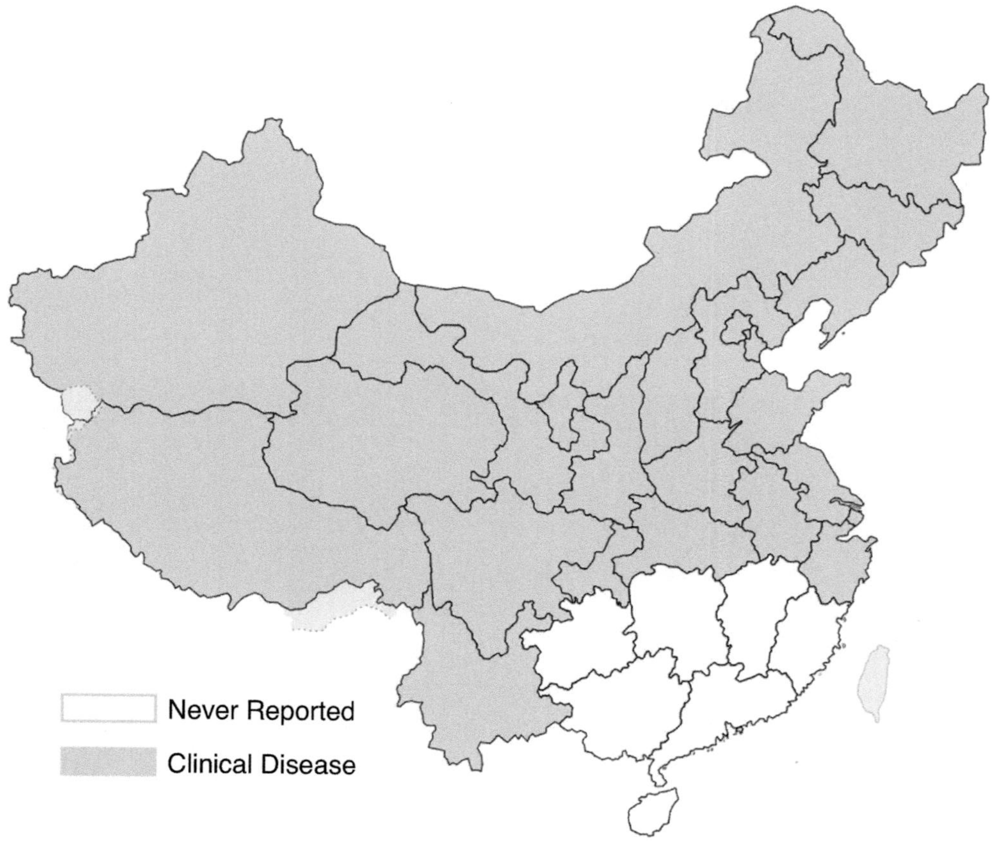

Fig. 8.1. CBPP spread to most parts of China between the 1950s and 1970s. (From Robin Nicholas.)

Yunnan, Qinghai, Xinjiang and Sichuan; 60,834 head of cattle were affected and 28,533 died representing a mortality rate of 47%. In addition, it was estimated in other areas of China that over 400,000 farm cattle were clinically infected and could not work on the farm. As China, in general, relied heavily on animal labour at this time, this was devastating for its agriculture.

Early Control Measures During the CBPP Epidemic

Due to these unacceptable losses, in the early 1950s, China urgently embarked on measures to control CBPP. This included vaccination using low virulent strains passaged in culture medium; surveillance and quarantine of infected cattle; and slaughtering of CBPP-infected and suspected cattle (Xin *et al.*, 2012). Although vaccination showed some success, these early vaccines were unstable and had short shelf lives because of the lack of freeze-drying equipment. So, from 1950 onwards, test and slaughter of seropositive cattle was the main control tool. Between 1952 and 1962, a total of 76,705 CBPP-infected cattle were culled, incurring huge financial burdens to the Chinese government at the time. These costs proved prohibitive for the complete control of CBPP, so cheaper and more effective methods were sought (Zhao and Jia, 1962).

Research and Development into Low-Virulent CBPP Vaccines

In 1956, following extensive research into suitable strains and possible animal models at

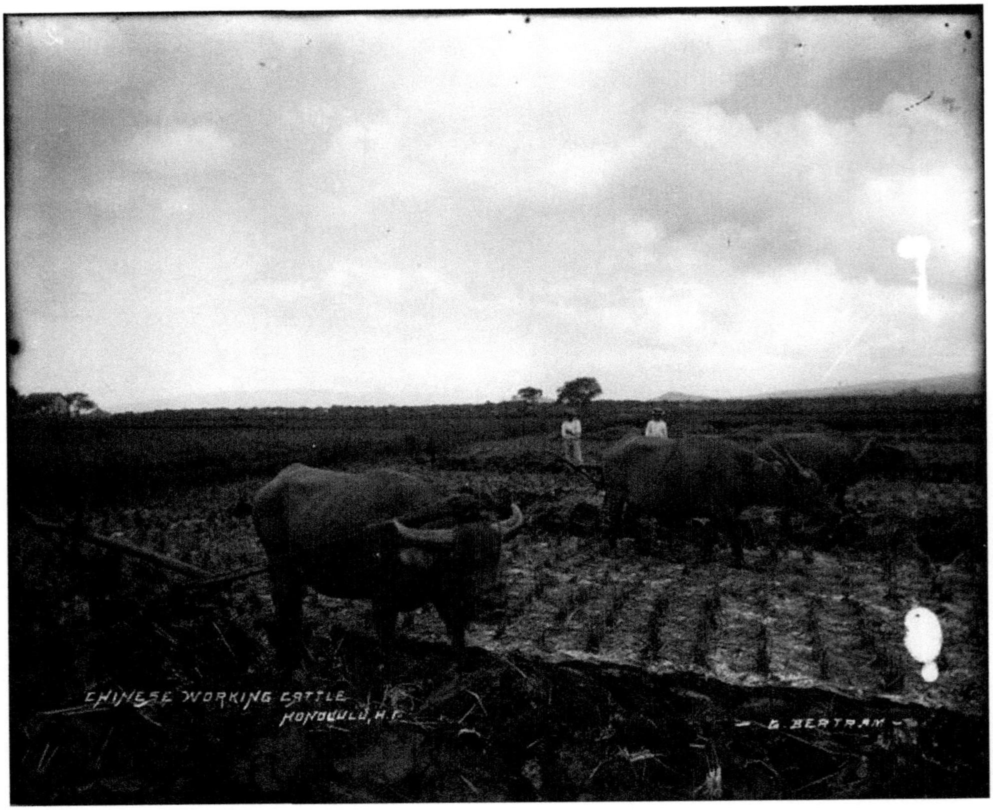

Fig. 8.2. The deaths of thousands of cattle between 1958 and 1970 were mostly due to CBPP, leading to starvation and loss of draft oxen. (From Bellinghausen, c.1883–1905; Brother Bertram Photo Collection, public domain via Wikimedia Commons.)

the Veterinary Research Institute at Gansu, an *M. m. mycoides* strain designated Ben-1 isolated from the lung of a CBPP-infected cow was inoculated into (perhaps surprisingly) the testicles of rabbits (Li *et al.*, 2009). The strain was re-isolated from the testes and inoculated into the thorax of rabbits; the subsequent isolates were continuously and exhaustively passaged 470 times in this same animal species. Though previously unreported elsewhere, infected rabbits showed increased body temperature, shortness of breath and fatigue, with an accompanying severe fibrinous pleuritis, catarrhal pneumonia and swollen parenchyma. *M. m. mycoides* could be isolated from most of the organs and blood. Gross examination of the rabbits showed that the Ben-1 strain had adapted to rabbits after 45 passages, as evidenced by reduced pathology which decreased further with continued passage. The mycoplasma titre in rabbit pleural fluid after 4th–6th passages was 10^{5-9} CFU/mL but increased after the 7th–44th passages to 10^{11} CFU/mL, which remained stable at this titre from the 45th generation onwards. Rabbit pleural fluid from the 191st to 204th passage was used to inoculate susceptible cattle then passaged for two generations in cattle; no clinical signs of CBPP or pathological changes were observed (Xin *et al.*, 2012).

It appeared that passaging *M. m. mycoides* in non-bovine animals had effectively reduced the virulence of the Ben-1 strain. However, the question remained as to whether the attenuated strain still retained the original immunogenicity. Experiments showed that the vaccine prepared from rabbit pleural fluid containing 10^9 CFU/mL, passaged between 120 and 359 times, could protect domestic cattle with high efficacy, i.e. four cattle vaccinated via the gluteal or subcutaneous tail tip route and challenged with the virulent Mu-1 strain of the *M. m. mycoides* did not show clinical signs or lung lesions; cattle in the challenged-control group that received no vaccine all showed signs of CBPP. An experiment on the duration of immunity using the 180th generation of pleural fluid containing 10^9 CFU/mL showed that the protection rate was still high with all four vaccinated cattle protected 28 months post-vaccination. However, after the Ben-1 strain was passaged in rabbits more than 406 times, its immunogenicity decreased, and its protection rate also dropped with only 2/4 of cattle being protected (Xin *et al.*, 2012).

Development and Application of Vaccines Prepared in Sheep and Tibetan Sheep

Unfortunately, the amount of vaccine antigen produced in rabbits was too small and insufficient for a nationwide vaccine campaign. Consequently, in 1957, in an effort to increase production, the 85th generation of pleural fluid containing the Ben-1 strain was inoculated into healthy sheep (Xin *et al.*, 2012). The sheep showed a rise in respiratory rate and an increase in temperature of 1°C within 3 days during which they became depressed and recumbent. Following euthanasia, the pleural fluid was then collected and continuously passaged in other healthy sheep. Vaccines prepared from diluted sheep pleural fluid of the 33rd–53rd generations reportedly achieved a 100% protection rate using 2 mL of vaccine containing 10^8 CFU/mL per animal via the intramuscular route; this immunity lasted for 27 months. The use of vaccines made from sheep pleural fluid significantly increased vaccine yield, reduced production costs and provided sufficient vaccines for the immunization programme.

While the sheep vaccine was safe in cattle, an unacceptable number of yaks and dzos (yak/cattle hybrids) were experiencing adverse vaccine reactions at a rate of 0.7% including a mortality rate of 0.08% (Xin *et al.*, 2012). Consequently, in 1959, after more investigations, the 155th generation of rabbit pleural fluid was inoculated into Tibetan sheep (Fig. 8.3). Vaccines made

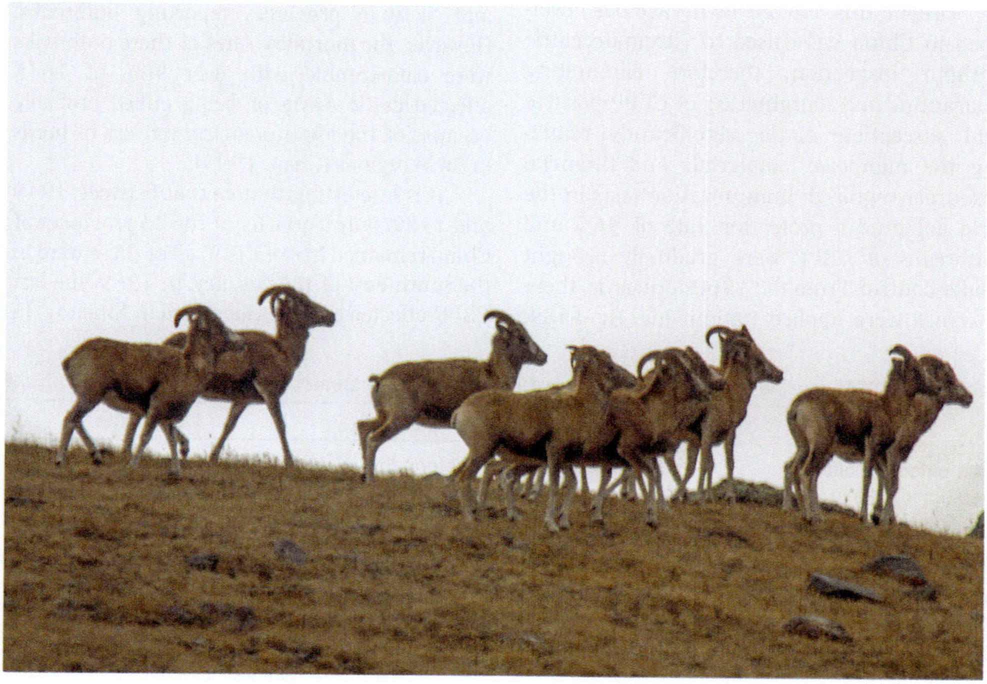

Fig. 8.3. Tibetan sheep, also known as argalis, were used to produce a safe CBPP vaccine. (From Bazdyrev, 2023, iNaturalist, Wikimedia Commons, CC BY 4.0.)

from the pleural fluid of Tibetan sheep at the 76th–150th passage, given intramuscularly, resulted in no adverse reactions in the yaks and dzos and were protective, although the duration of immunity was reduced to about 1 year. The Tibetan sheep-adapted vaccines were then used to immunize hundreds of thousands of yaks and dzos and proved to be safe and effective though the mechanism for the improved safety was not known.

In 1963, lyophilized vaccines were developed and were reported to give 100% protection with immunity lasting 2 years (Xin *et al.*, 2012). However, due to limited lyophilisation resources in the 1960s in China, these vaccines were not produced or applied on a large scale. Furthermore, there were few refrigerated transportation systems available. To overcome this difficulty, frozen pleural fluids from rabbits and sheep were sent to the regions where vaccination was to be applied and used to inoculate local rabbits and sheep to obtain pleural fluids for vaccine production (Zhao and Jia, 1962). A disadvantage of this, however, was that vaccines produced locally were rarely quality-controlled and consistency was variable.

Despite this, low-virulent vaccines developed in China were used to vaccinate cattle without inspection, therefore eliminating quarantine and slaughtering of CBPP-positive and susceptible cattle, significantly reducing the manpower, materials and financial resources required. Immunization tests in the field achieved a protection rate of 96% and outbreaks of CBPP were gradually brought under control. From the 1960s onwards, these vaccines were applied nationwide. By 1989, about 74.5 million cattle had been vaccinated, of which over a quarter were from Tibet and a fifth from Inner Mongolia (17.45 million) (Chen, 1993). Table 8.1 provides a summary of vaccine development in China between 1953 and 1963.

1963–1992: Impact of Vaccination on CBPP in China

As vaccines were gradually applied during the mid-1960s onwards, the CBPP epidemic began to abate as measured by reductions in gross pathology and positive serology (Chen, 1993). By 1965, it was estimated that only about 25,000 cattle were affected, 2000 of which had died showing a lower mortality rate than before. In the 1970s except for some counties in Xinjiang, Yunnan, Sichuan, Shanxi and Shannxi, where over 5000 cattle were affected of which nearly 40% died, CBPP occurrence in other provinces was sporadic. The number of CBPP outbreaks decreased further in the 1980s with only 22 counties in Xinjiang, Yunnan and Sichuan provinces reporting outbreaks. However, the mortality rates of these outbreaks were catastrophic with over 96% of 1648 affected cattle dying or being culled probably because of the immunological naivety of herds in these regions (Chen, 1993).

It is interesting to note that between 1949 and 1989, only a quarter of the 23 provinces of China remained free of CBPP, all of these were in the south-east of the country. In 1989, the last CBPP-affected cow was identified in Xinjiang, in

Table 8.1. CBPP vaccine development in China 1953–1963. (Table created by Robin Nicholas.)

Vaccine	Year	Institute	Comments
Attenuated in culture medium	1953	Harbin Veterinary Research Institute	Widely Used Before 1955
Attenuated in rabbits	1958	Harbin Veterinary Research Institute	Quality Control
Lapinized sheep adapted	1959	Harbin Veterinary Research Institute	Suitable for cattle and yaks, easy for large-scale vaccination, main vaccine in use
Lapinized Tibetan sheep adapted	1963	Lanzhou Veterinary Research Institute	Safer, adapted for yak and dzos

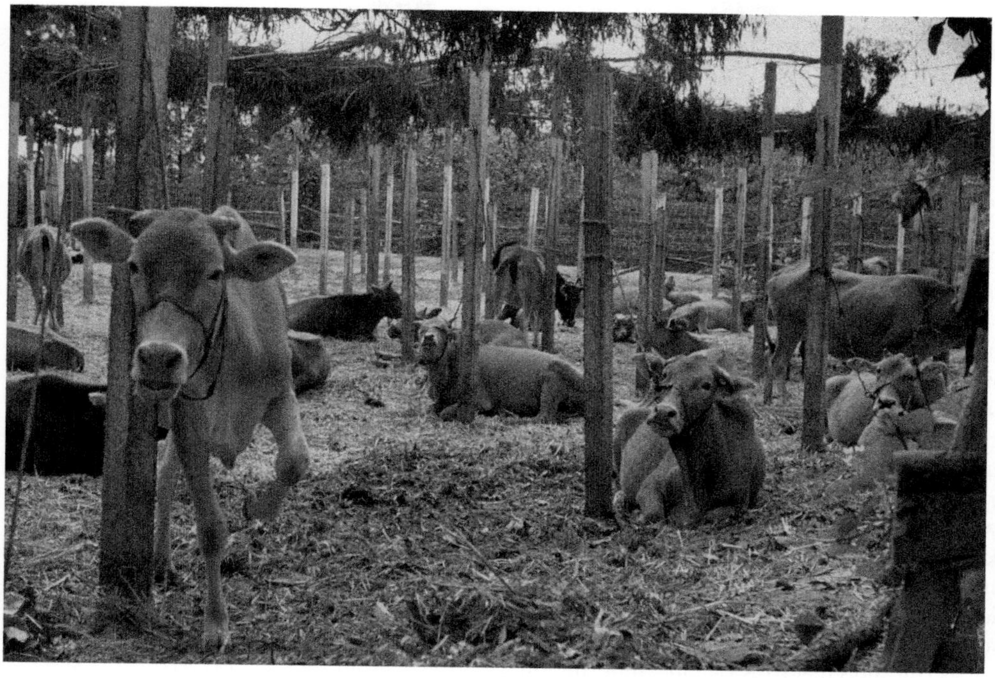

Fig. 8.4. The last case of CBPP was seen in cattle in Xinjiang in 1989. (From Wellmann, 1976, Wikimedia Commons, CC BY 4.0.)

the north-west of the country and slaughtered (Xin *et al.*, 2007) (Fig. 8.4).

Increased Surveillance for CBPP

In 1992, the Chinese ministry of agriculture stopped the use of all types of CBPP vaccines and started intensive surveillance for the disease by abattoir inspection and serological monitoring using complement fixation and micro-agglutination tests. During the next 4 years, although over 1200 seropositive cattle were detected, pathological examination and mycoplasma isolation tests on these cattle were all found to be negative for CBPP. As a result, in 1996 the Ministry announced the eradication of CBPP nationally (Xin *et al.*, 2007). However, the OIE's Terrestrial Animal Health Code (2008a) required further surveillance of the disease before China could completely achieve its goal of freedom from CBPP. In 2002, the Chinese agricultural department introduced a CBPP surveillance plan. Inner Mongolia, Sichuan, Jilin, Xinjiang, Henan, Heilongjiang, Shanxi, Yunnan, Shandong, Ningxia, Qinghai, Tibet and Hebei were identified as key provinces where both serology and clinical surveillance were implemented, while only clinical surveillance was required in the other provinces. Full investigations involving clinical surveillance, serological and pathological examination and mycoplasma isolation were carried out on all cattle in herds where CBPP was suspected. In the abattoir, samples from cattle with suspicious pathological lesions were taken for laboratory testing while other cattle from the same group were quarantined for serological and clinical surveillance. Veterinarians, cattle farmers and abattoir owners were encouraged to report suspicious cases to the National CBPP Reference Laboratory.

Serological Surveillance

According to the Terrestrial Animal Health Code (OIE, 2009), the most effective method of CBPP surveillance is meat inspection in abattoirs, followed by laboratory examination of the lungs of suspicious cattle. However, as not all cattle in China are slaughtered in abattoirs, serological surveillance of CBPP was found to be more suitable. In selected intensive surveillance areas, samples were randomly collected from coded sampling units (all the cattle kept in one village were considered as one sample unit) based on a known population sampling structure. About 26,000 bovine serum samples were collected nationwide annually and sent to CBPP laboratories appointed by the Chinese ministry of agriculture for diagnosis. Of these samples, 60% were from clinically normal cattle, 20% were from cattle with respiratory signs, and 20% came from cattle with pneumonic lesions seen at meat inspection. Animals with positive serological tests were re-sampled. If the second sample was again positive, the sampled animal was killed and examined post-mortem. Lung, lymph nodes and related tissues were taken for pathological and mycoplasma detection. Meanwhile, animals from herds under suspicion were subject to movement restriction, until the test results excluded CBPP infection. Between 2002 and 2007, 155,800 bovine serum samples were collected from 13 provinces and analysed by the CFT. In all, 375 serum samples were positive for CBPP. A second test was conducted on the seropositive cattle according to the guidelines of the 'Contagious Bovine Pleuropneumonia Surveillance Scheme' produced by the Chinese ministry of agriculture. All serum samples in the second test were negative except for one. The suspected animal was examined for clinical signs before it was killed for further analysis. Bacteriological testing of the lung, lymph nodes and hydrothorax eventually excluded the possibility of CBPP infection in that individual animal.

Pathogen Surveillance in the Abattoir

Between 1990 and 2012, 1.2 billion cattle underwent clinical examination for CBPP while 0.75 billion cattle were inspected in the abattoir. No cases of CBPP were diagnosed. From 2006 to 2007, 356 suspected lung samples and 1760 bovine serum samples from Xinjiang, Sichuan, Yunnan and Inner Mongolia were sent to the main reference laboratory in Harbin for testing. Serological and cultural analyses, performed using techniques such as mycoplasma isolation and mycoplasma-specific PCR, were negative for CBPP. Between March and June 2008, a handful of calves in Hubei, Tianjin, Heilongjiang and Anhui showed respiratory signs suggestive of CBPP. Serum samples and lungs from the calves were sent to the Harbin laboratory. Histopathological examination revealed pneumonic changes in five samples. Mycoplasma isolation, identification and serological analysis were then performed but results were all negative for CBPP. However, two strains of mycoplasma were isolated from diseased tissues of the Hubei and Tianjin samples. After 16S rRNA sequence comparison and specific PCR analysis, these two strains were identified as *Mycoplasma* bovis and unusually the small ruminant pathogen, *Mycoplasma agalactiae* (Xin *et al.*, 2008).

Risk from Outside China

China has many neighbouring countries, some of which, such as North Korea and Myanmar, do not report transboundary animal diseases to WOAH. India declared freedom in 2007 while concerns about the status of Pakistan have come into question since reports of clinical disease were reported in 2019 (Anjum *et al.*, 2019), which has yet to be reported officially. Mongolia last reported CBPP in 1973 but is not officially free (OIE, 2008b). Surveillance for CBPP in adjacent countries may not be sufficient to detect CBPP, so it is possible that the disease may exist in isolated regions of China. To minimize this risk and reduce illegal trade, China established 100 border control stations in cooperation with many of its neighbours where strict control measures are carried out including laboratory diagnosis, inspection and monitoring as well as information sharing and reporting.

Conclusion

CBPP once caused huge financial losses to agriculture in China causing great deprivation to its people who were starved of meat and draft oxen. Low virulent lapinized CBPP vaccines, lapinized sheep and Tibetan sheep-adapted vaccines, developed and used on over 74 million head of cattle in China, were effective in controlling and eventually eradicating CBPP after 60 years of infection. China's cattle population, which totals over 150 million head (OIE, 2008b), has now been free of CBPP for 30 years, and vaccination has not been used for about 25 years. After rinderpest, this is the second infectious animal disease eradicated from China. It has been widely accepted that the success of a vaccination campaign depends on four main factors: (i) good planning and organization; (ii) staff who are well trained, fully equipped and highly motivated; (iii) high-quality vaccines; and (iv) good international cooperation (Sylla *et al.*, 1995). CBPP was eradicated with the application of three of these factors but with minimum outside support though whether assistance was requested or rejected is a moot point. The vaccines used in China prepared in non-target species appear more efficacious than the T1/44 vaccine used widely throughout Africa, but today the preparation of the Ben-1 vaccine is unacceptable ethically and laborious requiring the use of living animals. Results of the trials of the Ben-1 vaccine in Africa have been well guarded, but it seems it did no better than the T1/44 though its preparation was modified to conform with ethical international standards which may account for its loss of efficacy (Jores *et al.*, 2020). Crucially, however, paramount in the success of China's war against CBPP was that it had the advantage of a centrally controlled surveillance and eradication programme enabling a high level of vaccine coverage.

Other Far East Countries

In 1991, Pierre-Charles Lefèvre (then the head of CBPP research at the internationally renowned IEMVT, Paris, Pierre), almost certainly based on clinical evidence, located the disease in a swathe of Asia running from Sinkiang, in the west of China, south-eastwards towards Thailand and Vietnam, covering Mongolia, Tibet, Bangladesh, Setchouan, Bhutan, Myanamar, Cambodia, Kampuchea and Assam (Lefèvre, 1991). Over 30 years later, it is highly likely many of those countries are now free of CBPP, though the official data relating to CBPP reported to the WOAH by countries in the Far East is sparse and unreliable; many countries do not report, do not have the technology or are not inquisitive. These include Myanmar, Vietnam, Thailand, Cambodia, Laos, both Koreas, Bhutan, the Philippines and Indonesia. Japan and Mongolia reported their last cases in 1941 and 1973, respectively.

The situation in Malaysia is more uncertain as, according to WOAH, the last case was reported in 2009. A paper published in 2016 gave a full account of the disease in peninsula Malaysia, locating it in two states on the north-eastern border with Thailand (Zarina *et al.*, 2016). While the authors could not isolate or detect the causative mycoplasma, serological detection using the highly reliable cELISA showed herd seroprevalence levels in over 3000 samples of 12 and 24% in the states of Terengganu and Kelantan, respectively. A photograph of a single diseased lung published in the paper was very suggestive of CBPP. The authors concluded that: 'this study indicated that low cattle populations in the Northeastern States of Peninsular Malaysia showed seroprevalence to CBPP. However, none revealed the presence of the pathogen, which was likely due to the absence of this organism in this country' (Zarina *et al.*, 2016).

This was a dangerous assumption. The high seroprevalence would strongly indicate the presence of the mycoplasma in these regions. Excessive antibiotic use in the field or poor culture technique could account for the negative response to detect the mycoplasma.

Writing early in the last century, Hutyra *et al.* (1938) reported that, while Japan became infected from Australia via imported cattle, the disease did not persist. The OIE, however, reported the last case in 1941, suggesting the likely persistence of the disease up until the beginning of the Second World War.

Korea, too, was infected though details are vague. Han (1965) writes: 'the occurrence of CBPP was not recognised until before the Second World War when it was found to occur in North Korea. The whole of the Republic of Korea is now free from the disease.' Given the animosity of the two countries, it is hard to tell whether this was true or merely propaganda. Whatever the truth, South Korea increased monitoring of its cattle on its side of the 38th parallel and remains free.

References

Anjum, A., Aslam, A., Akhtar, R., Yaqub, T., Naseer, J. *et al.* (2019) Seroprevalence of contagious bovine pleuropneumonia in cattle of Punjab, Pakistan and assessment of risk factors. *Indian Journal of Animal Research* 55, 101–104.

Chen, X.F. (1993) Pleuropneumonia contagiosa bovum; Contagious bovine pleuropneumonia. In: *History of Animal Disease in China*. Science Press, Beijing, China, pp. 349–355.

Han, K.Y. (1965) Contagious bovine pleuropneumonia in Korea. *Bulletin of the Office of International Epizooties 63*(1–2), 83–85.

Hou, A., Wei, Y.-S., Liu, X.-G., Li, Y.-L. and Lin, D. (1994) The eradication of CBPP in Henan Province, Henan. *Animal Husbandry and Veterinary Medicine 15*, 22–23.

Hudson, J.R. (1971) *Contagious Bovine Pleuropneumonia*. Food and Agriculture Organization (FAO) Agricultural Studies, No. 86, FAO, Rome.

Hutyra, F., Marek, J. and Manninger, R. (1938) *Special Pathology and Therapeutics of the Diseases of Domestic Animals*, 5th edition. Bailliere Tindall, USA, pp. 455–471.

Jores, J., Baldwin, C., Blanchard, A., Browning, G.F., Colston, A. *et al.* (2020) Contagious bovine and caprine pleuropneumonia: A research community's recommendations for the development of better vaccines. *NPJ Vaccines* 5, 66.

Lefèvre, P.C. (1991) Contagious bovine pleuropneumonia. In: *Atlas Des Maladies Infectieuses Des Ruminants*. IEMVT-CIRAD, Maison Alforts, Paris.

Li, Y., Xin, J.-Q., Gao, Y.-L., Zhang, J.-H., Nicholas, R.A.J. *et al.* (2009) Strains of *Mycoplasma mycoides* subsp. *mycoides* small colony type isolated in China between 1953 and 1960 show close similarity to strains of the Africa/Australia cluster. *The Veterinary Journal* 179, 137–141.

Newton, R.G. (1992) Contagious bovine pleuropneumonia in Australia: Some historic highlights from entry to eradication. *Australian Veterinary Journal* 69(12), 306–317.

OIE (2008a) *Terrestrial Animal Health Code*, Vol. 2. World Organisation for Animal Health, Paris, pp. 506–518.

OIE (2008b) *World Animal Health 2008*, Vol. 1. World Organisation for Animal Health, Paris, pp. 249–371.

OIE (2009) *Terrestrial Animal Health Code*, Vol. 2. World Organisation for Animal Health, Paris, pp. 618–625.

Provost, A., Perreau, P., Breard, A., Le Goff, C., Martel, J.L. *et al.* (1987) Contagious bovine pluropneumonia. *Revue Scientifique et Technique. Office International des Epizooties* 6(3), 565–679.

Sylla, D., Litamoi, J. and Rweyemamu, M.M. (1995) Vaccination strategies for contagious bovine pleuropneumonia in Africa. *Revue Scientifique et Technique. Office International des Epizooties* 14(3), 577–592.8593392

Xin, J., Li, Y., Nicholas, R.A.J., Chen, C., Liu, Y. *et al.* (2012) A history of the prevalence and control of contagious bovine pleuropneumonia in China. *The Veterinary Journal* 191(2), 166–170. 21439870

Xin, J.-Q., Gao, Y.-L., Li, Y., Wang, Y. and Qian, A.-D. (2007) Development of an indirect enzyme-linked immunosorbent assay for seromonitoring contagious bovine pleuropneumonia using recombinant lipoprotein LppQ of *Mycoplasma mycoides* subsp *mycoides* sc as antigen. *Agricultural Sciences in China* 6(1), 100–107.

Xin, J.Q., Li, Y., Guo, D., Song, N.-H., Chen, C. *et al.* (2008) First isolation of *mycoplasma bovis* from calf lung with pneumonia. *Chinese Journal of Preventive Veterinary Medicine* 30, 661–664.

Zarina, M., Zamri-Saad, M., Latiffah, H., Shahrom, M.S. and Norlida, O. (2016) Seroprevalence and detection of Contagious Bovine Pleuropneumonia (CBPP) in Northeast States of Peninsular Malaysia. *Pertanika Journal of Tropical Agricultural Sciences* 39, 257–265.

Zhao, X.-J. and Jia, S.-S. (1962) Field production and observation of lapinized or sheep-adapted vaccine. *Animal Husbandry and Veterinary Medicine* 9, 23–25.

9 CBPP: Passage to the Indian Subcontinent

Abstract

CBPP emerged first in Europe and then spread to Eastern Asia, including to Japan and China, from the Northern Territories of Australia at the end of the 19th century. Its route to India, however, is less well known as there is little evidence for large importations of cattle from Australia around this time. The lack of accurate diagnostic tests at this time meant veterinary authorities relied solely on clinical and pathological signs, many of which were non-specific. Consequently, any diagnoses of CBPP reported in the late 19th and early 20th centuries must be viewed with caution. More convincing reports of CBPP confirmed by laboratory tests were made in the 1930s and 1940s in the Indian state of Assam. Eradication campaigns began in the 1940s with immunization of live attenuated vaccines, and then more intensively in the 1950s and 1960s supplemented with serological screening and establishment of quarantine centres at international borders. The last case of CBPP reported to WOAH, was seen in 1990 but the launch of a new awareness campaign in Assam in 2002 and recent reports of disease in Pakistan suggest the disease has persisted in the Indian subcontinent well into the 21st century.

Introduction

Contagious bovine pleuropneumonia (CBPP), once a scourge of cattle worldwide, is now restricted to countries in sub-Saharan Africa, with Ethiopia, Ghana, Tanzania and Angola having the highest prevalence (WOAH, 2023). Very recent, though unofficial, reports have indicated it may also be present in the Punjab region of Pakistan. The true economic and social impact of CBPP is unknown in Africa because rigorous surveillance is not routinely carried out in all countries. Today, for the most part, CBPP is an enzootic disease with occasional serious outbreaks, still taking its toll on cattle with losses due to poor growth rates, fertility, emaciation and shortage of draft animals (Provost *et al.*, 1987).

The history of the worldwide spread of CBPP has been well documented (Egwu *et al.*, 1996). While it is not possible to completely exclude a CBPP-like disease in classical Roman times, it seems highly speculative given the lack of laboratory diagnosis and knowledge of disease pathology at the time. Descriptions of CBPP-like clinical signs were reported by Virgil but appeared to have had a much wider host range, including dogs and birds, than seen today (Blancou, 1996). Furthermore, his descriptions of cattle vomiting blood and froth do not sound much like CBPP. The consensus, backed by molecular studies (Dupuy *et al.*, 2012), is that the disease, known then as 'pulmona' first appeared in Middle Europe in the 16th century and was differentiated from other respiratory diseases by Bourgelat in 1765 (Provost *et al.*, 1987). It spread, through wars and trade, during the early 19th century throughout the continent, predominantly by movements of the favoured Swiss and Dutch cattle. The Netherlands became a 'hotbed of infection' (Blancou, 1996) with high mortality and morbidity rates. Britain, too, became infected through the importation of cattle from mainland Europe, resulting in huge losses. CBPP was then exported from Britain and the Netherlands via infected cattle to the USA, Australia and South Africa, respectively. From the latter, CBPP-affected cattle were trekked north by Boer farmers (Davies, 1991) and/or British troops (Tambi *et al.*, 2006), initially into East Africa and then via other cattle movements into the rest of Africa. One hypothesis suggests that CBPP may have been introduced even earlier to Africa, also by the British, during an 1868 military expedition into Abyssinia, now present-day Ethiopia (Provost *et al.*, 1987).

DOI: 10.1079/9781800627536.0009

Another theory is that it may already have been present in Africa, as the European explorer Thompson reported Masai cattle dying of a disease with signs similar to CBPP (Davies, 1991). Though not mutually exclusive, Dupuy *et al.* (2012) suggested another possible route of transmission: via cattle from Portuguese bases along the West African coast, possibly as early as the 17th century. However, the evidence for this speculation comes from molecular typing of the causative agent, *Mycoplasma mycoides* subsp. *mycoides*, which showed three separate genotypes in Central, Eastern and Western Africa (Yaya *et al.*, 2008). Unfortunately, the number of strains available is too few to provide a truly accurate assessment of the epidemiology of CBPP in Africa.

Various control measures, including slaughter, quarantine, movement restrictions and vaccination led eventually to eradication – first in the USA in 1892, Britain at the end of the 19th century, Australia in the 1960s, China in the 1980s, and Europe as a whole by the end of the 20th century. Other countries, including India and Pakistan, reported their last cases in 1990 and 1997, respectively (OIE, 2013). However, as will be seen later in this chapter, doubts exist about the complete disappearance of CBPP from the Indian subcontinent.

Asia

While the routes that CBPP took to the USA, Africa and Australia are well known, how and when it entered Asia has been scarcely reported. The possibility that it entered China from Russia was partly discounted by molecular typing which showed that Chinese strains of *M. m. mycoides* were identical to the African/Australian cluster (Xin *et al.*, 2011). Australia began shipping cattle to Hong Kong and Singapore in 1884 from the Northern Territories but trade was suspended because of disease outbreaks, almost certainly CBPP which was widespread in the region; trade suspensions occurred sporadically after that. This strongly suggests that CBPP may well have entered Asia at this time. Salmon (1896) writing about the origins of CBPP at the end of the 19th century described it, rather vaguely: ‘as existing in various parts of the continent of Asia though the time of its first appearance and extent of its distribution are very uncertain’.

In another contemporaneous account not long after CBPP had first reached Asia, Hutyra and Marek (1938)Hutyra *et al.* (1938) declared that it was widespread in Mongolia and Manchuria (now present-day China and parts of the Russian Far East) as well as India and China, though what these claims were based on other than word of mouth and speculation are also uncertain. Seventy years later, ter Laak (1992), using unnamed secondary sources, stated that New Zealand, mainland China, Mongolia, Myanmar, Bhutan, Nepal, Japan and India in the late 19th and early 20th centuries had also been infected from Australia. More authoritatively, Lefèvre (1991), in his *Atlas des Maladies Infectieuses des Ruminants*, located the disease in a swathe of Asia running from Sinkiang, in the west of China, south-eastwards towards Thailand and Vietnam covering Mongolia, Tibet, Bangladesh, Setchouan, Bhutan, Myanamar, Burma, Cambodia, Kampuchea and Assam; CBPP was also suspected in Pakistan and Nepal. However, despite the information deriving from the internationally renowned French Veterinary Institute in Alfort, Paris, there still must be doubt about the validity of some of the data as it would have been based, often, on unreliable clinical reports from Asian countries without diagnostic facilities.

India

The exact date of the arrival of CBPP in India has been hotly disputed and varies from the late 19th century to the early 1940s. Examining annual reports of the provincial civil veterinary department, Gopalakrishnan (1946) concluded that opinion up to the late 1930s was always divided as to the existence of the disease in India. The earlier proposal by Windsor that the horn of Africa was infected during a British military operation that began in India, is clearly unlikely as CBPP had almost certainly not reached India at the time of the expedition in 1868. Furthermore, donkeys, not bullocks, were the main beasts of burden for the invasion of Abyssinia (Nicholas, 2009). Additionally, there do not seem to have been any reports of major cattle imports from Australia around this time as trade did not begin for another 20 years (Anonymous, 1920). Indeed, had there been any importation of infected cattle to India in the late 19th and early 20th centuries, there would almost certainly have been reports by the British-run veterinary services of explosive and prolonged outbreaks in the immunologically naïve local herds such as those seen in Australia and Southern Africa (Egwu *et al.*, 1996). Curiously, Robert Wallace, professor of agriculture at Edinburgh University, in his book *India in 1887*, alluded briefly to the presence of pleuropneumonia in the north-west but said its effects were milder than in Britain and its action 'local' and present mainly in the north-west (now Pakistan) (Wallace, 1887). No other information is provided which must cast some doubt on the existence of CBPP at this time

This is not to say that there were no major outbreaks of respiratory disease in Indian cattle during the late period of British colonization. In 1892–1893, CBPP was included by the veterinary authorities in an annual list of diseases believed to occur in India although any diagnosis at that time would have been based solely on clinical and pathological signs. In the following decade, thousands of cattle died with lesions thought to be CBPP. In 1894–1895, the superintendent of South Punjab reported an outbreak of 'pleuropneumonia' in the Ferozepore area, comprising 138,000 cattle, of which 4000 died. Similar diseases were recorded in the remarkably detailed annual reports of the civil veterinary department between 1893 and 1904 in the same province, affecting 140,636 animals, of which 5631 died. However, there were doubts expressed by some authorities at the time, including those in Bengal, that this was not true CBPP and with hindsight was most likely to be bovine haemorrhagic septicaemia caused by *Pasteurella multocida*. Indeed, the veterinary superintendent at the time stated: 'It was much more likely that these were ordinary pneumonias with pleurisy' (Shirlaw, 1939).

Identification of diseases particularly multifactorial respiratory conditions in cattle in the late 19th century was not an exact science as seen with a transatlantic trade dispute between the USA and Great Britain. An argument had broken out over the ongoing diagnoses, 'of the insidious lung disease pleuropneumonia' in cattle imported from the USA in 1879 (Kastner *et al.*, 2005). Despite the irony of Great Britain having exported CBPP to the USA in the early half of the 19th century and at the time being heavily affected, British veterinary officials wanted to slaughter cattle imported from the USA believed to be affected by CBPP. However, these diagnoses were contested by both the US authorities and some experts in Britain, who believed it was a general non-contagious and less fatal bronchitis which had developed during a stressful transatlantic voyage known today as 'shipping fever'. While never satisfactorily resolved, the dispute accelerated US attempts to eradicate CBPP which it did in 1892. Great Britain suffered for a few years more.

In the early part of the 20th century, sporadic reports of CBPP-like disease were made near Karachi, the United Provinces, Berar, Jubbulpore and Nagpor districts, with high mortality although once again CBPP could not be confirmed. One convincing reason that these diseases may have been misdiagnosed was that there were few further reports of CBPP between 1905 and 1929; instead, a new category was inserted into the records, namely haemorrhagic septicaemia, suggesting doubts about the earlier diagnoses. As is well known, CBPP does not disappear so suddenly without strict control measures being put in place, for which there was no evidence in India. The reasons for these doubts must have been due to staff inexperienced at differentiating the various bovine pneumonias and the uncertainty of disease nomenclature at the time, compounded by the huge distances and difficulties encountered by veterinarians examining diseased cattle in the field.

Further arguments for the absence of CBPP up to that time came from two senior veterinary officers serving in India in the early 20th century. In 1927, Edwards said: 'India...for some reason has escaped infection' (as cited in Shirlaw, 1939).

A few years later, in 1939, Shirlaw stated, in no uncertain terms, after viewing reports dating back to the beginning of the century: 'There is no evidence that CBPP existed or has ever existed in British India' (Shirlaw, 1939).

While Shirlaw was probably correct about the historical reports, he believed that many of the later reports of CBPP-like disease in Assam, an isolated state in north-east India bordered by Bangladesh, Myanmar, Bhutan and China (Fig. 9.1) were caused by a fungal pathogen

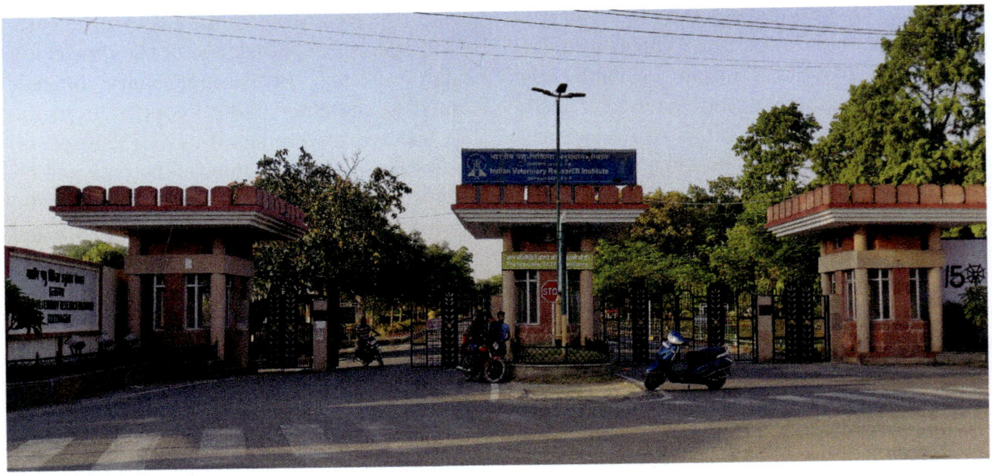

Fig. 9.1. Imperial Veterinary Research Institute, Izatnagar, Uttar Pradesh, where CBPP was first diagnosed. (From Abhimanyu7793, 2019, IVRI Izatnagar, Bareilly, Wikimedia Commons, CC BY 4.0.)

based on culture and histopathology. The mycotic-looking *Borrelomyces peripneumoniae*, later to be known as the bacterium *Asterococcus mycoides*, then renamed *Mycoplasma mycoides*, the definitive causative agent of CBPP, was later identified in pleural fluid from affected cattle. Five years after his pronouncement of its non-occurrence in India, Shirlaw had to admit that his fungal disease was in fact true CBPP and ravaging cattle in Assam (Shirlaw and Iver, 1946). His group was able to develop 'a medium of choice' for the *in vitro* culture of the 'Assam bovine pleuropneumonia organism' and showed that strains from this province were immunologically similar to confirmed CBPP pathogens from East Africa and Australia. It is interesting to note that despite taking 3 weeks and 10 weeks to arrive from Kenya and Australia, respectively, at the Imperial Veterinary Research Institute, Izatnagar, Uttar Pradesh (Fig. 9.2), the strains could be revived satisfactorily in the newly developed broth and still retained pathogenicity in cattle.

Assam

It is highly likely that the first true cases of CBPP in Assam were the deaths of 30 cattle reported between 1932 and 1933. Clear unambiguous descriptions were given of the pathology with all salient features of the disease known locally as 'Brahmaputra Valley Disease' were seen although the mycoplasma was not isolated or detected owing to the lack of culture facilities (Shirlaw and Iver, 1946). From then on, reports of CBPP were made annually. Laboratory investigations began seriously at the Imperial Veterinary Research Institute around 1936 with the isolation of the pathogen from pleural fluid and pieces of affected lung from cattle in Assam. Experimental subcutaneous inoculation of disease-free cattle with pleural fluid from infected animals led to large swellings at the inoculation site and, less frequently, CBPP-like lung lesions as seen in the field; this highlighted the difficulty in reproducing the clinical disease. Better results were seen when cattle inhaled or were intubated with large quantities of the mycoplasma though this was often inconsistent (Das, 1967). While intubation of mycoplasma directly into the bronchioles is often the most common method these days, contact infection of healthy cattle by animals incubating the disease is probably the best means of inducing natural infection (Huebschle *et al.*, 2006).

In March 1938, the disease was reported to be enzootic in certain areas surrounding the Brahmaputra River valley (Fig. 9.3). It was believed to be seasonal and observed more frequently during the monsoon period. In acute cases, the body temperature reached

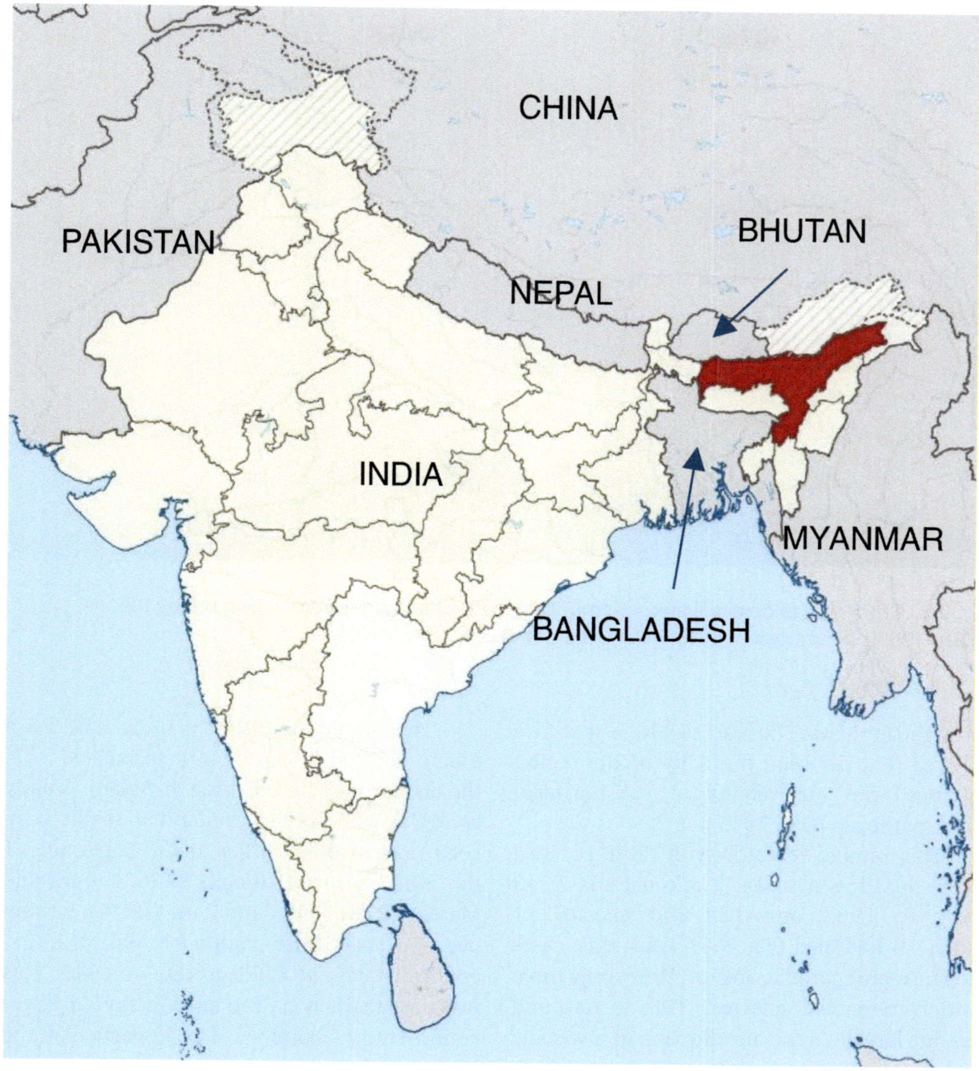

Fig. 9.2. Figure 9.2: Assam located in red with neighbours. (From Nicholas, 2023.)

40–41°C with both lungs showing lesions. However, in chronic cases, only one lung was usually involved. Post-mortem findings showed the lungs of infected cattle were hepatized and adhered to the chest wall which contained large amounts of sanguineous pleural fluid (Singh and Rana, 2014). All features described were classical CBPP lesions as seen today in sub-Saharan Africa. The disease was particularly prevalent in low-lying areas near the riverbank where many herds grazed. It was reported as spreading to domestic buffalo, but this species was much less susceptible and showed few clinical signs. The isolated nature of the area had two conflicting outcomes: first, control was clearly hampered by the remoteness of the region; and second, fortunately, apart from a single outbreak in the Sylhet district (in present-day Bangladesh), there was no detectable spread of the disease to the rest of India (Das, 1967). Other factors affecting the pace of control were the long incubation period of the disease which was reported to vary between 1 and 8 months and the insidious and silent spread of the disease

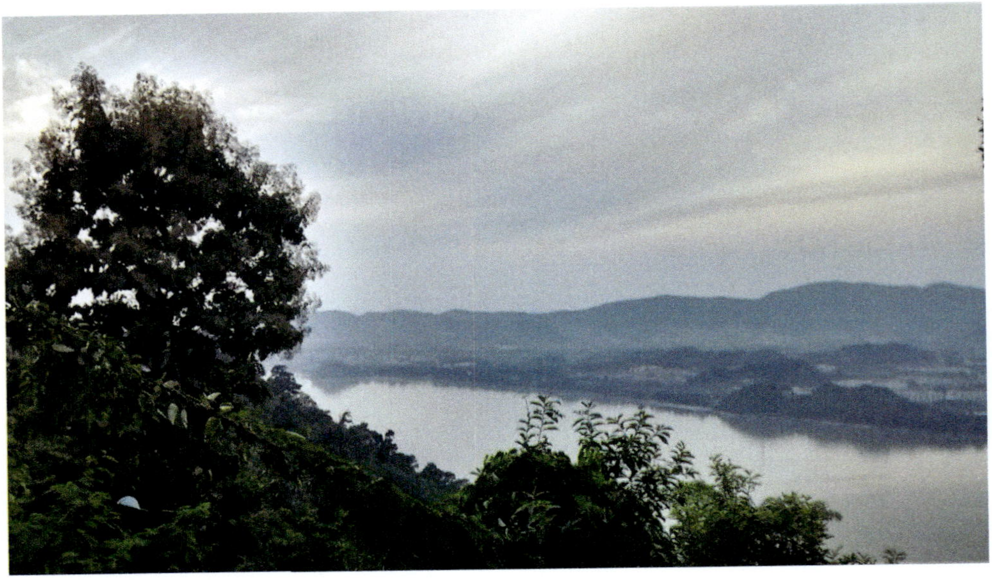

Fig. 9.3. CBPP was endemic in areas surrounding the Bramaputra river in Assam during the 1930s–1950s. (From Keshri, 2016, Wikimedia Commons, CC BY 4.0.)

through the herd (Shirlaw, 1939). It was also believed that the high humidity of the region enhanced the survivability of the normally fragile pathogen (Das, 1967).

The number of cattle with CBPP reached a peak in 1956 with 1471 affected and 1036 dying. By 1963, only 128 were affected, of which 10 had died (Fig. 9.4). After this, cases became more sporadic, and, by 1965, only three districts remained affected. This turnaround was due largely to the introduction of a vaccine made from a local strain of the pathogen which had been attenuated by serial passage in a broth medium and used as a vaccine after 12–25 subcultures. The vaccine was injected into the tail tip which often caused necrosis requiring treatment with the anti-inflammatory medication, sulphadiazine. Despite this, the tail tip site was adopted as the optimum route because fewer lung lesions occurred following experimental challenge with immunity lasting about 1 year. Vaccine records compiled by the veterinary authorities showed the number of animals vaccinated varied from 20,000 at the beginning of the 1950s to 86,000 towards the end of the decade with a gradual levelling off in 1962 as the disease came under control (Fig. 9.4).

The origins of CBPP in India have been much debated. Rao (1969) speculated that the disease may have existed in Assam as early as 1919 while others thought it might have been present even earlier at the beginning of the 20th century (Salmon, 1896; Hutyra and Marek, 1938). Singh and Rana (2014), writing over 70 years later, cautiously date the first confirmed case of CBPP as late as 1942. This was based largely on the introduction of better confirmatory laboratory tests, in particular, the agglutination test, and pathognomonic description of lesions recorded by veterinarians of the day. Das (1967) put the date of the first detection even later at 1944, but at this time, CBPP was already endemic in the Naga Hills and Manipur affecting at least eight districts containing, in all, 100,000 cattle belonging to about 1000 villages (Gopalakrishnan, 1946). It is perhaps not that surprising for the uncertainty of CBPP origin, given that the Japanese Imperial Army was attempting to invade India from Burma (now Myanmar) at this time; the fact that any animal health surveillance was going on close by was quite remarkable.

Clearly, the exact date of entry will never be known but it is difficult to understand where

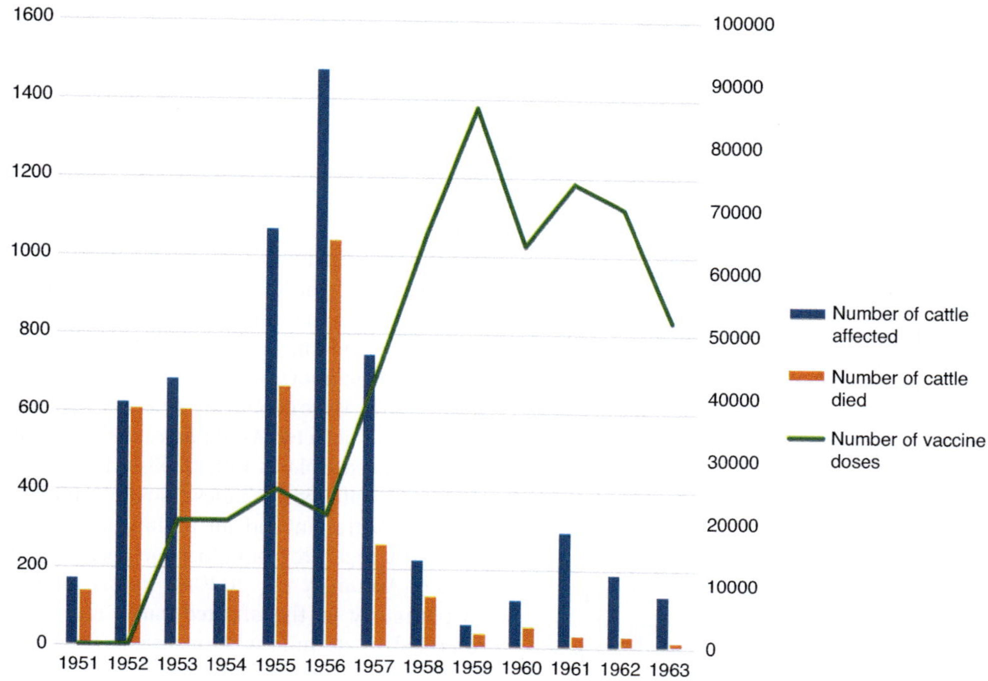

Fig. 9.4. Graph describing the number of cattle affected by, or diseased due to, CBPP, and vaccine doses administered, in the period between 1951 and 1963 in Assam. (Modified from Gopalakrishan, 1946.)

CBPP would have originated before Australian exports to Asia considering the isolated nature of the region. A more likely explanation is that CBPP entered Assam via affected cattle and yaks in the 1930s and 1940s from neighbouring countries of China, Bhutan and/or Burma where the disease was believed to have existed and its spread facilitated by the lack of border checkpoints. More precisely, the occurrence of the disease in the farmed areas of Lakhimpur, which is in the north-east corner of Assam, suggests the source of infection was most likely China. Indeed, it was well known that much of China, including provinces close to India, was affected by CBPP following its introduction into Shanghai from Australia (Xin *et al.*, 2011); indeed only six of the 23 provinces remained free of disease from 1949 to 1969, with nearly 200,000 reported to have died of CBPP, putting a great strain on the economy during the 'Great Leap Forward', which relied heavily on cattle for labour, meat and milk (Xin *et al.*, 2011).

To control animal movements, quarantine stations were established on the Bhutan border in the 1950s at the start of the eradication campaign; the health of cattle was then checked by veterinarians which included the use of the rapid agglutination tests for CBPP. No records have been found showing whether any positive animals were detected at these stations. While the last official case of CBPP was reported in Assam in 1990, a new eradication programme, which was a component of the rinderpest eradication project, was reported by the provincial newspaper *Sentinel* based in Guwahati (Anonymous, 2002). The programme was launched in March 2002 by Barooah, Assam's commissioner and secretary of the veterinary department, strongly suggesting that CBPP was continuing to cause problems and that greater awareness of the disease by cattle farmers was deemed necessary. No more information could be sourced on the outcome of the awareness campaign so it must be assumed no further cases of CBPP were reported to the authorities.

Freedom from CBPP

Three years after the last reported clinical case in 1987, India stopped vaccinating cattle for CBPP (Singh and Rana, 2014). Then, to show provisional freedom from disease required by WOAH, a programme was launched in 2001 by the department of animal husbandry and dairying within the ministry of agriculture, New Delhi; and the department of veterinary and animal husbandry, within the government of Assam. Bovine tissue samples were collected and tested for both the pathogen and its antibodies; this was undertaken jointly by the Mycoplasma Laboratory, IVRI, Izatnagar, and by the CBPP laboratory in Khanapara. No CBPP cases were detected, and India was declared provisionally free from disease taking effect from October 2003. Seven years later, on 26 May 2007, WOAH declared India free from CBPP infection as per OIE resolution number 17 (general session 82 of May 2014). Other countries, including Argentina, Australia, Botswana, Canada, China, Portugal, Singapore, Switzerland and the USA also obtained CBPP freedom status at that time.

Pakistan

It is tempting to speculate that the origins of CBPP in Pakistan were tied very closely to that of India as the countries only separated in 1947. However, while there have been no confirmed reports of CBPP in India, except in Assam, since Partition the disease looks to have continued to plague Pakistan, as evidenced by recent reports by Anjum *et al.* (2019, 2020a). To date, however, the extent of the disease in the country is not known. A recent series of clinical and seroprevalence studies have reported the presence of CBPP in several districts of the Punjab province, near the border with India (Anjum *et al.* 2019, 2020a, 2020b), but official notifications have not, at the time of writing (January 2025), been made to the EFSA Panel on Animal Health and Welfare at WOAH. In these studies, lung samples from over 500 cattle and nearly 300 buffalo, suspected clinically of having CBPP, were collected from abattoirs in three districts of Punjab namely Lahore, Kasur and Jhang. The results indicated that just over 9% of cattle were positive by a PCR detecting the 16S rRNA gene; all buffalo samples were negative for CBPP. These results were very similar to earlier studies which also showed a seroprevalence of 10% (Anjum *et al.*, 2019). This is surprising, perhaps, because antibodies are usually more widespread in herds than the pathogen itself. It should also be pointed out that the PCR used was not particularly specific as members of the *M. mycoides* cluster cross-react; however, the only other large ruminant member of the cluster is *M. leachii*, a rather rare organism more associated with mastitis and arthritis. More conclusive evidence that the authors had detected *M. m. mycoides* was that the sequenced isolates from Pakistan grouped phylogenetically with Chinese isolates and less so with Australian and an Italian isolate but are clearly separate from other members of the cluster (Anjum *et al.*, 2020a). Unfortunately, no pathology of the affected cattle has been described to determine whether lesions are acute or chronic. Incidentally, higher prevalence of disease was seen in cattle of more than 7 years of age, in female cattle, and in cross-bred cattle.

The above reports indicate that clinical disease is rife in the Punjab, an historical and politically sensitive area shared with India, though separated by an intensely monitored 3000-km border fence with only a single crossing point. Consequently, the risk to India of transboundary disease like CBPP from Pakistan that requires cattle movements to spread is low unless trade restrictions between the two countries change. Accepting the likelihood that CBPP is unknown to the main landmass of India then the origins in Pakistan must lie elsewhere, most probably in China. According to WOAH the last case officially reported in Pakistan was in 1997, which suggests that the disease has persisted in cattle since then but has been unreported. Indeed, it is well known that CBPP can exist in small herds silently with cattle exhibiting few clinical signs as it probably did in Europe in the late 20th century (Nicholas, 2009). While CBPP has only been reported to date in the state of Punjab, which constitutes the main cattle farming region of Pakistan, those areas like Khyber Pakhtunkhwa and Balochistan, which are closer to the Chinese border, may also be affected. Suspicion must also be cast on the occurrence of CBPP in adjacent countries like

Bhutan and Myanmar where little surveillance is carried out and borders are less secure.

Afghanistan

Little was known about the prevalence of animal diseases in Afghanistan until the establishment of the Central Veterinary and Diagnostic Research Laboratories (CVDRL) in 2009, which occupied newly constructed facilities in Kabul, funded by the EU and FAO. Despite considerable challenges within the country, the CVDRL, linked to a network of six regional and 12 provincial laboratories, had established diagnostic facilities for a range of bacterial, viral and protozoal diseases. The formation of a WOAH twinning programme with the Mycoplasma Group, Animal and Plant Health Agency (APHA) in the UK provided an opportunity to investigate the presence of important transboundary diseases, notably CBPP. Little targeted surveillance of the disease has taken place in Asia over the last few decades but freedom from CBPP was declared in India in 1990, and China in 1996. There have been no reports of CBPP in Afghanistan or its other neighbours, Iran, Turkmenistan, Tajikistan and Uzbekistan, although it is unlikely that these countries routinely monitor for the disease. The data presented by Bahir *et al.* (2017) provided a first assessment of the occurrence of CBPP in Afghanistan. From the results of the testing of cattle sera from most provinces, there was little evidence of the presence of CBPP in Afghanistan. The sample tested represented only 0.03% of the cattle population but had a good statistical chance of detecting disease at a prevalence of at least 1%. One province, Kunar, contained a high number of suspect ELISA-positive samples (nearly 20%) spread among four herds on first testing but these were found to be negative on retesting and by immunoblotting. Publicity including talks and posters were generated by the CVDRL staff describing the typical clinical signs and lesions of CBPP and should have helped the local veterinary staff to recognize the disease should it be present.

Tragically, the arrival of the Taliban in August 2021 led to the destruction of the state-of-the-art laboratory in Kabul and, consequently, all diagnostic and research activities came to a halt. It can thus be expected that a rise in animal disease will be seen across the country and the possible re-emergence of CBPP from neighbouring countries.

Conclusion

There are several possibilities for the origin of CBPP in Asia: direct arrival in cattle from Europe, most probably Great Britain; direct importation from Australia; or introduction from the neighbouring countries of China, Bhutan or Myanmar, which would also have had origins in Australia. A final possibility is importation through China from Russia which was affected in the 19th and early 20th centuries though the geopolitics suggests this is the least likely route (Xin *et al.*, 2011). Experience from Africa showed that, without attempts to stamp out CBPP immediately on arrival in South Africa from the Netherlands, it spread progressively north, marked by large outbreaks with high mortality when infected cattle came in contact with immunologically naïve local breeds. It has been reported that over 100,000 cattle died within 2 years of its introduction (Egwu *et al.*, 1996). In Australia too, the lack of control when the disease was first identified led to a century of CBPP characterized by large and episodic outbreaks. There appear to be no similar descriptions of prolonged CBPP-like disease in India in the late 19th and early 20th centuries. While there were reports of respiratory cattle disease with high mortality at this time, it seems very likely that these reported CBPP outbreaks were misdiagnosed and were, in fact, haemorrhagic septicaemia caused by *Pasteurella multocida* which does not persist so stubbornly. Indeed, some experts at the time, including Shirlaw, were convinced that CBPP had never infected India until the confirmed cases in Assam in the late 1930s and early 1940s. Due to the isolated nature of this Indian province and the lack of trade with the rest of India, it is highly likely that CBPP was introduced with cattle and buffalo from China, or the neighbouring countries mentioned earlier.

References

Anjum, A., Aslam, A., Akhtar, R., Yaqub, T., Naseer, J. *et al.* (2019) Seroprevalence of contagious bovine pleuropneumonia in cattle of Punjab, Pakistan and assessment of risk factors. *Indian Journal of Animal Research* 55(1), 101–104.

Anjum, A., Aslam, A., Akhtar, R., Yaqub, T., Khan, M.R. *et al.* (2020a) Molecular detection and pathological investigation of contagious bovine pleuropneumonia in selected districts of Punjab, Pakistan. *Pakistan Journal of Zoology* 52(2), 797–800.

Anjum, A., Usman, S., Aslam, A., Faiz, M., Usman, S. *et al.* (2020b) Prevalence and molecular detection of contagious bovine pleuropneumonia in large ruminants in Punjab, Pakistan. *Tropical Biomedicine* 37(2), 273–281.

Anonymous (2002) CBPP eradication programme launched in Assam. Sentinel (Guwahati) 18/3/2002. Available at: www.indiaenvironmentportal.org.in/content/140831/bovine-pleuropneumonia/ (accessed 4 August 2024).

Anonymous (1920) Parliamentary Departments Library. Available at: www.aph.gov.au/about_parliament_departments_library/pubs/rp/rp1920/chronology/liveexport (accessed 14 August 2024).

Bahir, W., Omar, O., Rosales, R.S., Hlusek, M., Ziay, G. *et al.* (2017) Search for OIE-listed ruminant mycoplasma diseases in Afghanistan. *BMC Veterinary Research* 13(1), 149.

Blancou, J. (1996) Early methods of surveillance and control for contagious bovine pleuropneumonia. *Revue Scientifique et Technique. Office International des Epizooties* 15(4), 1241–1282.

Das, C. (1967) Bovine contagious pleuropneumonia in Assam. *Study of Its Epizootiological Aspect Indian Veterinary Journal* 44, 109–113.

Davies, G. (1991) Contagious bovine pleuropneumonia: What every veterinarian ought to know. *State Veterinary Journal* 1, 9–11.

Dupuy, V., Manso-Silván, L., Barbe, V., Thebault, P., Dordet-Frisoni, E. *et al.* (2012) Evolutionary history of contagious bovine pleuropneumonia using next generation sequencing of *Mycoplasma mycoides* subsp. mycoides 'small colony'. *PLOS ONE* 7(10), e46821.

Egwu, G., Nicholas, R.A.J., Ameh, J.A. and Bashiruddin, J.B. (1996) Contagious bovine pleuropneumonia: An update. *Veterinary Bulletin* 66, 195–208.

Gopalakrishnan, V.R. (1946) Preliminary note on vaccination against bovine contagious pleuropneumonia in Assam. *Indian Journal of Veterinary Science and Husbandry* 16, 209–210.

Huebschle, O.J.B., Ayling, R.D., Godinho, K., Lukhele, O., Tjipura-Zaire, G. *et al.* (2006) Danofloxacin (Advocin™)reduces the spread of contagious bovine pleuropneumonia to healthy in-contact cattle. *Research in Veterinary Science* 81(3), 304–309.

Hutyra, F. and Marek, J. (1938) Contagious pleuropneumonia. In: *Special Pathology and Therapeutics of the Diseases of Domestic Animals*, Vol. 1. Alexander Eger, Chicago, pp. 455–471.

Kastner, J., Powell, D., Crowley, T. and Huff, K. (2005) Scientific conviction amidst scientific controversy in the transatlantic livestock and meat trade. *Endeavour* 29(2), 78–83.

Lefèvre, P.C. (1991) Contagious bovine pleuropneumonia. In: *Atlas Des Maladies Infectieuses Des Ruminants*. IEMVT-CIRAD, Maison Alforts, Paris.

Nicholas, R.A.J. (2009) Contagious bovine pleuropneumonia: In search of the origins and virulence of lung sickness. *Microbiologist* 10, 41–43.

OIE (2013) *World Animal Health in 2012*. World Organisation for Animal Health, Paris.

Provost, A., Perreau, P., Breard, A., Le Goff, C., Martel, J.L. *et al.* (1987) Contagious bovine pleuropneumonia. *Revue Scientifique et Technique. Office International des Epizooties* 6(3), 565–679.

Rao, C.K. (1969) Contagious bovine pleuropneumonia in India. *Bulletin of the Office of International Epizooties* 71, 1309–1312.

Salmon, J. (1896) *Diseases of Cattle and on Cattle Feeding*. Government Printing Office, Washington, DC, pp. 376–379.

Shirlaw, J.F. (1939) Observations on the existence of contagious bovine pleuropneumonia in British India. *Journal of Veterinary Science and Animal Husbandry* 9, 139–150.

Shirlaw, J.F. and Iver, P.R.K. (1946) Studies on contagious bovine pleuropneumonia in Assam. *Indian Journal of Veterinary Science and Animal Husbandry* 16, 191–208.

Singh, V.P. and Rana, R. (2014) Contagious bovine pleuropneumonia infection and eradication. *Indian Farming* 64, 15–18.

Tambi, N.E., Maina, W.O. and Ndi, C. (2006) An estimation of the economic impact of contagious bovine pleuropneumonia in Africa. *Revue Scientifique et Technique. Office International des Epizooties* 25(3), 999–1011.

ter Laak, E.A. (1992) Contagious bovine pleuropneumonia a review. *Veterinary Quarterly* 14(3), 104–110.

Wallace, R. (1887) India in 1887 as seen by Robert Wallace. Available at: https://archive.org/details/indiainasseenby00wallgoog (accessed 12 December 2024).

World Organisation for Animal Health (2023) *Annual Report*. OIE, Paris. Available at: https://www.oie.int/scientific-expertise/reference-laboratories/annual-reports/ (accessed 5 November 2024).

Xin, J., Li, Y., Nicholas, R.A.J., Chen, C., Liu, Y. *et al*. (2011) History of the prevalence and control of CBPP in China. *Veterinary Journal* 191, 166–170.

Yaya, A., Manso-Silván, L., Blanchard, A. and Thiaucourt, F. (2008) Genotyping of *Mycoplasma mycoides* subsp. *mycoides* SC by multilocus sequence analysis allows molecular epidemiology of contagious bovine pleuropneumonia. *Veterinary Research* 39(2), 39.

10 Re-Emergence of CBPP in Europe

Abstract

CBPP had persisted in Europe for the first half of the 20th century before appearing to die out in the late 1960s. Then, the disease reappeared in France in 1980, Spain in 1981, Portugal in 1983 and, finally, Italy in 1990. The isolates from these new outbreaks were almost identical. Furthermore, comparative analysis of the new European isolates with African strains showed that the former were biochemically and immunologically quite different. Subsequently, genetic analysis revealed a genomic segment of 8.8 kb, present in African strains, which was completely missing in these new European strains; within this region was a copy of the *lppB* gene, a potential virulence factor, and the glycerol uptake gene. A single European strain from outbreaks in France in 1967 before the re-emergence did not have this deletion. This section will explore the implications and source of these re-emergent strains.

The Re-Emergence in Southern Europe

After nearly 25 years absence of disease to date (in 2025), it is probably safe to say that it is unlikely that CBPP will ever be seen in Europe again. There is no live cattle trade with endemic areas of sub-Saharan Africa, and though European borders now stretch well into Asia, there is little confirmed evidence of pockets of CBPP existing there. CBPP was largely eradicated from Europe in the early 20th century, but sporadic outbreaks occurred somewhere in Europe every decade of the first half of the 20th century (Nicholas *et al.*, 2000). Portugal and Spain reported eradicating the disease in 1957 and 1961, respectively (Anonymous, 1967). Sporadic outbreaks, however, continued on the French–Spanish borders in 1967 (Poumarat and Solsona, 1995) and, such was the seriousness of these, the OIE called for urgent attention referring to the cases as 'event[s] of extreme gravity' (Anonymous, 1967). Whether action was taken by countries at risk is uncertain, but CBPP seemed to go quiet in the 1970s although possibly surveillance was not thorough enough to detect subclinically affected herds in mountainous regions. But in October 1980, not unexpectedly perhaps, the disease was noticed first in the cattle-breeding region in the Eastern Pyrenees in a dairy herd outside the village of Palau de Cerdagne in the French Département des Pyrénées Orientales (Fig. 10.1); then, following the instigation of serological monitoring, six more herds were found nearby, some serologically but not always clinically positive. It appeared that the first animal to show respiratory signs in Palau de Cerdagne had done so the previous March but was not suspected of having CBPP. In the following 2 years, seven CBPP-infected herds were identified followed in 1984 by another four positive herds. In the same year, four herds, technically in Spain but in fact within the Spanish enclave of Llivia (Fig. 10.2), a few miles within France where cattle from both countries could mingle freely, were eventually diagnosed with CBPP (ter Laak, 1992). Deaths were reported in only three of the 21 positive herds but one unusually lost half its cattle and showed 90% morbidity. Seropositivity in the affected herds ranged from 10% to 60% seropositive as measured by the complement fixation test (CFT) (ter Laak, 1992).

Early on, CBPP had not been recognized because of the low mortality and morbidity, probably due to the suppression of clinical signs by the rapid use of antimicrobials and corticosteroids. It is also possible that strains of low virulence had been circulating on the Spanish–French border over the last couple of decades and were not detected until changes occurred, such as the introduction of more susceptible or naïve cattle. Furthermore, unfamiliarity with the macroscopic CBPP lesions by

DOI: 10.1079/9781800627536.0010

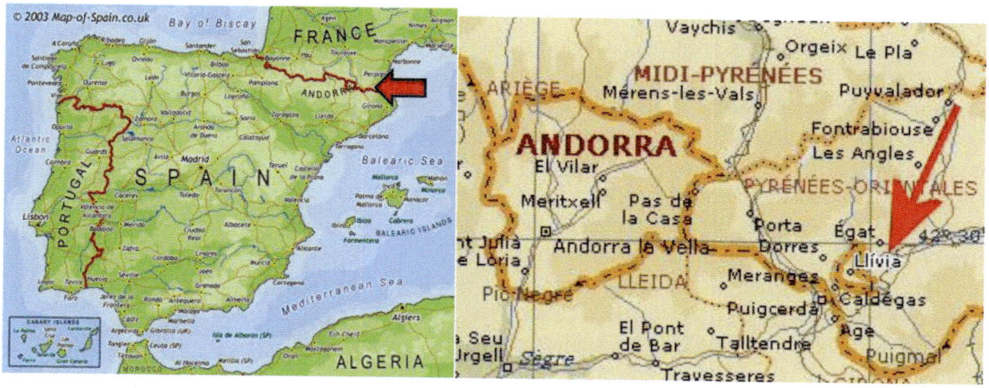

Fig. 10.1. Location of Llivia where outbreaks of CBPP broke out in the 1980s. (From Robin Nicholas.)

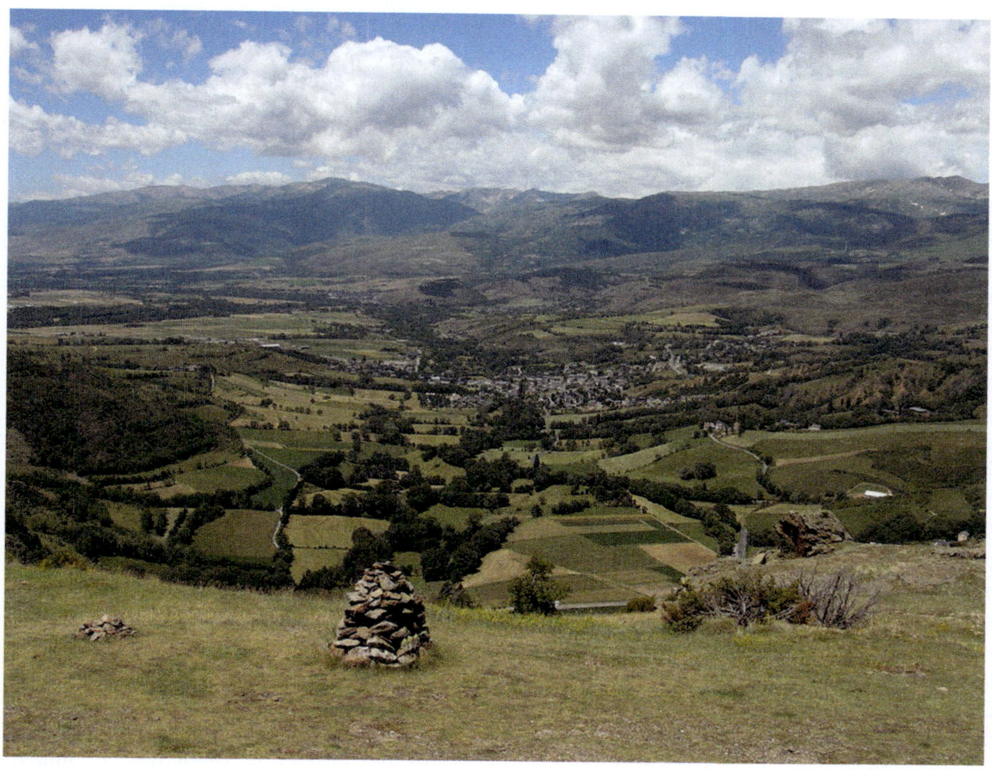

Fig. 10.2. The Spanish enclave, Llivia, within French territory. (From MarkCat, n.d., Wikimedia Commons, CC BY 4.0.)

the veterinarians charged with carrying out the post-mortems delayed diagnosis further. Once recognized, a total of 1200 cattle were killed in the whole region to prevent possible spread.

Portugal

In January 1983, nearly 1000 km away from Llivia at an abattoir in the picturesque medieval

Portuguese border town of Monção, CBPP was suspected in a tuberculosis-positive cow belonging to a farm in the village of Poldras, about 10 km from the Spanish border (Regalla, 1984). According to one account, this animal had been introduced illegally from Spain (Regalla *et al.*, 1996). In the same month, four sera from cattle in the same region with suspected CBPP tested positive. It was thought at the time that the disease had returned to Portugal after an absence of over 30 years. The truth, in fact, following extensive serological surveillance begun immediately after the first positive cases, was that CBPP was widespread throughout the country, with increasing prevalence from south to north, and with the majority of the infection concentrated in the region of Entre Douro and Minho and Beira Litoral. But some cases were even detected deep in the south in lower Alentejo (Regalla, 1984).

It appeared that the disease had been present in Portugal possibly as early as August of the previous year and had just not been noticed, due to low morbidity and negligible mortality. So, clearly the Monção animal had not been the only source of the outbreaks. In 1983, over 1500 outbreaks were reported – the high number was due to the small size of northern Portuguese farms, typically containing two or three cows, with the use of common milking parlours within villages facilitating the spread of the disease (Fig. 10.3). Serological testing, followed by the slaughter of infected and contact cattle, quickly brought the disease under control in the central and southern regions of Portugal, enabling the resumption of exports from those parts (Fig. 10.4). In the north, however, the slow payment of compensation often led private veterinarians to delay reporting cases because of the economic hardship it caused poorer farmers. Consequently, outbreaks continued there until the end of the 20th century. It was also thought that the damper conditions of the wooded north provided better conditions for the mycoplasmas to persist in the environment and spread, even through a green barrier, but firm evidence for this is difficult to find. As will be seen later in Italy, the illegal movement of cattle was more often the cause of disease transmission.

The heavy lifting for the testing of thousands of bovine sera during the eradication campaign was performed by the CFT which was

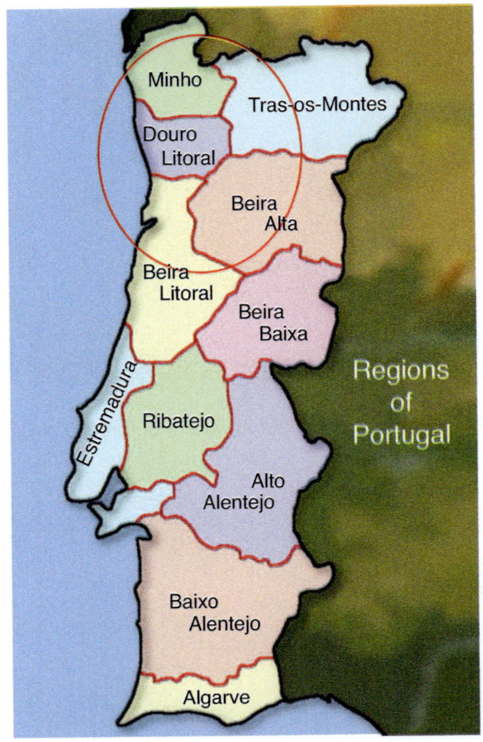

Fig. 10.3. Showing CBPP-endemic regions of Portugal 1985 (circled). (From Robin Nicholas.)

modified to a more convenient microtitre format at the Laboratorio di Investigação Nationicial Veterinária (LNIV) in Lisbon. Despite the accuracy of the test, concerns were raised about the large number of dubious and suspicious results leading to delays and uncertainties. For that reason, a highly sensitive and specific centrally located western blotting test was introduced for confirmation, though it required a high level of skill to interpret. This certainly improved the confidence of the serological results provided by the LNIV. In 2004, Portugal was declared free of CBPP by WOAH.

On the face of it, there was a remarkable homogeneity among the strains isolated in Portugal and, indeed, those from France and Spain. Digging a little deeper, Varela *et al.* (2010) conducted some genetic analysis on 65 strains of the causative mycoplasma isolated during the outbreaks in Portugal between 1993 and 1998. The researchers could differentiate the majority of strains from the Entre Douro-Minho region from those isolated in the Beira Litoral

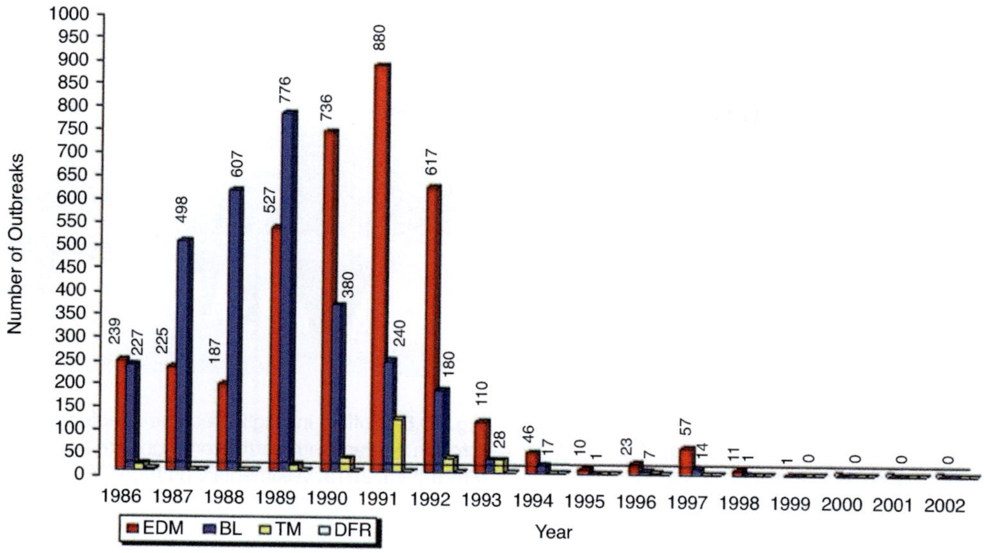

Fig. 10.4. CBPP outbreaks in Portugal between 1983 and 1999. (From Nicholas *et al.*, 2008.)

region, suggesting that there may have been two re-emergence events in Portugal. This may help explain the commonly held and conflicting belief that CBPP was introduced from Spain via Monção in 1983, when in fact the disease had already been present the previous year, though where that came from remains unknown.

Spain

It could have been predicted that CBPP would arrive in Spain, maybe not for the first time, with the vast hordes of cattle supplying the Napoleonic armies in the early 19th century during the Peninsula Wars, as happened in the rest of Europe. However, no evidence exists for this, and it was not until 1853 that there were reports of the disease in imported French cattle, which quickly infected the provinces of Barcelona, Lérdia and Gerona (Garcia, 1990). The following year, new outbreaks appeared in Navarre, Santander and Vizkaya, later spreading to Madrid. Little more information is available on the outcome of these outbreaks, and CBPP likely plagued Spain in some capacity during most decades of the 20th century before it appeared to have been eradicated by the end of the 1960s.

The detection of a CBPP-positive cow on the Spanish–Portuguese border in 1983 was believed by the Portuguese to have originated in Spain; consequently, it was strongly suspected that areas of Spain, other than the Pyrenees, were also infected. It was widely known that Spain had been battling CBPP in the 1960s and had even resorted to vaccination because of its economic and welfare impact (Nicholas *et al.*, 2000). This, however, was eventually stopped because it contravened European policy on CBPP of stamping out as vaccine antibodies detected in cattle would lead to interference with detection, particularly in countries where Spanish cattle were exported. For reasons still puzzling, it was not until 1989, 6 years after the start of the Portuguese outbreaks, that CBPP was detected on four farms in the province of Madrid, and then 1 year later on 13 farms in Segovia. More outbreaks were located in the northern coastal regions of Asturias and Galicia. In response, a Surveillance and Control Programme was developed in accordance with EEC legislation against CBPP with the zoning of the country into: high-risk areas including the municipalities of Madrid, Segovia, Zamora, Salamanca and Cantabria; medium-risk areas comprising neighbouring municipalities or within 10 km from outbreaks; and low-risk areas covering the rest of the country (Ministerio de Agricultura, Pesca y Alimentación, 2006). The frequency of surveillance of herds was based on the level of perceived risk. Those herds in high-risk areas were monitored every 6 months while those herds in medium-risk areas were examined every year. In low risk areas, 10% of herds were surveyed annually. A rise in infection was seen between 1990 and 1991, with seropositivity of 2.57% of herds mainly in Madrid, Cantabria and the Basque Country. Control measures, including clinical and abattoir surveillance and mandatory reporting, led to a steep decline in positivity between 1992 and 1993 but there was a resurgence between 1993 and 1997, peaking in 1995 probably due to the partial slaughter of clinically affected herds (ter Laak, 1992). No cases were reported in 1998 and continued surveillance by the Spanish Authorities well into the 21st century indicates the complete eradication of the disease.

Italy

A century after its last recorded outbreak, CBPP was diagnosed in October 1990 in a herd of nearly 600 dairy cattle in Martinengo close to Bergamo in Lombardy's Po Valley in northwest Italy. The outbreak initially appeared as a severe enzootic respiratory disease a few months earlier but was suppressed by intensive antibiotic therapy. However, the disease reappeared in the autumn killing 15 cows, many showing suspicious lesions not immediately recognized as CBPP (Martel *et al.*, 1991). Laboratory testing in Lyon, at the request of the IZS Brescia, confirmed CBPP. A month later, the disease was detected in meat cattle in the village of Valgrana, Cuneo, some 300 km away near the French border, though there appeared to be no connection between the two infected farms; indeed the dairy herd had not introduced cattle for over 20 years (Barale *et al.*, 1990). The Valgrana herd had received some 6-month-old French calves the previous year but tracing them to their home farm in France revealed no infection (Martel *et al.*, 1991). It is impossible to say which farm became infected first but the disease had probably been present in the region for up to 2 years spreading quickly into Lombardy, the main bovine dairy region; however, because of antimicrobial usage and lack of familiarity with the pathology of the pneumonic cows by inspecting veterinarians, it remained hidden. Experts from the OIE and EU could not solve this mystery.

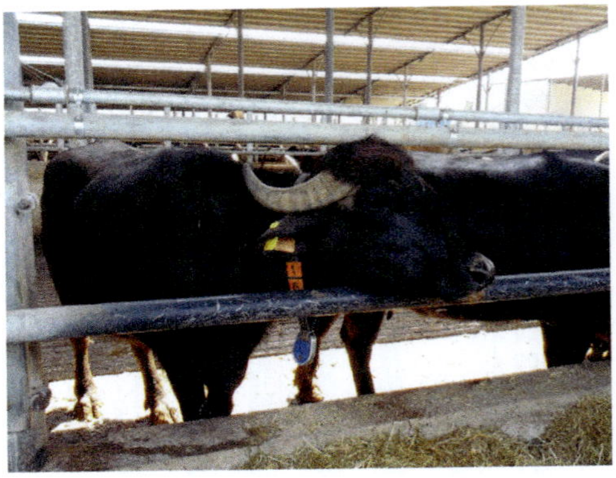

Fig. 10.5. Buffalo in Puglia became infected through contact with cattle from northern Italy. (From d'Itri, 2013, Wikimedia Commons, CC BY 2.0.)

Between October 1990 and September 1993, there were 94 outbreaks (66% in Lombardy) affecting nearly 23,000 cattle and buffaloes. The majority of outbreaks that occurred outside Lombardy were linked to movements of animals from this region extending to Puglia in the south where 2000 buffaloes became infected through contact with affected cattle from the north, though clinical and pathological signs in this species were slight (Fig. 10.5). Epidemiological analysis indicated strongly that spread was via cattle movements and direct animal-to-animal transmission (Fig. 10.6); suggestions that there may have been indirect routes such as infected fodder and machinery and water and wind-borne means were much more likely explained by illegal cattle movements (Giovanini *et al.*, 2000).

The Deletion Event

The question that no one wanted to answer or, indeed, even ask was: Where did the disease come from? CBPP has always been someone else's disease: had Spanish cattle infected French cattle high up in the Pyrenees, or vice versa, and had Spanish cattle infected Portuguese

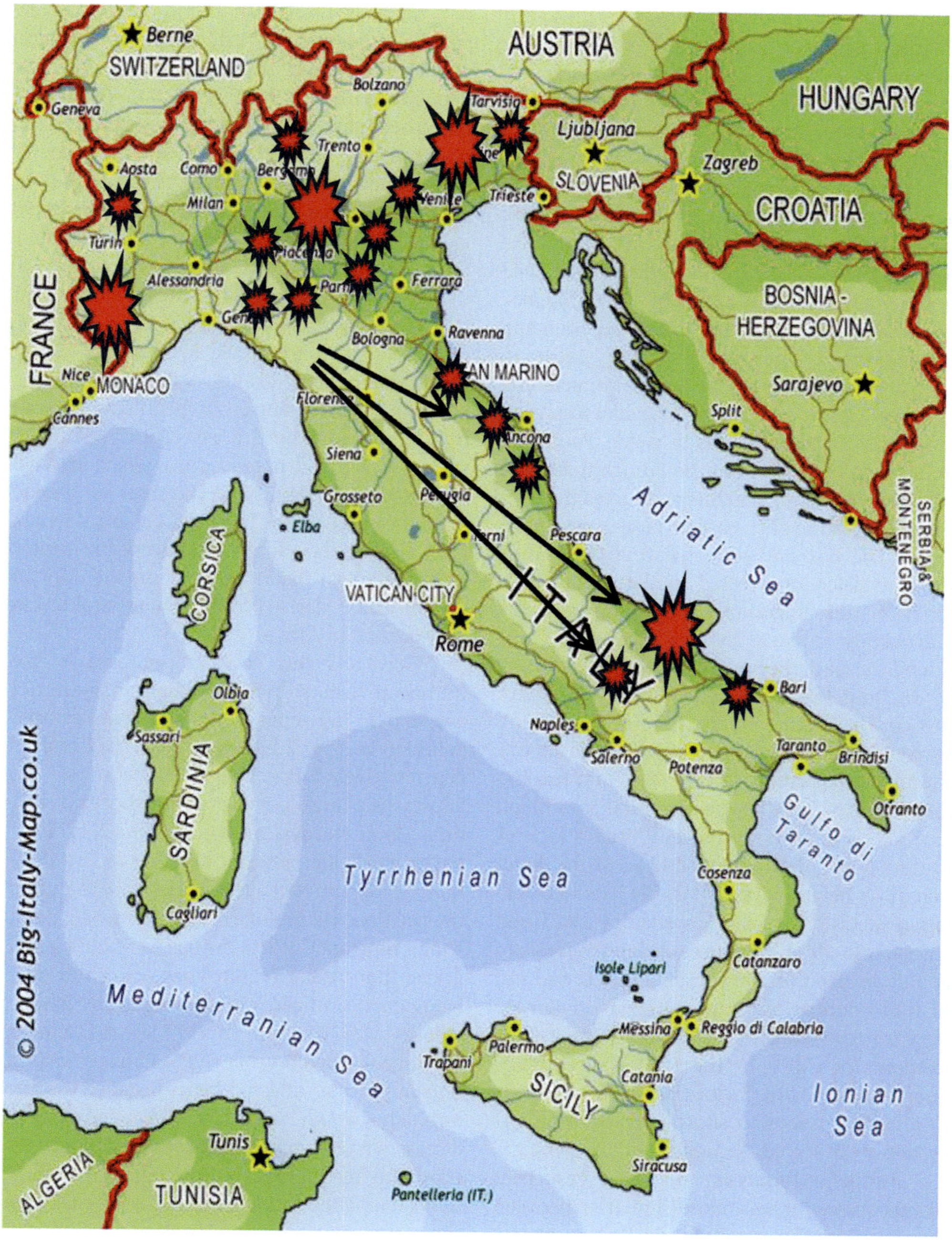

Fig. 10.6. Spread of CBPP through Italy 1980–1983 showing main outbreak areas and cattle movements. (From Robin Nicholas.)

ones, though this seemed highly unlikely given the seropositivity throughout Portugal at the time of the 'Monção incursion'? And now Italy! The timing was also unfortunate as trade with members of the European Community was now in full swing and borders were open to all. Cattle could be bought in one country and transported to another. Farmers could now, for example, take high-quality calves from northern Italy to their farms in Northumberland, in England, in a trailer.

Attempting to answer the question but increasing the confusion, Giovanini *et al.* (2000) identified five outbreaks in Italy arising from direct importation from France (two outbreaks); and, surprisingly, Poland (two) and Germany (one). Poland and Germany's last outbreaks were in 1936 and 1926, respectively, so seemed unlikely sources. At the time of the outbreaks, Spain and Portugal had been experiencing outbreaks but were not exporting cattle to Italy during this period (E. Scanziani, personal communication). In France there had also been outbreaks in the previous 5 years. Poumarat and Solsona (1995) from the French Reference laboratory in Lyon, who had conducted the confirmatory testing of the Italian cases, were quick out of the box and proposed that CBPP may have persisted undetected in the Italian Alps for years; this suggestion was both diversionary and highly unlikely as Italian veterinarians attend the slaughtering of all cattle in abattoirs throughout Italy so would probably not have missed the pathognomic lesions (Scanziani, personal communication). Moreover, France is the largest exporter of live cattle to Italy, sending an average of 900,000 head annually (as much as 85% of imports) because of Italy's lack of grazing land (Anonymous, 2024). Of the direct and close neighbours to Italy, Switzerland had last seen CBPP in 1895, Austria in 1921 and Hungary in 1901. Of course, a claim of freedom is only as good as the surveillance carried out in that country and few countries in Europe were carrying sufficient screening to guarantee freedom for CBPP in the late 20th century. Subsequently, both Switzerland and Hungary conducted surveys to show they were almost certainly CBPP-free (Nicholas *et al.*, 2000).

Antigenic analysis of these resurgent strains showed a very close similarity between them, all with the exception of a 98 kda protein not expressed by the majority of Italian strains and almost certainly represented a clonal variant (Goncalves *et al.*, 1998). This did not rule out France as the source of the infection as very few strains were examined. Despite this minor discrepancy, further comparative analysis of the new European isolates with African and Australian strains showed that the former did not oxidize glycerol, resulting in little hydrogen peroxide production attributable to the lack of the enzyme L-α glycerol phosphate oxidase (Houshaymi *et al.*, 1997); African strains, on the other hand, produced copious amounts of this toxic oxygen radical. Subsequently, genetic analysis revealed a genomic segment of 8.8 kb, present in African strains, which was completely lacking in these new European strains (Vilei and Frey, 2001); within this region was a copy of the *lppB* gene, a potential virulence factor, and the glycerol uptake gene. The 70 kDa product of this gene was not detected by immunoblotting in the re-emerging strains. A final piece of the jigsaw was that a single European strain stored from the outbreaks in France in 1967, before the re-emergence, did not have this deletion. Vilei *et al.*, 2000) concluded that the observed genetic difference was caused by a deletion event which gave rise to the cluster of European strains, rather than an insertion event in the African cluster and is derived from an ancestral strain now present in Africa.

How had this deletion occurred in the European strains? While mycoplasmas are not averse to losing genes – a process that has been going on for over 2 billion years as they evolved degeneratively from cell-walled ancestors – the latest was a huge loss over a very short space of time. Could natural mutation perhaps brought on by antibiotic pressure have led to this deletion? Unfortunately, the events surrounding the deletion will probably remain a mystery, but concerns about CBPP in Europe were sufficiently grave that research into new vaccines was being carried out in some commercial Spanish laboratories. This was not widely known, as official policy to control CBPP in Europe centred on slaughter of affected herds because vaccine antibody would adversely affect serological disease surveillance. Did European laboratories have the technology at the time to attempt molecular attenuation or could serial passage, the most widely practised method, bring about such massive loss of genetic material? And, most alarmingly, how could such a strain appear in cattle in four European countries in such a short space of time? It has been speculated that the movement of cattle 'immunized' with this so-called attenuated strain may have been responsible for these new outbreaks, but no evidence exists to support this. A highly informed source who wished to remain anonymous wrote to one of the authors (RN) in 2009:

> Since there is no [adequate] explanation how the disease spread in Europe by a strain that is somewhat attenuated, some persons speculated that the strain was perhaps produced by passaging a virulent strain in the attempt to attenuate it and produce a new live vaccine that was then spread by selling 'immunized' cattle. (Anonymous, 2009, personal communication)

An experimental infection in cattle in Switzerland, which compared a single new European strain with an African strain, provided some evidence to support the view that this deletion produced strains that were less virulent than African ones (Abdo *et al.*, 1998). However, some doubts remained in those who saw the lesions in the unexpected outbreaks in Portugal in 1983–1999, and those in Italy in the early 1990s, because of the severity of the lesions, particularly early in the epidemic (Nicholas *et al.*, 2008). In fact, mortality was reported in three French herds (up to 50% in one small herd) in the Pyrenees in 1980 (ter Laak, 1992). While clinical signs were often absent because of the close confinement of the cattle and, of course, the widespread use of antibiotics in Europe, lung lesions were often spectacular, completely destroying whole lungs, although usually only one, a differential diagnostic characteristic of CBPP. Moreover, exercising these normally stationary animals could readily stimulate coughing. It was evident that, as the disease progressed over time in Europe, it became more chronic in nature with the sequestrum becoming the dominant lesion, but this was also true in cattle in parts of Africa where CBPP was endemic. In addition, there was no evidence to suggest that strains in Europe before 1967 were particularly virulent. This cyclical nature of CBPP outbreaks was well known to researchers in Africa 40–50 years ago: as the epidemic progresses, the disease becomes milder (Egwu *et al.*, 1996). Although a great deal of work has been done on the pathogenicity mechanisms of *M. m. mycoides*, there is still much to know.

References

Abdo, E.M., Nicolet, J., Miserez, R., Gonçalves, R., Regalla, J. *et al.* (1998) Humoral and bronchial immune responses in cattle experimentally infected with *Mycoplasma mycoides* subsp. *mycoides* small colony type. *Veterinary Microbiology* 59(2–3), 109–122.

Anonymous (1967) Contagious bovine pleuropneumonia in the Pyrenees. *Veterinary Record* 80, 141.

Anonymous (2009) Correspondence from unnamed source to R.A.J. Nicholas.

Anonymous (2024) Beef production in italy (inrae.fr). Available at: https://sustainbeef.hub.inrae.fr/project/wp2.1-description-of-beef-production-systems/wp2.1.1-beef-production-national-statistics/beef-production-in-italy (accessed 20 September 2024).

Barale, G., Moda, G. and Valpreda, M. (1990) Description of an outbreak of contagious bovine pleuropneumonia. *Nuovo Progresso Veterinario* 46(3), 91–95.

Egwu, G., Nicholas, R.A.J., Ameh, J.A. and Bashiruddin, J.B. (1996) Contagious bovine pleuropneumonia: An update. *Veterinary Bulletin* 66, 195–208.

Garcia, M.I.C. (1990) Peripneumonia bovina. *Mundo Gunadero* 2, 54–55.

Giovanini, A., Bellini, S., Salman, M.D. and Caporale, V. (2000) Spatial risk factors related to outbreaks of contagious bovine pleuropneumonia in Northern Italy (1990–1993). *Revue Scientifique et Technique. Office International des Epizooties* 19(3), 764–772.

Goncalves, R., Regalla, J., Nicolet, J., Frey, J., Nicholas, R. *et al.* (1998) Antigen heterogeneity among *Mycoplasma mycoides* subsp. *mycoides* SC isolates: Discrimination of major surface proteins. *Veterinary Microbiology* 63(1), 13–28.

Houshaymi, B., Miles, R.J. and Nicholas, R.A.J. (1997) Oxidation of glycerol differentiates African from European isolates of *Mycoplasma mycoides* subsp. *mycoides* SC (small colony). *Veterinary Record* 140, 182–183.

Martel, J.L., Bellini, P., Perrin, M., Poumarat, F., Dannacher, G. *et al.* (1991) En 1991 dans le sud de L'Europe. *Le Pointe Veterinaire* 23(138), 27–32.

Ministerio de Agricultura, Pesca y Alimentación (2006) Programa nacional de vigilancia de la perineumonía contagios bovina 2021–2025 1–13. Available at: https://www.mapa.gob.es/es/ganaderia/temas/

sanidad-animal-higiene-ganadera/programadevigilanciapcb_tcm30-561130.pdf (accessed 15 March 2025).

Nicholas, R.A.J., Ayling, R.D. and McAuliffe, L. (2008) Contagious bovine pleuropneumonia. In: *Mycoplasma Diseases of Ruminants*. CABI, Wallingford, UK, pp. 69–97.

Nicholas, R.A.J., Bashiruddin, J.B., Ayling, R.D. and Miles, R. (2000) Contagious bovine pleuropneumonia: A review of recent developments. *Veterinary Bulletin* 70, 821–838.

Poumarat, F. and Solsona, M. (1995) Molecular epidemiology of *Mycoplasma mycoides* subsp. *mycoides* biotype small colony, the agent of contagious bovine pleuropneumonia. *Veterinary Microbiology* 47, 305–315.

Regalla, J. (1984) Epidemiological aspects of the contagious bovine pleuropneumonia in Portugal. *Repositório de Trabalhos Do Laboratorio Nacional de Investigação Veterinaria* XVI, 13–18.

Regalla, J., Caporale, V., Giovannini, A., Santini, F., Martel, J.L. *et al.* (1996) Manifestation and epidemiology of contagious bovine pleuropneumonia in Europe. *Revue Scientifique et Technique. Office International des Epizooties* 15(4), 1309–1329.

ter Laak, E.A. (1992) Contagious bovine pleuropneumonia: A review. *Veterinary Quarterly* 15, 104–110.

Varela, F., Inacio, J. and Botelho, A. (2010) Molecular diversity assessed by VNTR and IS1296 typing of historical *Mycoplasma mycoides* subsp. *mycoides* SC strains. *Veterinary Microbiology* 146, 295–302.

Vilei, E.M. and Frey, J. (2001) Genetic and biochemical characterization of glycerol uptake in *Mycoplasma mycoides* subsp. *mycoides* SC: Its impact on H_2O_2 production and virulence. *Clinical and Diagnostic Laboratory Immunology* 8(1), 85–92.

Vilei, E.M., Abdo, E.-M., Nicolet, J., Botehlo, A., Goncalves, R. *et al.* (2000) Genomic and antigenic differences between the European and African/Australian clusters of *Mycoplasma mycoides* subsp. *mycoides* SC. *Microbiology* 146, 477–486.

11 Appliance of Science: Technological Advances in Diagnosis of CBPP

Abstract

Diagnosis of CBPP until the early 20th century could only be achieved definitively by post-mortem examination and, even then, lesions were not always pathognomonic, particularly in the early stages of disease. Although isolation of the causative mycoplasma was achieved in 1898, colony morphology could not be relied on as later other mycoplasmas with similar appearance began to be isolated. Agglutination tests were quickly developed providing the possibility of a positive diagnosis on a living animal for the first time but were superseded by the complement fixation test, which is still in use in many reference laboratories today. The development of enzyme immunoassays in the early 1980s allowed the serological screening of large numbers of samples and enabled the automation of testing essential for eradication programmes. Nucleic acid amplification assays like PCR developed in the late 1980s revolutionized the detection and identification of mycoplasmas enabling diagnosis in hours rather than days or weeks and were soon adopted as approved tests by regulatory bodies like WOAH. Isolation and propagation of mycoplasmas are still important for antigen production needed in serological tests and vaccine production and the development of specific fully defined media for high growth remains a goal.

Laboratory Diagnosis

The isolation and culture of the CBPP pathogen in cell-free nutrient media at the Pasteur Institute by Nocard and Roux (1990) was a major advance in mycoplasmology: the study of small wall-less degenerate bacteria. However, at the time, there was a great deal of uncertainty about the nature of these microbes, which were able to pass through filters that normally retained all known micro-organisms and were consequently known as filterable viruses. The *in vitro* growth of these mycoplasmas now offered the possibility to study their morphology, produce purer vaccines and develop diagnostic tests capable of detecting CBPP in cattle.

The first *in vitro* test involved culturing diluted, filtered lung fluid from an infected animal in broth containing up to 10% cattle or horse serum. Within 2 to 3 days, a turbidity would be seen in the broth which, when inoculated onto a nutrient solid medium, would give rise to the characteristic fried egg colonies. Direct application of the lung fluid onto the solid medium was also shown to be successful and quicker (Hutyra and Marek, 1912). This test was not truly specific, as later many more mycoplasmas were isolated with similar fried egg appearance, but the isolation of these colonies from CBPP-affected herds was confirmation enough for many. Histological examination of lung material from dead cattle also proved useful though not all were convinced at the time that the detection of the organising perivascular foci in the middle of necrotic tissue and peribronchial foci were pathognomonic for CBPP as they later were shown to be (Nunes Petisca *et al.*, 1988).

Various media based on the work of Nocard and Roux was reported by European workers during the early 20th century but, with eradication well on its way mainly by stamping out (and war not far off), research efforts to develop improved media and methods of detection moved to Australia, where CBPP was still rampant. Backed by funding from the ultimately short-lived and unsuccessful Empire Marketing Board (set up in 1926 by British colonial secretary, Leo Amery, to boost intra-Empire trade), along with the cattle industry and the Queensland government, a research laboratory was set up in Oonoonba, Townsville on the Queensland coast (Newton, 1992). A talented team of scientists that included Arthur Turner and Andrew Campbell began work on CBPP

DOI: 10.1079/9781800627536.0011

and soon developed a medium based on one that they had used to grow anaerobic organisms (Turner *et al.*, 1935). It was composed of a pig stomach acid digest of bovine muscle and liver and enriched with 10% of calf or other mammalian serum. In this medium, named BVF-OS, the pleuropneumonia organisms could reach maximum growth within 48 hours and remain virulent for calves through many subcultures. A vaccine they developed from 4-day-old cultures eventually led to the V5 strain, isolated in Victoria, and was used throughout the vaccine campaign.

A test that could determine the CBPP-status of living animals enabling the identification of infected from non-infected animals was urgently required. The first attempt was to use similar technology that had been used for tuberculosis testing in which concentrated lung fluid from a CBPP-affected cow was inoculated subcutaneously. A rise in temperature of 1–2°C indicated the animal had been exposed but results were inconsistent. Improvements in reliability were later reported when concentrated culture-grown material was used instead of clinical material, but the test never went into routine use (Hutyra *et al.*, 1938).

Serological Tests

A major tool missing from the fight against CBPP was a test that could detect the presence of the mycoplasma in cattle. Tests to detect 'precipitins' and 'precipitogens' (antigens that induce the precipitin antibodies) in the serum of affected cattle were reported early in the 20th century in France and Belgium but were soon abandoned because of poor sensitivity though their combined use, while a little cumbersome, could increase that significantly (Hutyra *et al.*, 1938). Subjective interpretation of the test was another problem that was not so evident with agglutination tests which resulted in a very visible clumping on a glass slide following the mixing of culture-grown organisms with a positive serum. Many years later a modified agglutination test that used a latex bead-bound polysaccharide antigen extracted from culture-grown mycoplasma to detect antibodies in blood or serum was shown to be highly convenient and rapid for testing cattle in the field (Fig. 11.1) (Nicholas *et al.*, 2008).

A major drawback to the serological tests described above was their inability to screen large numbers of sera that would be required in any eradication programme. This was rectified when Campbell modified a serological test that had been developed by the German bacteriologist August Wasserman to detect antibodies against syphilis at the turn of the 20th century (Turner *et al.*, 1935). The complement fixation test (CFT) was used immediately to test cattle in Western Australia and Queensland and was shown to detect nearly all acute and subacute cases and most chronic cases. The test also proved remarkably specific confirming the CBPP-free status of 3000 cattle from an uninfected region.

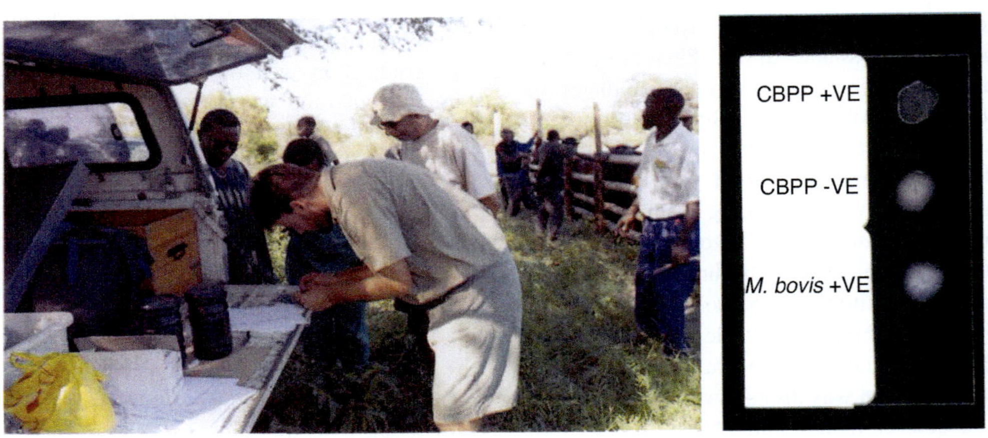

Fig. 11.1. Latex agglutination test and its use in the field. (From Robin Nicholas.)

Originally boiled antigen from pleural exudate was used in the CFT but soon *in vitro*-grown antigen was substituted improving production and standardization. Like all tests, it is only as good as the technicians performing it, but one of its other advantages is that if it does fail, it is possible to identify the problem quickly from the range of test controls used. Perhaps with the advent of enzyme-based assays, it is surprising that the CFT is still used because of its relatively laborious preparation but its accuracy and precision make it the test of choice in many reference laboratories today.

Enzyme Immunoassays

The advent of the enzyme-linked immunosorbent assays revolutionized serological testing across biomedical and veterinary medical fields which enabled the rapid and automated testing of large numbers of sera. The tests are generally sensitive and specific and ultimately cost-effective. The first commercial test to appear was the highly specific competitive test developed at the CIRAD-EMVT in Montpellier (Le Goff and Thiaucourt, 1998) which quickly became the OIE-approved test along with the long-established CFT. Many comparative assays have been carried out show that, while CFT is more sensitive in the early stages of infection, the cELISA is better able to detect chronic carriers in the later stages. Neither test detects all positive cattle. In-house indirect ELISAs using whole cell or extracted antigens are often the most sensitive but conversely tend to detect more false positive sera at the beginning of an eradication campaign when there are many infected herds. These tests do, however, become a problem when there are fewer positive herds. These issues can be overcome by the use of a confirmatory test like the immunoblotting test to be carried out on sera where results are suspicious. Though complex, time-consuming and requiring well-trained staff, highly sensitive and specific immune (western) blotting tests (IBT) were described by Gonçalves *et al.* (1998) in which the simultaneous presence of five antigens (110, 98, 95, 62/60 and 48) are diagnostic for sera from infected cattle (Fig. 11.2). This test was used in the latter stages of the Portuguese eradication campaign when increasing numbers of CFT-positives were seen in clinically-free regions thus reducing the time to declare herds free of CBPP.

Immunocytochemistry (ICC) is a very useful confirmatory test for CBPP, particularly where the causative organism *M. m. mycoides* is not recoverable (often following long transport distances or antibiotic treatment) where the animal has died of acute disease or where serology is not possible or unclear (Scanziani *et al.*, 1997).

Molecular Diagnosis

It is hard to overestimate the impact of nucleic acid amplification tests like the polymerase chain reaction (PCR) on mycoplasma diagnosis. These slow-growing bacteria can take days, if not weeks, to identify using culture and serological tests. Powerful diagnostic systems based on PCR have been developed for the rapid detection, identification, and differentiation of members of the *M. mycoides* cluster and the specific identification of *M. m. mycoides* over the last few decades. The first reported test was based on a gene probe, CAP 21, which could distinguish *M. m. mycoides*, and the closely related *M. m. capri*, from other mycoplasmas (Taylor *et al.*, 1992). Primers were designed that amplified a 0.5 kb region of the gene of both *mycoides* subspecies. Identification of the CBPP pathogen was achieved by digesting the amplified fragment with the restriction enzyme *Asn*1 to give a characteristic banding pattern (Bashiruddin *et al.*, 1994). The test was used immediately after development to detect CBPP-infected cattle during the re-emergent outbreaks on isolated strains and clinical material, most effectively in pleural fluid (Nicholas *et al.*, 1994). It was then used for a period to check all cattle imported into the UK from Italy with negative results.

Since its introduction, PCRs have been used for the detection and identification of *M. m. mycoides* from culture and clinical materials including nasal mucous, pleural fluid, tissue from lungs, lymph node, kidney, spleen and semen from cattle, the milk and respiratory tract of small ruminants (Nicholas *et al.*, 2008). In some cases, they had superior diagnostic sensitivities compared to conventional diagnostic

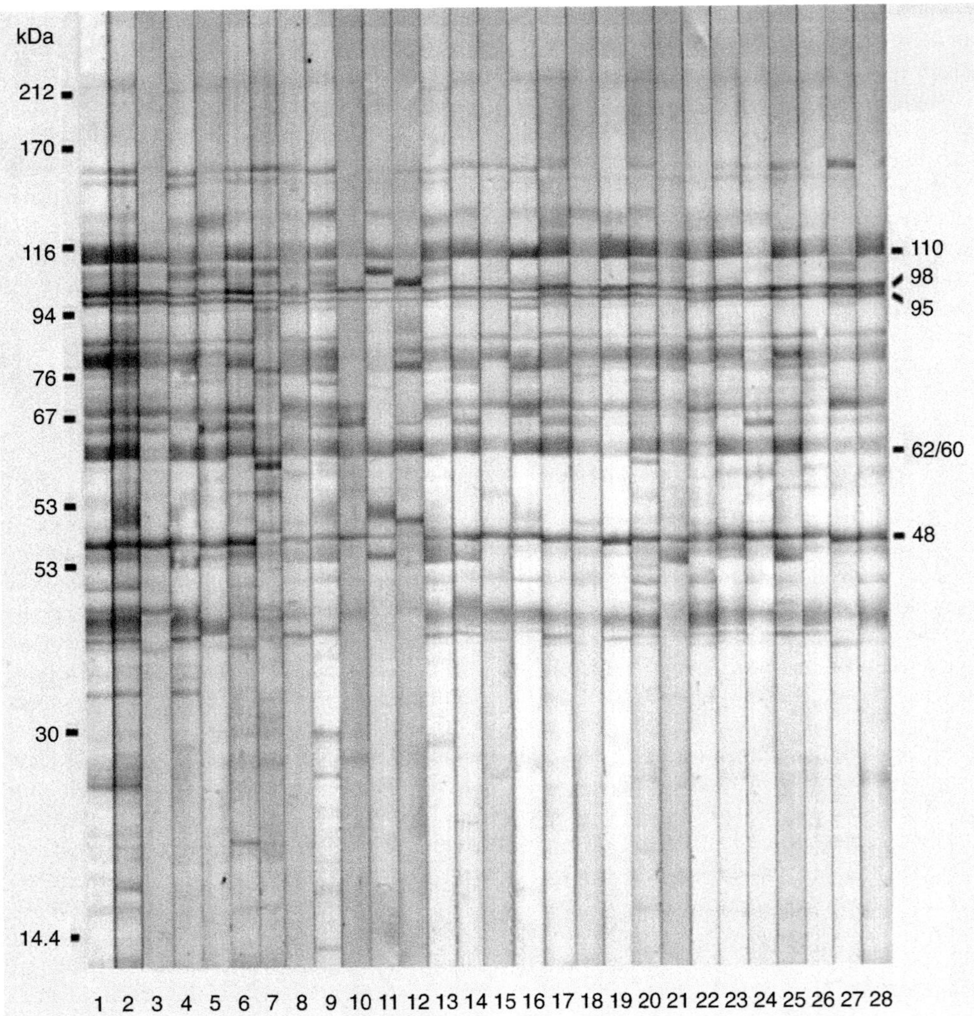

Fig. 11.2. Immunoblot of samples from cattle. Positive sera showing the five major bands. Molecular markers on left. (Photo courtesy of Dr Rosario Gonçalves.)

tests. Particularly sensitive nested and real-time PCR systems have been used for the detection of *M. m. mycoides* from culture and clinical material where the target organism may be in low numbers such as in nasal swab samples.

Most published PCRs and multiplex systems only detect one or a small number of mycoplasmas at a time. The publication of a PCR/denaturing gradient gel electrophoresis (DGGE) test with universal primers based on the 16S RNA gene enabled the detection of over 70 different mycoplasmas including those of the *Mycoides* cluster even in mixed culture (McAuliffe *et al.*, 2005; Nicholas *et al.*, 2008). This test provided a much larger intelligence as to what co-infecting mycoplasmas were present in a tissue or organ. While the migration patterns of the two *mycoides* subspecies were similar in the DGGE, confirmatory PCRs could be applied quickly. Sadly, microarray tests, while promising in development, have not yet gone into routine diagnostic service (Schnee *et al.*, 2012).

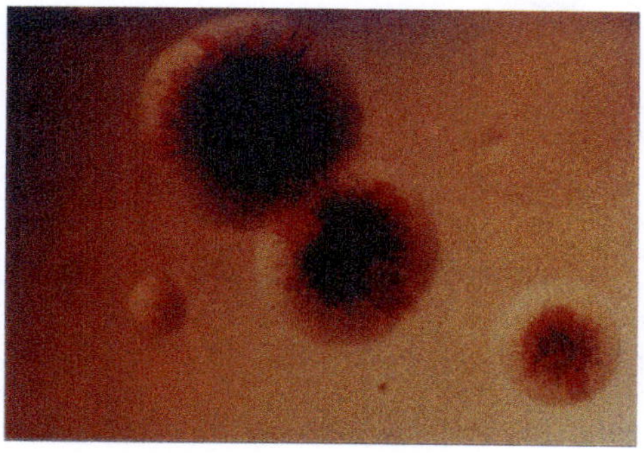

Fig. 11.3. Showing stained colonies of *Mycoplasma mycoides* subsp. *mycoides* with diagnostic medium. (Photo courtesy of Dr Helena Windsor.)

Biochemical Tests

With the introduction of PCR, many biochemical tests became redundant but are still useful for comparing strain differences. A diagnostic commercially available solid medium based on tetrazolium reduction was developed in which *M. m. mycoides* colonies became red after a few days (Fig. 11.3) This medium is useful in the primary isolation from clinical material, enabling immediate identification of colonies for subsequent confirmation by standard and molecular methods (Mycoplasma Experience Ltd, Reigate, UK).

The use of colorimetric assays to measure the production of hydrogen peroxide, confirmed for the first time that the re-emergent European *M. m. mycoides* strains did not oxidise glycerol (Houshaymi *et al.*, 1997) and showed that they had not originated from Africa.

Other Tests

A major recommendation in the report of the Gap Analysis Meeting for CBPP, held in 2023 and, indeed, other recent reports (EU Discontools; WOAH Group of experts etc.), is the development and validation of a rapid, cost-effective diagnostic assay able to be performed in the field. Presently, only a latex agglutination test satisfies these criteria but lacks both sensitivity and specificity on individual animals. Loop-mediated isothermal amplification (LAMP) is an innovative and economic gene amplification tool based on its ability to amplify a target gene with high efficiency under isothermal conditions, unlike PCR, in the range of 60–65°C. In comparison to conventional PCR and real-time PCR, the LAMP technique is less sensitive to inhibitors present in biological samples. It does not require temperature cycling and can be performed using a simple heating device such as a water bath; therefore, it can potentially be used for tests in the field. LAMP is more specific and faster than PCR and real-time PCR because it employs four oligonucleotide primers, namely FIP (forward inner primer), BIP (backward inner primer), F3 (forward primer) and B3 (backward primer) to recognize six different regions of the target gene. Two extra primers, LF (loop forward) and LB (loop backward), are also incorporated in order to accelerate the amplification of reaction as well as enhance the specificity. LAMP has been shown to be a sensitive and specific method for the detection of veterinary pathogens. The detection of *M. m. mycoides* by LAMP was first reported by Mair *et al.* (2013) more than a decade ago but was never commercialized or used in the field. Furthermore, the method was not validated on field samples. It is understood that presently (2025) the teams led by USDA are developing the technology with colleagues in Kenya.

Final Remarks

In Olorunshola *et al.*, 2017, Olorunshola *et al* argued that the diagnostic tests available today are more than sufficient to detect affected herds and that the race to develop increasingly more sensitive tests will only confuse diagnoses. PCRs are capable of detecting infinitesimal quantities of organisms and one must ask, what is the significance of detecting fractions of a pathogen in the absence of clinical or pathological signs when a simple tool like a latex agglutination test will do the job?

References

Bashiruddin, J.B., Nicholas, R.A., Santini, F.G., Ready, R.A., Woodward, M.J. *et al.* (1994) Use of the polymerase chain reaction to detect mycoplasma DNA in cattle with contagious bovine pleuropneumonia. *Veterinary Record* 134(10), 240–241.

Gonçalves, R., Regalla, J., Nicolet, J., Frey, J., Nicholas, R. *et al.* (1998) Antigen heterogeneity among *Mycoplasma mycoides* subsp. *mycoides* SC isolates: Discrimination of major surface proteins. *Veterinary Microbiology* 63(1), 13–28.

Houshaymi, B.M., Miles, R.J. and Nicholas, R.A. (1997) Oxidation of glycerol differentiates African from European isolates of *Mycoplasma mycoides* subsp. *mycoides* SC (small colony). *Veterinary Record* 140(7), 182–183.

Hutyra, F. and Marek, J. (1912) *Contagious Bovine Pleuropneumonia. Special Pathology and Therapeutics of the Diseases of Domestic Animals*, American edition. Bailliere Tindall, USA, pp. 389–391.

Hutyra, F., Marek, J. and Manninger, R. (1938) Contagious bovine pleuropneumonia. In: *Special Pathology and Therapeutics of the Diseases of Domestic Animals*, 5th edition. Bailliere Tindall, USA, pp. 455–458.

Le Goff, C. and Thiaucourt, F. (1998) A competitive ELISA for the specific diagnosis of contagious bovine pleuropneumonia (CBPP). *Veterinary Microbiology* 60(2–4), 179–191.

Mair, G., Vilei, E.M.W., Frey, A. and Unger, M. (2013) Isothermal loop-mediated amplification for CBPP. *BMC Veterinary Research* 9, 108–112.

McAuliffe, L., Ellis, R., Lawes, J., Ayling, R.D. and Nicholas, R.A.J. (2005) 16S rDNA and DGGE: A single generic test for detecting and differentiating mycoplasma species. *Journal of Medical Microbiology* 54, 1–9.

Newton, L.G. (1992) Contagious bovine pleuropneumonia in Australia: Some historic highlights from entry to eradication. *Australian Veterinary Journal* 69(12), 306–317.

Nicholas, R., Ayling, R. and McAuliffe, L. (2008) Contagious bovine pleuropneumonia. In: *Mycoplasma Diseases of Ruminants*. CABI Publishing, Wallingford, UK, pp. 69–97.

Nicholas, R.A.J., Bashiruddin, J.B., Santini, F.G., Regalla, J. and Taylor, T.K. (1994) Evaluation of a polymerase chain reaction for contagious bovine pleuropneumonia in naturally infected cattle. *IOM Letters* 3, 15–16.

Nocard, E. and Roux, E. (1990) The microbe of pleuropneumonia. 1896. *Reviews of Infectious Diseases* 2, 354–358. Available at: https://www-jstor-org.er.lib.k-state.edu/stable/pdf/4455506.pdf?refreqid=fastly-default%3A2ba70aaea06d16af0c778db70b5041d6&ab_segments=&initiator=&acceptTC=1 (accessed 5 January 2025).

Nunes Petisca, J.L., Duraco, J.F.C., Lage, M., Gonçalves, J.M.M., Ramos, M.J.A. *et al.* (1988) [Pathogenesis and pathology of contagious bovine pleuropneumonia in Portugal.] Patogenia e anatomia atologica de peripneumonia contagiosa dos bovinos (PPCB) em Portugal. In: *Repositorio Des Trabalhos Do Laboratorio Nacional de Investigacão Veterinaria (Lisbon)*. Numero Special, pp. 1–10.

Olorunshola, I.D., Peters, A.R., Scacchia, M. and Nicholas, R.A.J. (2017) CBPP: never out of Africa. *Veterinary Bulletin* 12, 1–7. DOI: 10:1079/PAVSNNR201712019.

Scanziani, E., Paltrinieri, S., Boldini, M., Grieco, V., Monaci, C. *et al.* (1997) Histological and immunohistochemical findings in thoracic lymph nodes of cattle with contagious bovine pleuropneumonia. *Journal of Comparative Pathology* 117(2), 127–136.

Schnee, C., Schulsse, S., Hotzel, H., Ayling, R.D., Nicholas, R.A.J. *et al.* (2012) A novel rapid DNA microarray assay enables identification of 37 mycoplasma species and highlights multiple mycoplasma infections. *PLOS ONE* 7, e33237.

Taylor, T.K., Bashiruddin, J.B. and Gould, A.R. (1992) Application of a diagnostic DNA probe for the differentiation of the two types of *Mycoplasma mycoides* subsp. *mycoides*. *Research in Veterinary Science* 53(2), 154–159.

Turner, A.W., Campbell, A.D. and Dick, A.T. (1935) Recent work on Pleuro-pneumonia Contagiosa Boum in Northern Queensland. *Australian Veterinary Journal* 11(2), 63–71.

12 Future Prospects and Lessons Learnt

Lessons Learnt

In his excellent scholarly account of the origins of CBPP, the former director general of the OIE, Jean Blancou (2000), using secondary sources chiefly from 19th-century French researchers including Delafond and Leclainche, examined the evidence for descriptions of CBPP-like diseases in classical literature. His first reference was to a clinically similar disease that broke out in the eastern Sicily in 212 BCE during the Greek wars but, with closer inspection, seems unlikely as its host range of birds, dogs, humans and cattle was too wide for what we now know as CBPP. Virgil, writing in Latin in the first century BCE, was also believed to be referring to a bovine respiratory disease in which the coughing of blood and fever are noticeable features. Later descriptions in the 4th century AD of chronic lung disease are more likely to be caused by tuberculosis, a much more ancient disease.

The search for the birth of a disease such as CBPP is, of course, a largely futile task as definitive evidence was not available until diagnostic tests could confirm clinical and pathological signs, even allowing for very clear descriptions of the disease by 18th-century pathologists such as Haller. Even more recently, reports of CBPP-like disease in Asia in the late 20th century were largely conjecture and speculation and not based on accurate diagnosis.

However, the scientific landscape has shifted significantly in the last decade or two with the introduction of powerful tools capable of measuring small genetic mutations in an organism's genome with these changes acting as molecular evolutionary clocks. In 2012, Fischer *et al.* partially sequenced important housekeeping genes from over 100 strains of members of the *M. mycoides* cluster, including over 30 isolates of the CBPP pathogen; they then analysed the data to estimate the timing of the origin of each member of the cluster and correlate the estimated demographic history of the pathogens with that of their hosts. Results were striking: the common ancestor of the cluster dated to about 8000 BCE, which, according to Zeder and Hesse (2000), coincided with the paleolithic domestication of livestock when large herds of livestock (often mixed) were established, favouring the spread and diversification of these mycoplasmas to different hosts. Drilling down into the results it is clear that *M. m. mycoides* emerged relatively recently, as genetic variation among strains is minimal compared to the caprine pathogen *M. m. capri* from which it evolved (Fig. 12.1). The latter appears to have emerged over 3000 years ago, possibly following some further change in livestock husbandry, and shows, as one would expect, extensive genetic heterogeneity. Using next-generation sequencing technology exclusively on 20 widely occurring strains of *M. m. mycoides*, Dupuy *et al.* (2012) went one step further and dated the most recent common ancestor to around 1700, give or take 100 years. This would comfortably coincide with the reports of clinical CBPP in Europe and bring us closer to being able to identify the date of its first emergence. This recent emergence of the CBPP pathogen would also account for its virulence for cattle as its new host is still in the process of adapting to the new infection. A similar scenario is seen with the goat pathogen *M. capricolum* subsp. *capripneumoniae*, the cause of contagious caprine pleuropneumonia, which emerged a little before the time of its bovine cluster relative. It also shows little genetic variation and is highly virulent (Fig. 12.1).

At the time of writing (February, 2025) Europe has been free of CBPP for a quarter of a century and, despite the disease's ability to reside unnoticed in small herds, as it appears to have done in the Pyrenees in the 1970s, it is highly unlikely to have survived this long undetected. Furthermore, it is hoped that improved awareness and surveillance of mycoplasma

DOI: 10.1079/9781800627536.0012

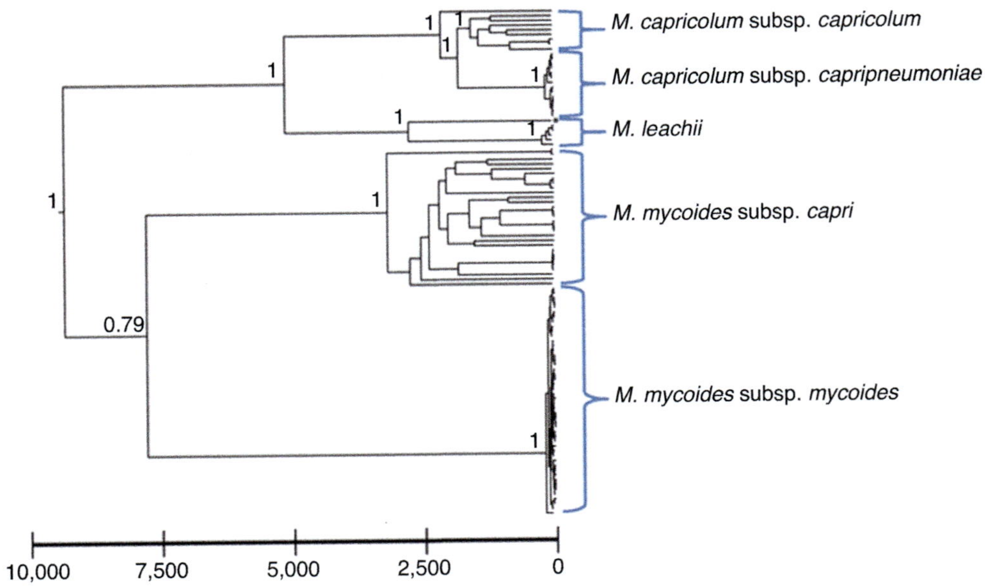

Fig. 12.1. Molecular evolution of the Mycoides cluster showing *M. mycoides* subsp. *mycoides* emerging relatively recently. (Fischer *et al.*, 2012.)

diseases should rapidly locate future outbreaks. Of course, memories fade and resources dwindle, but the present period of CBPP silence is unprecedented for Europe. On the other hand, European borders have extended further east to areas where surveillance may be less rigorous, but little evidence exists for forgotten pockets of CBPP. Bovine respiratory disease, caused by a variety of viruses and bacteria (in particular the relatively new kid on the block, *Mycoplasma bovis*), may from time to time cause confusion but laboratory tests today are both fast and specific. The threat from other areas like Africa is negligible as only CBPP-free Botswana (presently) has any trade links with the EU, but that is exclusively for beef which poses no risk from CBPP. But such was the concern of the impact on trade of the CBPP outbreaks that Botswana slaughtered nearly 400,000 cattle to protect its lucrative markets in the early 1990s.

The resurgence of CBPP in Europe, however, still requires explanation. While in the end, careful examination of the European outbreaks shows that the disease remained hidden for less than a decade, it was clear that it was present in most of the affected countries during this time but had been unforgivingly missed by veterinarians and diagnostic laboratories. But what cannot be so easily explained is that the strain that re-emerged in all affected countries was deficient in a large chunk of its genome. Was this Europe's COVID-19 laboratory escape, or were these changes spontaneous? Whichever, the deletion conveniently took out some important virulence genes which may have had some effect on virulence, though this is by no means proven.

At the end of the 19th century, Daniel E. Salmon, chief of the Bureau of Animal Industry (BAI), confidently predicted that the USA would not see CBPP again; after a century and a quarter, his prediction still holds. Recently, there has been renewed interest in North America in the disease, where previously research was highly restricted for fears of escape of the pathogen. Today US collaboration with East Africa may help resolve the intractable problems of CBPP following the failure of previous attempts by the Food and Agriculture of the United Nations, WOAH, and European and African laboratories to have any impact on its prevalence.

Hutyra *et al.* (1938) mysteriously claimed that CBPP was 'not unknown' to South America but provided no evidence for the claim. If it was known there, perhaps brought in by the conquering Portuguese or Spanish or by later traders, it never established, unlike other ruminant mycoplasmas including the closely related goat pathogen *M. mycoides* subsp. *capri*. CBPP's failure to infect cattle must be a great relief to the livestock industry in Brazil, Argentina and neighbouring countries which today provide a quarter of the world's beef.

The threat of re-infection of Australia and New Zealand must be considered far less likely than in Europe, mostly because of their strict import controls, especially New Zealand which has not allowed livestock imports for over a decade. Despite this, New Zealand has just experienced an expensive and politically and socially divisive eradication campaign for *Mycoplasma bovis* which could only have arrived in imported semen from Europe; consequently, restrictions on this sample have been greatly strengthened. Credit must be given to the New Zealand veterinary authorities for eradicating this widely occurring non-statutory disease particularly as the form of the disease seen was, on the whole, clinically mild. The approaches to the eradication of CBPP between Australia and New Zealand make for an interesting comparative study and reflect the host of different factors between the two countries including geography, husbandry, climate and approaches to vaccination. These conditions enabled New Zealand to rid itself of CBPP, probably within two decades, while Australia suffered for over a century.

From sources studied in this book, it is clear that Australia, itself a victim of an infected heifer from Britain, then spread the disease during an export drive beginning in the 19th century to the rest of the Pacific nations and Asia. It made some impact on Japan and Korea, but little information exists on other countries, suggesting it never established itself. China, however, was a closed book until the 1990s when communication was first established with the then AHVLA in the UK. The impact of CBPP was huge, greatly impeding the development of agriculture in China in the 1950s and 1960s. Fortunately, a united approach involving research, culling and vaccination with detailed record-keeping saw the last case in 1989. It is highly likely that the disease spread from China to neighbouring countries including Assam, a small state in north-east India. Despite the war with Japan raging close by, British and Indian scientists in the 1940s were able to study the disease, carry out experimental infections, establish diagnostic tests and develop a vaccine with a local strain and effectively control the disease within 30 years – an impressive achievement! The isolated region where Assam is situated meant CBPP was unable to spread further into India. Examining the Imperial veterinary records stretching back to the end of the 19th century, we believe India was never infected though other bacterial respiratory diseases like haemorrhagic septicaemia may have confused some veterinarians at the time. Consequently, General Napier could not have taken CBPP from India to the Horn of Africa in the mid-19th century as is sometimes believed, because it was not there. Furthermore, journalist-turned-explorer Henry Morton Stanley, who accompanied Napier's expedition, made no mention of any diseases in the cattle though he was aware of glanders in the donkeys, which were the primary beasts of burden.

Are other parts of Asia infected with CBPP? Well, according to published reports (admittedly in undistinguished journals) in the last decade, both Malaysia and Pakistan have described CBPP, though official bodies like WOAH, FAO and CIRAD do not appear to have recognized these outbreaks. Certainly, no mycoplasma strains or photos have been presented to the CBPP community so we must wait for confirmation. Should these reports prove to be true then surveillance in neighbouring countries should be intensified.

Over 20 years ago, an OIE Committee met in Paris to draw up plans to eradicate CBPP from the world although, in fact, this primarily meant Africa. It was based on a template for foot-and-mouth disease, which has also stubbornly resisted attempts of control. It is true to say that hopes of eradication are further away than when the committee met. Unlike Europe where a single strategy of movement control, test and slaughter was imposed enabling the eradication of CBPP at the end of the 20th century, the lack of sustained cooperation between countries in sub-Saharan Africa seriously inhibits control of this transboundary disease. In addition, a panoply of other factors compounds control efforts including a need for an improved safer and more robust vaccine and greater national coverage, a lack of versatile diagnostic field test, greater awareness of the socio-economic impact of CBPP, poor private and public funding, climate change, wars and terrorist activities. Moreover, the COVID-19 pandemic has exacerbated the problem further by drastically reducing the submission of country reports of CBPP by 70% from 2017 to 2022, resulting in the reporting of only 20 outbreaks in 2022 from two countries compared to a peak of 273 in 2019 before the beginning of the pandemic. Moreover, the number of countries reported to be vaccinating against CBPP has dropped drastically from 25 in 2015, to only four in 2022. Clearly, this alarming situation will have serious impacts on attempts to control CBPP. It is hard not to see that a meeting organized by the USDA and an international consortium called STAR-IDAZ held near Cambridge in 2023 to identify gaps in CBPP research will not be needed again soon.

This book, a contribution to the wider literature on animal diseases generally, and CBPP specifically, reinforces the lesson that disease is a matter of both health and, importantly, economics. Economic considerations have been decidedly influential in motivating proper disease-control responses throughout the history of CBPP. Although not the only example, that of the USA and Great Britain during the 19th century provides evidence. Committed to free trade principles for both food supply and ideological reasons, and uniquely invested in both US agriculture and the transatlantic livestock and meat trade, Great Britain was motivated by economic considerations to reject an outright ban on American cattle imports despite the discovery of CBPP in a January 1879 shipment landed at Liverpool. Indeed, the so-called 'immediate slaughter order', a regulatory tool that enabled Britain to continue to import American livestock, albeit slaughtered at ports of entry, came as a relief to those from the USA, who were still able to export cattle. Yet the USA, keen to resume access to the lucrative store cattle market, was, again, economically motivated to come up with regulatory approaches that controlled this disease. Thanks to forward-thinking (and economically minded) veterinarians like James Law and Charles Lyman, *both* the domestic as well as international economic cost of livestock diseases would become important reasons for the US government to undertake more aggressive animal disease regulation. Fortunately, these and other US veterinary leaders had colleagues in Great Britain and Europe from whom they could draw helpful advice. While progress was held up at times by scientific confusion regarding the microbiology and diagnosis of CBPP, by the 1890s a robust transatlantic cross-fertilization of scientific and regulatory insights enabled the two countries to similarly understand, appreciate and manage livestock diseases. While the store cattle trade itself was not restored, this cooperation led to both countries successfully eradicating the disease from their shores by the end of the 19th century.

The cooperation modelled over a century ago by our own US and British forebears is just one small episode in the wider, international story with many characters speaking and writing in many different languages. With fascination, we have found CBPP to be a disease that has demanded the involvement of a diverse heritage of scholarly, thoughtful and persistent individuals. While 'individuals', their efforts have proved successful not because of individualism but rather cooperation. Therefore, a final lesson we offer is, if we might be so bold, a mandate: that, through fora like WOAH, scientists from all nations continue to partner together in the science of CBPP.

References

Blancou, J. (2000) Contagious bovine pleuropneumonia. In: *History of the Surveillance and Control of Transmissable Animal Diseases*. OIE, Paris, pp. 133–134.

Dupuy, V., Manso-Silván, L., Barbe, V., Thebault, P., Dordet-Frisoni, E. *et al.* (2012) Evolutionary history of contagious bovine pleuropneumonia using next generation sequencing of *Mycoplasma mycoides* subsp. mycoides 'small colony'. *PLOS ONE* 7(10), e46821. DOI: 10.1371/journal.pone.0046821.

Fischer, A., Shapiro, B., Muriuki, C., Heller, M., Schnee, C. *et al.* (2012) The origin of the '*Mycoplasma mycoides* cluster' coincides with domestication of ruminants. *PLOS ONE* 7(4), e36150. DOI: 10.1371/journal.pone.0036150.

Hutyra, F., Marek, J. and Manninger, R. (1938) *Special Pathology and Therapeutics of the Diseases of Domestic Animals*, 5th edition. Bailliere Tindall, USA, pp. 455–458.

Zeder, M.A. and Hesse, B. (2000) The initial domestication of goats (*Capra hircus*) in the Zagros mountains 10,000 years ago. *Science* 287(5461), 2254–2257. DOI: 10.1126/science.287.5461.2254.

Index

Locators in *italics* and in **bold** indicate *figures* and **boxes**, respectively

Printed and bound by CPI Group (UK) Ltd, Croydon, CR0 4YY
13/09/2026
14961117-0008